Resuscitation of the Fetus and Newborn

Editors

PRAVEEN KUMAR
LOUIS P. HALAMEK

CLINICS IN PERINATOLOGY

www.perinatology.theclinics.com

Consulting Editor

LUCKY JAIN

December 2012 • Volume 39 • Number 4

ELSEVIER

Elsevier, Inc. • 1600 John F. Kennedy Blvd. • Suite 1800 • Philadelphia, PA 19103-2899

http://www.theclinics.com

CLINICS IN PERINATOLOGY Volume 39, Number 4
December 2012 ISSN 0095-5108, ISBN-13: 978-1-4557-4921-8

Editor: Kerry Holland
Developmental Editor: Donald Mumford

Clinics in Perinatology (ISSN 0095-5108) is published quarterly by Elsevier Inc., 360 Park Avenue South, New York, NY 10010-1710. Months of issue are March, June, September, and December. Business and Editorial Offices: 1600 John F. Kennedy Blvd., Ste. 1800, Philadelphia, PA 19103-2899. Customer Service Office: 3251 Riverport Lane, Maryland Heights, MO 63043. Periodicals postage paid at New York, NY and additional mailing offices. Subscription prices are $273.00 per year (US individuals), $401.00 per year (US institutions), $326.00 per year (Canadian individuals), $509.00 per year (Canadian institutions), $400.00 per year (foreign individuals), $509.00 per year (foreign institutions), $130.00 per year (US students), and $187.00 per year (Canadian and foreign students). Foreign air speed delivery is included in all Clinics subscription prices. All prices are subject to change without notice. **POSTMASTER:** Send address changes to *Clinics in Perinatology*, Elsevier Health Sciences Division, Subscription Customer Service, 3251 Riverport Lane, Maryland Heights, MO 63043. **Customer Service: Telephone: 1-800-654-2452** (U.S. and Canada); **1-314-447-8871** (outside U.S. and Canada). **Fax: 1-314-447-8029. E-mail: journalscustomerservice-usa@elsevier.com** (for print support); **journalsonlinesupport-usa@elsevier.com** (for online support).

Reprints. For copies of 100 or more, of articles in this publication, please contact the Commercial Reprints Department, Elsevier Inc., 360 Park Avenue South, New York, NY 10010-1710. Tel. (212) 633-3812; Fax: (212) 482-1935; E-mail: reprints@elsevier.com.

Clinics in Perinatology is also pubilshed in Spanish by McGraw-Hill Interamericana Editores S.A., P.O. Box 5-237, 06500 Mexico D.F., Mexico.

Clinics in Perinatology is covered in *MEDLINE/PubMed (Index Medicus) Current Contents, Excepta Medica, BIOSIS and ISI/BIOMED.*

Printed in the United States of America.

Contributors

CONSULTING EDITOR

LUCKY JAIN, MD, MBA
Richard W. Blumberg Professor and Executive Vice Chairman, Department of Pediatrics, Emory University School of Medicine, Atlanta, Georgia

GUEST EDITORS

PRAVEEN KUMAR, MBBS, DCH, MD, FAAP
Professor of Pediatrics, Division of Neonatology, Department of Pediatrics, Northwestern University Feinberg School of Medicine, Ann and Robert H Lurie Children's Hospital of Chicago, Northwestern Memorial Hospital, Chicago, Illinois

LOUIS P. HALAMEK, MD, FAAP
Professor and Associate Chief, Education and Training, Division of Neonatal and Developmental Medicine, Department of Pediatrics, Stanford University; Director, Fellowship Training Program in Neonatal–Perinatal Medicine, Director, Center for Advanced Pediatric and Perinatal Education; Attending Neonatologist, Lucile Packard Children's Hospital, Palo Alto, California

AUTHORS

BREE ANDREWS, MD, MPH
The University of Chicago, Chicago, Illinois

KHALID AZIZ, MA, MEd(IT), FRCPC
Associate Professor, Department of Pediatrics, University of Alberta, DTC5027 Royal Alexandra Hospital, Edmonton, Alberta, Canada

RAMA BHAT, MD
Professor of Pediatrics, Department of Pediatrics, Children's Hospital of Wisconsin, Medical College of Wisconsin, Wauwatosa, Wisconsin

YAIR J. BLUMENFELD, MD
Clinical Assistant Professor of Obstetrics and Gynecology, Division of Maternal-Fetal Medicine, Department of Obstetrics and Gynecology, Lucile Packard Children's Hospital, Stanford University School of Medicine, Palo Alto, California

WILLIAM A. CAREY, MD
Assistant Professor, Department of Pediatrics, Neonatal Medicine, Mayo Clinic, Rochester, Minnesota

CHRISTOPHER E. COLBY, MD
Assistant Professor, Department of Pediatrics; Division Chair, Neonatal Medicine, Mayo Clinic, Rochester, Minnesota

NEIL N. FINER, MD
Professor of Pediatrics, Director, Division of Neonatology, Department of Pediatrics, University of California San Diego Medical Center, University of California San Diego School of Medicine, San Diego, California

JAY P. GOLDSMITH, MD
Clinical Professor, Department of Pediatrics, Tulane University, New Orleans, Louisiana

LOUIS P. HALAMEK, MD, FAAP
Professor and Associate Chief, Education and Training, Division of Neonatal and Developmental Medicine, Department of Pediatrics, Stanford University; Director, Fellowship Training Program in Neonatal–Perinatal Medicine, Director, Center for Advanced Pediatric and Perinatal Education; Attending Neonatologist, Lucile Packard Children's Hospital, Palo Alto, California

NOAH H. HILLMAN, MD
Division of Pulmonary Biology, Cincinnati Children's Hospital Medical Center, University of Cincinnati, Cincinnati, Ohio

SUSAN R. HINTZ, MD, MS Epi
Professor of Pediatrics, Division of Neonatal and Developmental Medicine, Department of Pediatrics, Stanford University School of Medicine; Medical Director, The Center for Fetal and Maternal Health, Lucile Packard Children's Hospital, Palo Alto, California

ALAN H. JOBE, MD, PhD
Division of Pulmonary Biology, Cincinnati Children's Hospital Medical Center, University of Cincinnati, Cincinnati, Ohio

SUHAS G. KALLAPUR, MD
Division of Pulmonary Biology, Cincinnati Children's Hospital Medical Center, University of Cincinnati, Cincinnati, Ohio

VISHAL KAPADIA, MD
Assistant Professor of Pediatrics, Division of Neonatal-Perinatal Medicine, Department of Pediatrics, The University of Texas Southwestern Medical Center at Dallas, Dallas, Texas

JOHN KATTWINKEL, MD
Professor, Department of Pediatrics, University of Virginia, Charlottesville, Virginia

JOANNE LAGATTA, MD, MA
Assistant Professor, Medical College of Wisconsin, Wauwatosa, Wisconsin

JOHN LANTOS, MD
Director of Pediatric Bioethics, Professor of Pediatrics, University of Missouri, Kansas City School of Medicine, Children's Mercy Hospital, Kansas City, Missouri

TINA A. LEONE, MD
Director, Neonatal-Perinatal Medicine Training Program, Associate Clinical Professor of Pediatrics, University of California San Diego Medical Center, University of California San Diego School of Medicine, San Diego, California

WILLIAM MEADOW, MD, PhD
Professor of Pediatrics, Co-Section Chief, Neonatology, Director, Neonatology Fellowship Program, The University of Chicago, Chicago, Illinois

SUSAN NIERMEYER, MD, MPH, FAAP
Professor of Pediatrics, Section of Neonatology, Children's Hospital Colorado, University of Colorado School of Medicine, Aurora, Colorado

COLM P.F. O'DONNELL, MB, FRCPI, MRCPCH, FRACP, PhD
Department of Neonatology, The National Maternity Hospital; Department of Neonatology, Our Lady's Children's Hospital; National Children's Research Centre; School of Medicine and Medical Science, University College Dublin, Dublin, Ireland

ALAN M. PEACEMAN, MD
Professor, Chief of Maternal Fetal Medicine, Department of Obstetrics and Gynecology, Feinberg School of Medicine, Northwestern University, Chicago, Illinois

JEFFREY M. PERLMAN, MB, ChB
Professor of Pediatrics, Division Chief, Division of Newborn Medicine, Weill Cornell Medical College, New York Presbyterian Hospital, New York, New York

TONSE N.K. RAJU, MD, DCh
Program Officer, Eunice Kennedy Shriver National Institute of Child Health and Human Development, National Institutes of Health, Bethesda, Maryland

WADE RICH, RRT, CCRC
Clinical Research Coordinator, Division of Neonatology, Department of Pediatrics, University of California San Diego Medical Center, University of California San Diego School of Medicine, San Diego, California

STEVEN A. RINGER, MD, PhD
Assistant Professor, Department of Newborn Medicine, Brigham and Women's Hospital, Harvard Medical School, Boston, Massachusetts

GEORG M. SCHMÖLZER, MD, PhD
Department of Pediatrics, University of Alberta, Edmonton, Canada; Division of Neonatology, Department of Pediatrics, Medical University Graz, Graz, Austria; Neonatal Research Group, Murdoch Childrens Research Institute, Melbourne, Australia

SEETHA SHANKARAN, MD
Professor of Pediatrics, Wayne State University School of Medicine; Director, Division of Neonatal/Perinatal Medicine, Children's Hospital of Michigan and Hutzel Women's Hospital, Detroit, Michigan

NALINI SINGHAL, MD, DCh
Professor Pediatrics, University of Calgary, Calgary, Alberta, Canada

DHARMAPURI VIDYASAGAR, MD
Professor Emeritus, Department of Pediatrics, University of Illinois at Medical Center at Chicago, Chicago, Illinois

JANELLE R. WALTON, MD
Assistant Professor of Obstetrics and Gynecology, Department of Obstetrics and Gynecology, Feinberg School of Medicine, Northwestern University, Chicago, Illinois

GARY M. WEINER, MD, FAAP
Associate Clinical Professor, Department of Pediatrics, St. Joseph Mercy Hospital, Ann Arbor, Michigan; Wayne State University School of Medicine, Detroit, Michigan

MYRA H. WYCKOFF, MD
Associate Professor of Pediatrics, Division of Neonatal-Perinatal Medicine, Department of Pediatrics, The University of Texas Southwestern Medical Center at Dallas, Dallas, Texas

Contents

Foreword: The Neonatal Golden Hour   xiii

Lucky Jain

Preface: Resuscitation of the Fetus and Newborn   xv

Praveen Kumar and Louis P. Halamek

Erratum   xvii

Identification, Assessment and Management of Fetal Compromise   753

Janelle R. Walton and Alan M. Peaceman

The main goals of fetal surveillance are to avoid fetal death and to recognize the fetus that will benefit from early intervention with resuscitation or delivery. Surveillance can occur in the antepartum or intrapartum period. Continuous fetal heart rate monitoring is the most common form of surveillance in the intrapartum period. Several techniques are used in the antepartum period, including nonstress test, biophysical profile, and contraction stress test. Multiple techniques are used once distress is noted in the fetus, with the ultimate resuscitation effort being delivery.

Physiology of Transition from Intrauterine to Extrauterine Life   769

Noah H. Hillman, Suhas G. Kallapur, and Alan H. Jobe

The transition from fetus to newborn is the most complex adaptation that occurs in human experience. Lung adaptation requires coordinated clearance of fetal lung fluid, surfactant secretion, and onset of consistent breathing. The cardiovascular response requires striking changes in blood flow, pressures, and pulmonary vasodilation. Energy metabolism and thermoregulation must be quickly controlled. The primary mediators that prepare the fetus for birth and support the multiorgan transition are cortisol and catecholamine. Abnormalities in adaptation are frequently found following preterm birth or cesarean delivery at term, and many of these infants need delivery room resuscitation to assist in this transition.

Cellular Biology of End Organ Injury and Strategies for Prevention of Injury   785

Jeffrey M. Perlman

The interruption of placental blood flow induces circulatory responses to maintain cerebral, cardiac, and adrenal blood flow with reduced renal, hepatic, intestinal, and skin blood flow. If placental compromise is prolonged and/or severe, total circulatory failure is likely with cerebral hypoperfusion and resultant hypoxic ischemic cerebral injury with collateral renal, cardiac, and hepatic injury. Management strategies should be targeted at restoring cerebral perfusion and oxygen delivery and minimizing the extent of secondary injury. Specifically, the focus should include the judicious use of supplemental oxygen, avoidance of hypoglycemia and elevated temperature in the delivery room, and the early administration of therapeutic hypothermia to high-risk infants.

The Role of Oxygen in the Delivery Room   803

Jay P. Goldsmith and John Kattwinkel

As recently as the year 2000, 100% oxygen was recommended to begin resuscitation of depressed newborns in the delivery room. However, the most recent recommendations of the International Liaison Committee on Resuscitation counsel the prudent use of oxygen during resuscitation. In term and preterm infants, oxygen therapy should be guided by pulse oximetry that follows the interquartile range of preductal saturations of healthy term babies after vaginal birth at sea level. This article reviews the literature in this context, which supports the radical but judicious curtailment of the use of oxygen in resuscitation at birth.

Delivery Room Management of Meconium-Stained Infant   817

Rama Bhat and Dharmapuri Vidyasagar

This article discusses the historical background, epidemiology, and pathophysiology of meconium-stained amniotic fluid and provides current concepts in delivery room management of meconium-stained neonate including the current Neonatal Resuscitation Program guidelines.

Chest Compressions for Bradycardia or Asystole in Neonates   833

Vishal Kapadia and Myra H. Wyckoff

When effective ventilation fails to establish a heart rate of greater than 60 bpm, cardiac compressions should be initiated to improve perfusion. The 2-thumb method is the most effective and least fatiguing technique. A ratio of 3 compressions to 1 breath is recommended to provide adequate ventilation, the most common cause of newborn cardiovascular collapse. Interruptions in compressions should be limited to not diminishing the perfusion generated. Oxygen (100%) is recommended during compressions and can be reduced once adequate heart rate and oxygen saturation are achieved. Limited clinical data are available to form newborn cardiac compression recommendations.

Medications in Neonatal Resuscitation: Epinephrine and the Search for Better Alternative Strategies   843

Gary M. Weiner and Susan Niermeyer

Epinephrine remains the primary vasopressor for neonatal resuscitation complicated by asystole or prolonged bradycardia not responsive to adequate ventilation and chest compressions. Epinephrine increases coronary perfusion pressure primarily through peripheral vasoconstriction. Current guidelines recommend intravenous epinephrine administration (0.01–0.03 mg/kg). Endotracheal epinephrine administration results in unpredictable absorption. High-dose intravenous epinephrine poses additional risks and does not result in better long-term survival. Vasopressin has been considered an alternative to epinephrine in adults, but there is insufficient evidence to recommend its use in newborn infants. Future research will focus on the best sequence for epinephrine administration and chest compressions.

Resuscitation of Preterm Infants: Delivery Room Interventions and Their Effect on Outcomes   857

Colm P.F. O'Donnell and Georg M. Schmölzer

> Despite advances in neonatal care, the rate of oxygen dependence at 36 weeks' postmenstrual age or bronchopulmonary dysplasia has not fallen. Neonatologists are increasingly careful to apply ventilation strategies that are gentle to the lung in the neonatal intensive care unit. However, there has not been the same emphasis applying gentle ventilation strategies immediately after birth. A lung-protective strategy should start immediately after birth to establish a functional residual capacity, reduce volutrauma and atelectotrauma, facilitate gas exchange, and improve oxygenation during neonatal transition. This article discusses techniques and equipment recommended by international resuscitation guidelines during breathing assistance in the delivery room.

Infants with Prenatally Diagnosed Anomalies: Special Approaches to Preparation and Resuscitation   871

Christopher E. Colby, William A. Carey, Yair J. Blumenfeld, and Susan R. Hintz

> When a fetal anomaly is suspected, a multidisciplinary approach to diagnosis, counseling, pregnancy management, surveillance, delivery planning, and neonatal care is critical to creating a comprehensive management plan. This article provides a basic framework for integrating prenatal diagnostic and maternal-fetal care considerations, delivery planning, special resuscitation needs, and immediate and later neonatal care and evaluation into developing a thoughtful management plan for infants with prenatally diagnosed complex anomalies including congenital heart disease, intrathoracic masses, fetal airway obstruction, neural tube defects, abdominal wall defects, and skeletal dysplasia.

Optimal Timing for Clamping the Umbilical Cord After Birth   889

Tonse N.K. Raju and Nalini Singhal

> This article provides a brief overview of pros and cons of clamping the cord too early (within seconds) after birth. It also highlights evolving data that suggest that delaying cord clamping for 30 to 60 seconds after birth is beneficial to the baby, with no measurable negative effects either the baby or the mother.

Neonatal Stabilization and Postresuscitation Care   901

Steven A. Ringer and Khalid Aziz

> Neonatal mortality is a major health care concern worldwide. Neonatal resuscitation alone does not address most causes of neonatal mortality; caregivers need to be trained in both neonatal resuscitation and stabilization. Neonatal stabilization requires caregivers to evaluate whether babies are at-risk or unwell, to decide what interventions are required, and to act on those decisions. Several programs address neonatal stabilization in a variety of levels of care in both well-resourced and limited health care

environments. This article suggests a shift in clinical, educational, and implementation science from a focus on resuscitation to one on the resuscitation-stabilization continuum.

Hypoxic-ischemic Encephalopathy and Novel Strategies for Neuroprotection   919

Seetha Shankaran

This article covers the outcome of full-term infants with encephalopathy due to hypoxic-ischemia and pathophysiology of brain injury following hypoxic-ischemia. Clinical and imaging evidence for hypothermia for neuroprotection is presented. The outcome of infants with hypothermia for encephalopathy due to hypoxic-ischemia from recent trials is summarized. Facts regarding the clinical application of cooling obtained from the randomized trials and knowledge gaps in hypothermic therapy are presented. The review concludes with the future of hypothermia for neuroprotection.

The Delivery Room of the Future: The Fetal and Neonatal Resuscitation and Transition Suite   931

Neil N. Finer, Wade Rich, Louis P. Halamek, and Tina A. Leone

Despite advances in the understanding of fetal and neonatal physiology and the technology to monitor and treat premature and full-term neonates, little has changed in resuscitation rooms. The authors' vision for the Fetal and Neonatal Resuscitation and Transition Suite of the future is marked by improvements in the amount of physical space, monitoring technologies, portable diagnostic and therapeutic technologies, communication systems, and capabilities and training of the resuscitation team. Human factors analysis will play an important role in the design and testing of the improvements for safe, effective, and efficient resuscitation of the newborn.

The Mathematics of Morality for Neonatal Resuscitation   941

William Meadow, Joanne Lagatta, Bree Andrews, and John Lantos

This article discusses the ethical issues surrounding the resuscitation of infants who are at great risk to die or survive with significant morbidity. Data are introduced regarding money, outcomes, and prediction. Gestational age influences some of the outcomes after birth more than others do. Prediction is possible at four stages of the resuscitation process. Data suggest that antenatal and delivery room predictions are inadequate, and prediction at the time of discharge is too late. The predictive value (>95%) for the outcome of death or survival with neurodevelopmental impairment is discussed.

Index   957

GOAL STATEMENT

The goal of *Clinics in Perinatology* is to keep practicing neonatologists and maternal-fetal medicine specialists up to date with current clinical practice in perinatology by providing timely articles reviewing the state of the art in patient care.

ACCREDITATION

The *Clinics in Perinatology* is planned and implemented in accordance with the Essential Areas and Policies of the Accreditation Council for Continuing Medical Education (ACCME) through the joint sponsorship of the University of Virginia School of Medicine and Elsevier. The University of Virginia School of Medicine is accredited by the ACCME to provide continuing medical education for physicians.

The University of Virginia School of Medicine designates this enduring material activity for a maximum of 15 *AMA PRA Category 1 Credit*(s)™ for each issue, 60 credits per year. Physicians should only claim credit commensurate with the extent of their participation in the activity.

The American Medical Association has determined that physicians not licensed in the US who participate in this CME enduring material activity are eligible for a maximum of 15 *AMA PRA Category 1 Credit*(s)™ for each issue, 60 credits per year.

Credit can be earned by reading the text material, taking the CME examination online at http://www.theclinics.com/home/cme, and completing the evaluation. After taking the test, you will be required to review any and all incorrect answers. Following completion of the test and evaluation, your credit will be awarded and you may print your certificate.

FACULTY DISCLOSURE/CONFLICT OF INTEREST

The University of Virginia School of Medicine, as an ACCME accredited provider, endorses and strives to comply with the Accreditation Council for Continuing Medical Education (ACCME) Standards of Commercial Support, Commonwealth of Virginia statutes, University of Virginia policies and procedures, and associated federal and private regulations and guidelines on the need for disclosure and monitoring of proprietary and financial interests that may affect the scientific integrity and balance of content delivered in continuing medical education activities under our auspices.

The University of Virginia School of Medicine requires that all CME activities accredited through this institution be developed independently and be scientifically rigorous, balanced and objective in the presentation/discussion of its content, theories and practices.

All authors/editors participating in an accredited CME activity are expected to disclose to the readers relevant financial relationships with commercial entities occurring within the past 12 months (such as grants or research support, employee, consultant, stock holder, member of speakers bureau, etc.). The University of Virginia School of Medicine will employ appropriate mechanisms to resolve potential conflicts of interest to maintain the standards of fair and balanced education to the reader. Questions about specific strategies can be directed to the Office of Continuing Medical Education, University of Virginia School of Medicine, Charlottesville, Virginia.

The faculty and staff of the University of Virginia Office of Continuing Medical Education have no financial affiliations to disclose.

The authors/editors listed below have identified no professional or financial affiliations for themselves or their spouse/ partner:
Bree Andrews, MD, MPH; Khalid Aziz, MA, MEd(IT), FRCPC; Rama Bhat, MD; Yair J. Blumenfeld, MD; Robert Boyle, MD (Test Author); William A. Carey, MD; Christopher E. Colby, MD; Neil N. Finer, MD; Jay P. Goldsmith, MD; Noah H. Hillman, MD; Susan R. Hintz, MD, MS Epi; Kerry Holland, (Acquisitions Editor); Lucky Jain, MD, MBA (Consulting Editor); Vishal Kapadia, MD; John Kattwinkel, MD; Praveen Kumar, MBBS, DCH, MD, FAAP (Guest Editor); Joanne Lagatta, MD, MA; John Lantos, MD; Tina A. Leone, MD; William Meadow, MD, PhD; Susan Niermeyer, MD, MPH; Colm P.F. O'Donnell, MB, FRCPI, MRCPCH, FRACP, PhD; Alan M. Peaceman, MD; Jeffrey M. Perlman, MB, ChB; Tonse N.K. Raju, MD, DCh; Wade Rich, RRT, CCRC; Steven A. Ringer, MD, PhD; Georg M. Schmölzer, MD, PhD; Seetha Shankaran, MD; Nalini Singhal, MD, DCh; Dharmapuri Vidyasagar, MD; Janelle R. Walton, MD; and Gary M. Weiner, MD.

The authors/editors listed below identified the following professional or financial affiliations for themselves or their spouse/partner:
Louis P. Halamek, MD, FAAP (Guest Editor) is a consultant for Laerdal Medical.
Alan H. Jobe, MD, PhD is on the Advisory Board for and receives supplies of surfactant for animal studies from Chiesi Pharm - Parma Italy; and receives research support from Research Tech Inc.
Suhas G. Kallapur, MD receives research support from Merck and is on the Speakers' Bureau for Ikaria.
Myra H. Wyckoff, MD receives research support from Ikaria.

Disclosure of Discussion of Non-FDA Approved Uses for Pharmaceutical Products and/or Medical Devices.
The University of Virginia School of Medicine, as an ACCME provider, requires that all faculty presenters identify and disclose any off-label uses for pharmaceutical and medical device products. The University of Virginia School of Medicine recommends that each physician fully review all the available data on new products or procedures prior to clinical use.

TO ENROLL
To enroll in the Clinics in Perinatology Continuing Medical Education program, call customer service at 1-800-654-2452 or visit us online at www.theclinics.com/home/cme. The CME program is available to subscribers for an additional fee of $196.00.

CLINICS IN PERINATOLOGY

FORTHCOMING ISSUES

March 2013
Necrotizing Enterocolitis
Patricia Denning, MD, and
Akhil Maheshwari, MD, *Guest Editors*

June 2013
Retinopathy of Prematurity
Graham E. Quinn, MD, and
Alistair Fielder, MD, *Guest Editors*

September 2013
Management in the Peripartum Period
James Hebl, MD, and
Randall Flick, MD, *Guest Editors*

RECENT ISSUES

September 2012
Advances in Respiratory Care
of the Newborn
Judy L. Aschner, MD, and
Richard A. Polin, MD, *Guest Editors*

June 2012
Innovations in Fetal and Neonatal Surgery
Hanmin Lee, MD, and
Ronald B. Hirschl, MD, *Guest Editors*

March 2012
Evidence-Based Neonatal Pharmacotherapy
Alan R. Spitzer, MD, and
Dan L. Ellsbury, MD, *Guest Editors*

RELATED INTEREST

Pediatric Clinics of North America, Volume 59, Issue 5 (October 2012)
Neonatal and Pediatric Clinical Pharmacology
John N. van den Anker, MD, PhD, FCP, FAAP, Max Coppes, MD, and
Gideon Koren, MD, *Guest Editors*

Foreword

The Neonatal Golden Hour

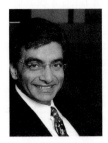

Lucky Jain, MD, MBA
Consulting Editor

In his bestselling book *Better,* Atul Gawande[1] provides us with a startling description of how serious trauma is managed in modern day wars and how medical teams have managed to lower mortality among injured soldiers to remarkably low levels. They have done so despite the significantly higher fire power of the weaponry they face and the lack of any major medical or technologic advances to assist them. "How the military medical teams have achieved this is important to think about, it is the simple, almost banal changes that have produced enormous improvements," says Gawande in his book.[1] Key changes with the most impact include emphasis on the Golden Five Minutes, not the Golden Hour, as the most critical time to respond. This is because battlefield injuries are often much more severe than civilian trauma, and the concept of the Golden Hour proved to be less relevant when a bleeding soldier ran the risk of dying in minutes.[2,3] The army responded by assembling "Forward Surgical Teams," small teams of just 20 or so medical personnel who travel directly behind the troops with makeshift hospital rooms that can be assembled from "drash" tents and portable supply packs. Medical teams focus less on definitive repair, more on stabilization and damage control, with rapid transport to the nearest support hospital via helicopters. Once there, mortality drops rapidly since definitive repair can be addressed without the pressure of time and resource constraints.

As one reads this captivating story, it is hard not to draw parallels to recent advances in neonatal resuscitation with a substantial impact on birth asphyxia and neonatal deaths. These gains have been made not through any major breakthrough in technology, but through the rapid deployment of trained personnel, whose main job is to stabilize the neonate using minimal equipment and standardized checklists. Much too often, these teams also have only a few golden minutes to respond. The concept of Golden Hour is still relevant though; it allows additional focus on postresuscitation care, thermoregulation, hypoglycemia management, and attention to other issues such as hypovolemia and sepsis management.

Clin Perinatol 39 (2012) xiii–xiv
http://dx.doi.org/10.1016/j.clp.2012.10.002
0095-5108/12/$ – see front matter © 2012 Elsevier Inc. All rights reserved.

perinatology.theclinics.com

The Neonatal Resuscitation Program (NRP) has made, and continues to make, an enormous impact on newborn care in the critical initial period. In a recent report from China, more than 110,659 professionals received NRP training from 2004 to 2009 in 20 target provinces; delivery room deaths related to intrapartum events subsequently dropped by more than 50%.[4] Yet, in countries where this has not been a priority, the human cost of delayed resuscitation is enormous; death and permanent brain injury resulting from delayed or inadequate resuscitation sadly are still a big problem in many developing nations. In a study[5] from Tanzania, birth asphyxia was the leading cause (26.8%) of admission to the neonatal care unit and directly responsible for nearly half of the deaths. As expected, most of the deaths occurred within the first day of life. Worldwide, of the nearly 136 million babies born each year, an estimated 814,000 term infants die from intrapartum-related events.[6] The presence of trained personnel at these deliveries with minimum equipment can prevent a vast majority of these deaths.

In this issue of the *Clinics in Perinatology*, Drs Kumar and Halamek have assembled an impressive array of authors who provide us state-of-the-art information about important aspects of neonatal resuscitation. It is our hope that through NRP and offerings like this, neonatal resuscitation will become a top priority for health care systems worldwide.

Lucky Jain, MD, MBA
Department of Pediatrics
Emory University School of Medicine
2015 Uppergate Drive
Atlanta, GA 30322, USA

E-mail address:
ljain@emory.edu

REFERENCES

1. Gawande A. Casualties of war. In: Better. New York: Picador Books; 2007.
2. Murdock D. Trauma: when there's no time to count. AORN J 2008;87:322–8.
3. Murad MK, Issa DB, Mustafa FM, et al. Prehospital trauma system reduces mortality in severe trauma: a controlled study of road traffic casualties in Iraq. Prehosp Disaster Med 2012;27(36):41.
4. Xu T, Wang HS, Ye HM, et al. Impact of a nationwide training program for neonatal resuscitation program in China. Chin Med J 2012;125:1448–56.
5. Mmbaga BT, Lie RT, Olomi R, et al. Cause specific mortality in a neonatal care unit in Northern Tanzania: a registry based cohort study. BMC Pediatr 2012;12:116.
6. Lee AC, Cousens S, Wall SN, et al. Neonatal resuscitation and immediate newborn assessment and stimulation for the prevention of neonatal deaths: a systematic review, meta-analysis and Delphi estimation of mortality effect. BMC Public Health 2011;11:S12.

Preface

Resuscitation of the Fetus and Newborn

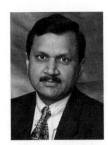 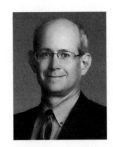

Praveen Kumar, MBBS, DCH, MD, FAAP   Louis P. Halamek, MD, FAAP
Guest Editors

Advances in obstetric and neonatal care have led to significant improvement in perinatal outcomes worldwide. Significant reduction in fetal as well as neonatal morbidity and mortality is partly due to close attention to fetal well-being prior to delivery and a coordinated team approach to neonatal resuscitation at birth. To be able to deliver a healthy infant to parents is what drew us all to obstetrics and neonatology. Whether it be the basic processes that characterize fetal and neonatal physiology, the technologies and methodologies that allow delivery of effective care to the newborn transitioning from an intrauterine to an extrauterine existence, the techniques that facilitate optimal human performance during situations as stressful as neonatal resuscitation, or the ethical challenges inherent in dealing with the uncertainties associated with an extremely preterm birth, we find these topics captivating, challenging, and rewarding.

This edition of *Clinics in Perinatology* is devoted to the topic of resuscitation of the fetus and newborn. The authors that have contributed to this edition represent some of the most prominent basic scientists, clinical investigators, and clinicians in the field of neonatal–perinatal medicine. Their articles, on topics that are core to the field, provide state-of-the-art insight into the challenges that face everyone who assumes responsibility for caring for a compromised fetus and the neonate in the first minutes of life. Recently revised clinical guidelines for neonatal resuscitation are discussed in detail

Clin Perinatol 39 (2012) xv–xvi
http://dx.doi.org/10.1016/j.clp.2012.10.001
perinatology.theclinics.com

and current gaps in knowledge are acknowledged. This edition will serve as a reference for all of us who care for neonates in need of resuscitation. Our hope as coeditors is that not only will you find this issue to be engaging and enjoyable reading but also that it will stimulate you to contribute to the field and potentially be one of the next authors when neonatal resuscitation is again chosen as a topic for *Clinics in Perinatology*.

Praveen Kumar, MBBS, DCH, MD, FAAP
Division of Neonatology
Department of Pediatrics
Northwestern University Feinberg School of Medicine
Ann and Robert H Lurie Children's Hospital of Chicago
Northwestern Memorial Hospital
Chicago, IL 60611, USA

Louis P. Halamek, MD, FAAP
Division of Neonatal and Developmental Medicine
Department of Pediatrics
Stanford University
Fellowship Training Program in Neonatal-Perinatal Medicine
Center for Advanced Pediatric and Perinatal Education
Lucile Packard Children's Hospital
Suite 315, 750 Welch Road
Palo Alto, CA 94305, USA

E-mail addresses:
p-kumar@northwestern.edu (P. Kumar)
halamek@stanford.edu (L.P. Halamek)

Erratum

An article entitled "Maternal-Fetal Surgery: History and General Considerations" published in the June 2012 issue of *Clinics in Perinatology* (39:2). It was learned after publication that the guidelines for fetal repair of myelomeningocele, which appeared in this article, were presented as being published by the NIH, but they were neither supplied by the NIH nor published by them. To prevent this information from being erroneously cited, the article was removed.

Clin Perinatol 39 (2012) xvii
http://dx.doi.org/10.1016/j.clp.2012.10.003
0095-5108/12/$ – see front matter Published by Elsevier Inc.

perinatology.theclinics.com

Identification, Assessment and Management of Fetal Compromise

Janelle R. Walton, MD*, Alan M. Peaceman, MD

KEYWORDS

- Fetal monitoring • Antepartum surveillance • Intrapartum surveillance
- Intrapartum fetal resuscitation

KEY POINTS

- Antepartum and intrapartum surveillance techniques provide an opportunity to monitor fetal well being. The current gold standard, continuous fetal heart rate monitoring allows for identification of the compromised fetus.
- In the antepartum period several surveillance techniques are employed: fetal movement assessment, nonstress test, biophysical profile, modified biophysical profile, contraction stress test and Doppler velocimetry. These techniques can be used for both low risk and high risk pregnancies.
- A standardized classification system for electronic fetal heart rate monitoring, developed by the Eunice Kennedy Shriver National Institute of Child Health and Human Development, the American College of Obstetricians and Gynecologists, and the Society for Maternal-Fetal Medicine allows for more uniform diagnosis of the fetus in potential distress.
- A number of resuscitative therapies are available to resuscitate the potentially compromised fetus. The ultimate technique available to is delivery.
- Additional research is necessary and underway to develop new monitoring techniques.

INTRODUCTION

The main goals of fetal surveillance are to avoid fetal death and promptly recognize the fetus that will benefit from early intervention with resuscitation or delivery. The fetus can be assessed in the antepartum and the intrapartum periods. The authors will review physiology, examine the different modalities for fetal surveillance, and assess techniques for fetal resuscitation. The mainstay of techniques for fetal resuscitation include maternal repositioning, oxygen administration, discontinuation of induction

Department of Obstetrics and Gynecology, Feinberg School of Medicine, Northwestern University, 250 East Superior Avenue, Suite 05-2191, Chicago, IL 60611, USA
* Corresponding author. Department of Obstetrics and Gynecology, Division of Maternal Fetal Medicine, Northwestern University, 250 East Superior Avenue, Suite 05-2191, Chicago, IL 60611.
E-mail address: Janelle.walton@northwestern.edu

Clin Perinatol 39 (2012) 753–768
http://dx.doi.org/10.1016/j.clp.2012.09.001
0095-5108/12/$ – see front matter © 2012 Elsevier Inc. All rights reserved.

agents, tocolysis, and even amnioinfusion. The ultimate resuscitation effort would be delivery—accomplished either via operative vaginal delivery or cesarean section. These will be discussed in detail in the text.

PHYSIOLOGY

Various surveillance techniques can identify the fetus that is suboptimally oxygenated or acidemic. The fetal heart rate (FHR) pattern, level of activity, and degree of muscular tone are all sensitive to hypoxemia and acidemia.[1,2] The FHR is normally controlled by the fetal central nervous system and mediated by sympathetic or parasympathetic nerve impulses originating in the fetal brainstem. Therefore, the presence of intermittent FHR accelerations associated with fetal movement is believed to be an indicator of adequate oxygenation sufficient to maintain normal fetal autonomic nervous system function.

The range of normal umbilical blood gas parameters has been established by cordocentesis performed in pregnancies in which a healthy infant was ultimately born.[3] The lower 2.5 centile for fetal venous pH was 7.37 in normal infants. Fetuses with nonreactive nonstress tests were found to have mean umbilical vein pH of 7.28 ($\pm$0.11). Cessation of fetal movement was associated with a mean umbilical vein pH of 7.16 ($\pm$0.08).[4] These correlations inform the basis for surveillance currently.

Factors besides acid-base and oxygenation status can impact biophysical parameters. These include prematurity, fetal sleep-wake cycle, maternal medications, and fetal central nervous system abnormalities.

FETAL MONITORING
History

Auscultation of fetal heart tones was first described in Europe in the 17th century by placing the ear on the maternal abdomen.[5] Subsequently, DeLee and Hillis developed the fetoscope in 1917.[6] In 1958, Hon reported the use of continuous recording of FHR using a fetal electrocardiographic monitor placed on the maternal abdomen. Electronic fetal monitoring became widely used in practice in the United States soon after its introduction in the early 1970s.[7] It was used among 45% of laboring women in 1980, 62% in 1988, 74% in 1992, and 85% in 2002.[8]

Despite its widespread use, limitations of monitoring include poor interobserver and intraobserver reliability, uncertain efficacy, and high false-positive rates. FHR monitoring can be performed externally or internally. Most external monitors use a Doppler device with computerized logic to interpret and count the Doppler signals. Internal FHR monitoring is accomplished with a fetal electrode (first described in 1963) that is attached to the scalp or other presenting part. Tracings from currently used external monitoring devices are now thought to be of equivalent quality for interpretation as those obtained internally.

Interpreting the FHR

In 2008, the Eunice Kennedy Shriver National Institute of Child Health and Human Development partnered with the American College of Obstetricians and Gynecologists and the Society for Maternal-Fetal Medicine to sponsor a workshop focused on electronic FHR monitoring.[9] Its goals were to (1) review and update the definitions for FHR pattern categorization from the prior workshop, (2) assess existing classifications systems for interpreting specific FHR patterns and make recommendations about a system for use in the United States, and (3) make recommendations for research priorities for EFM. Necessary terms are defined and described later.

Uterine activity

Uterine contractions are quantified as the number of contractions present in a 10-minute window, averaged during a 30-minute period. Contraction frequency, duration, intensity, and relaxation time between contractions are important to clinical practice. Normal uterine activity is defined as 5 contractions or less in 10 minutes, averaged during a 30-minute window. Tachysystole is defined as greater than 5 contractions in 10 minutes, averaged during a 30-minute window. Tachysystole should be qualified regarding the presence or absence of associated FHR decelerations. In addition, tachysystole applies to both spontaneous and stimulated labor. The terms "hyperstimulation" and "hypercontractility" are not defined and should no longer be used in clinical practice.

Baseline

A normal FHR baseline is 110 to 160 beats per minute (bpm). Tachycardia is defined as FHR baseline greater than 160 bpm, whereas bradycardia is defined as FHR baseline less than 110 bpm. The mean FHR is rounded to increments of 5 bpm during a 10-minute segment, excluding periodic or episodic changes, periods of marked FHR variability, or segments of baseline that differ by greater than 25 bpm. The baseline must be for a minimum of 2 minutes in any 10-minute segment or the baseline is indeterminate. In this case, one may use the prior 10-minute window to determine baseline.

Fetal tachycardia is most frequently caused by maternal fever and is a normal response to hyperthermia. However, tachycardia can also be seen before maternal fever, as in chorioamnionitis, as well as in response to certain drugs (parasympatholytic or sympathomimetic agents). A serious cause of fetal tachycardia is fetal hypoxemia, likely caused by β-adrenergic stimulation. Fetal bradycardia with preserved FHR variability is not a sign of fetal asphyxia and a baseline of 90 to 110 FHR may be normal for some fetuses. Fetal bradycardia can reflect hypoxemia when the FHR has previously been higher and there is absent FHR variability.

Variability

Variability is defined as fluctuations in the baseline FHR that are irregular in amplitude and frequency. It is visually quantitated as the amplitude of peak-to-trough in beats per minute. Classification is as follows:

Absent—amplitude range undetectable
Minimal—amplitude range detectable but 5 bpm or less
Moderate (normal)—amplitude range 6 to 25 bpm
Marked—amplitude range greater than 25 bpm

The presence of baseline FHR variability is a useful indicator of fetal central nervous system integrity. Moderate FHR variability is strongly associated with an umbilical pH greater than 7.15.[10] In most cases, normal FHR variability can provide reassurance about fetal status. In the absence of maternal sedation, magnesium sulfate administration, chronic β-blockade, or extreme prematurity, decreased or absent variability can serve as a barometer of the fetal response to hypoxia.

Accelerations

An acceleration is defined as a visually apparent abrupt increase (onset to peak in <30 seconds) in the FHR. At 32 weeks of gestation and beyond, an acceleration has a peak of 15 bpm or greater higher than baseline, with a duration of 15 seconds or longer but less than 2 minutes from onset to return. Before 32 weeks of gestation, an acceleration has a peak of 10 bpm or greater higher than baseline, with duration of 10 seconds or longer but less than 2 minutes from onset to return. A prolonged acceleration lasts 2 minutes or longer but less than 10 minutes in duration. If an acceleration lasts 10 minutes or longer, it is a baseline change.

The presence of FHR accelerations in the intrapartum period is always reassuring, but the absence of accelerations is not necessarily reflective of fetal hypoxemia.

Decelerations

These are episodic decreases to lower than the baseline and are mediated by the fetal chemoreflex in response to hypoxia. They are classified next. They are defined as "recurrent" if they occur with at least 50% of the contractions.

Early deceleration

This is defined as a visually apparent usually symmetric gradual decrease and return of the FHR associated with a uterine contraction. A gradual FHR decrease is defined as from the onset to the FHR nadir of 30 seconds or longer. The decrease in FHR is calculated from the onset to the nadir of the deceleration. The nadir occurs at the same time as the peak of the contraction. Often, the onset, nadir, and recovery of the deceleration are coincident with the beginning, peak and ending of the contraction, respectively.

Early deceleration is typically reassuring and not associated with fetal compromise. The physiology is thought to be central vagal stimulation caused by altered cerebral blood flow (ie, compression of the fetal head).

Late deceleration

This is defined as a visually apparent, usually symmetric gradual decrease and return of the FHR associated with a uterine contraction. The decrease is defined and calculated in the same manner as in an early deceleration. However, the deceleration is delayed in timing, with the nadir of the deceleration occurring after the peak of the contraction. In most cases, the onset, nadir, and recovery of the deceleration occur after the beginning, peak, and ending of the contraction, respectively.

Late decelerations are a reflection of stress associated with uterine contractions. In the normally oxygenated fetus, the FHR is generally unaffected by contractions. However, in suboptimal conditions, the Po_2 during a contraction may be driven to less than a critical level and subsequently the FHR slows. This follows a characteristic pattern, described earlier. The occasional late deceleration does not necessarily indicate compromise, but recurrent late decelerations are considered to be nonreassuring.

Variable deceleration

This is defined as a visually apparent abrupt decrease in FHR. An abrupt FHR decrease is defined as from the onset of the deceleration to the beginning of the FHR nadir within less than 30 seconds. The decrease in FHR is calculated from the onset to the nadir of the deceleration. The decrease in FHR is 15 bpm or greater, lasting 15 seconds or greater, and less than 2 minutes in duration. When variable decelerations are associated with uterine contractions, their onset, depth, and duration commonly vary with successive uterine contractions.

Variable decelerations are the most common form of intrapartum decelerations. They are frequently preceded and followed by small accelerations in the FHR. Variable decelerations are often associated with umbilical cord compression and favorable outcome if brief, shallow, and episodic. However, recurrent, prolonged, and deep variable decelerations may result in progressive hypoxemia and acidemia.

Prolonged deceleration

This is defined as a visually apparent decrease in the FHR to less than the baseline. Decrease in FHR from the baseline is 15 bpm or greater, lasting 2 minutes or longer but less than 10 minutes in duration. If a deceleration lasts 10 minutes or longer, it is a baseline change.

Sinusoidal pattern

This is a visually apparent, smooth, sine wave–like undulating pattern in FHR baseline with a cycle frequency of 3 to 5 per minute that persists for 20 minutes or longer. This rare pattern can be associated with severe chronic anemia, hypoxia, and acidosis. In addition, pseudosinusoidal patterns can be observed with certain medications (opiates).

Classification of FHR Tracings (3-Tier System)

Category I (normal) FHR tracings are strongly predictive of normal fetal acid-base status at time of observation.[9] These tracings can be monitored in a routine manner and no specific action is required. They include all of the following:

Baseline rate: 110 to 160 bpm
Baseline FHR variability: moderate
Late or variable decelerations: absent
Early decelerations: present or absent
Accelerations: present or absent

Category II (indeterminate) FHR tracings are not predictive of abnormal fetal acid-base status, yet presently there is not adequate evidence to classify these as category I or III tracings. These require evaluation and continued surveillance and reevaluation, taking into account clinical circumstances. Ancillary tests or resuscitation may need to be used at times. Some examples can include any of the following:

Baseline rate
    Bradycardia not accompanied by absent baseline variability
    Tachycardia
Baseline FHR variability
    Minimal baseline variability
    Absent baseline variability with no recurrent decelerations
    Marked baseline variability
Accelerations
    Absence of induced accelerations after fetal stimulation
Decelerations
    Recurrent variable decelerations accompanied by minimal or moderate baseline variability
    Prolonged deceleration greater than 2 minutes but less than 10 minutes
    Recurrent late decelerations with moderate baseline variability
    Variable decelerations with other characteristics such as slow return to baseline, overshoots, or "shoulders"

Category III (abnormal) FHR tracings are associated with abnormal fetal acid-base status at the time of observation. These tracings require prompt evaluation and management to resolve the pattern. These tracings include either

Absent baseline FHR variability and any of the following:
    Recurrent late decelerations
    Recurrent variable decelerations
    Bradycardia
Sinusoidal pattern

When EFM is used intrapartum, it should be reviewed frequently. In the low-risk patient, the FHR tracing should be reviewed every 30 minutes in the first stage of labor and every 15 minutes in the second stage. High-risk patients (hypertension, growth restriction, etc) should be monitored every 15 minutes in the first stage and every 5 minutes in the second stage of labor.

ANTEPARTUM FETAL SURVEILLANCE

The primary goal of fetal surveillance is to prevent fetal death. An additional and equally important goal of both antepartum and intrapartum fetal surveillance is to identify the compromised fetus before irreversible hypoxic damage to vital organs occurs. Although the fetal mortality rate has declined steadily, it has been relatively stable at approximately 6 deaths per 1000 births since 2003.[11] Antepartum surveillance can significantly reduce the risk of antepartum death. There are several well-recognized maternal conditions and pregnancy-associated conditions that place pregnancy at increased risk for intrauterine fetal death (**Box 1**). These patients are appropriate for surveillance in that it is hoped the compromised fetus can be identified in a timely manner to allow for intervention. In contrast, there are several causes (cord prolapse, placental abruption) that are unpredictable in nature. Fetal surveillance would not be helpful in trying to prevent these situations. There are various techniques for surveillance that will be reviewed here.

Box 1
Conditions that require fetal surveillance

Maternal Conditions

    Pregnancy-related conditions

Antiphospholipid syndrome

    Preeclampsia

Hyperthyroidism

    Decreased fetal movement

Diabetes mellitus

    Oligohydramnios

Cyanotic heart disease

    Intrauterine growth restriction

Systemic lupus erythematosus

    Multiple gestation

Hypertension

    Postterm pregnancy

Chronic renal disease

    Previous fetal demise

Hemoglobinopathies

    Isoimmunization

    Preterm premature rupture of membranes

    Unexplained third-trimester bleeding

Fetal Movement Assessment

In general, the presence of fetal movement is a marker for reassuring fetal well-being. Conversely, decreased movement often, although not always, precedes fetal death. Thus, maternal perception of movement is the cheapest, simplest, and oldest method of surveillance. Several methods have been described. There is no consensus on the optimal number of movements or duration of monitoring. Nevertheless, there are 2 popular approaches. One describes the woman lying on her side to count movement.[12] The perception of 10 distinct movements during a 2-hour period is considered reassuring. Another approach has the woman count movements for 1 hour 3 times per week.[13] The count is considered reassuring if it is at least equal to the previously established baseline count. As in all types of surveillance, additional evaluation is needed if the count is not reassuring.

Nonstress Test

The nonstress test (NST) is frequently the first line in fetal surveillance. The NST is based on the premise that the heart rate of the noncompromised fetus will temporarily accelerate with fetal movement. The association between FHR and fetal movement was described as early as 1975.[14] Although FHR reactivity is a good indicator of normal fetal autonomic function, the absence of such is not necessarily pathologic. Loss of reactivity is most commonly associated with sleep cycle but can also be caused by fetal acidosis.

The patient is typically placed in the semirecumbent, tilted position and the FHR is monitored with an external transducer. A reactive test is defined as one in which there are at least 2 accelerations that peak (but do not have to remain) 15 bpm higher than baseline and last at least 15 seconds before returning to baseline. Most NSTs are reactive within 20 minutes. For those that do not meet criteria, the test can be extended for 40 minutes to account for the fetal sleep-wake cycle. A nonreactive test is defined as one in which 2 such accelerations do not occur in 40 minutes.

NSTs in noncompromised preterm fetuses are often nonreactive: from 24 to 28 weeks, up to 50% of NSTs are nonreactive[15]; from 28 to 32 weeks, 15% of NSTs are not reactive.[16] Vibroacoustic stimulation can be used to elicit accelerations; this safely reduces testing time without compromising the test.[17] Acoustic stimulation is performed by placing an artificial larynx on the maternal abdomen and applying the stimulus for 1 to 2 seconds. This can be repeated 3 times to elicit accelerations.

In general, 15% of all NSTs will be nonreactive. Of these, 25% will have a positive contraction stress test (CST), described later. In the largest series of NSTs the stillbirth rate (corrected) was 1.9 per 1000.[18] Thus, its negative predictive value is 99.8%. The NST also has a high false-positive rate (75%–90%) associated with nonreactive NST.

Biophysical Profile

The biophysical profile (BPP), initially described by Manning in 1980, combines the NST with 4 sonographic observations.[19] Criteria are as follows:

1. NST (can be omitted if all 4 ultrasound components are normal)
2. Fetal breathing movements ($\geq$1e episodes lasting at least 30 seconds in a 30-minute time period)
3. Fetal movement ($\geq$3 discrete body or limb movements in 30 minutes)
4. Fetal tone ($\geq$1 episode of extension of a fetal extremity with return to flexion or opening and closing of fetal hand)
5. Amniotic fluid volume (single vertical pocket of $\geq$2 cm)

Each component is assigned a score of 2 (present and normal) or 0 (absent, insufficient, abnormal). A score of 8 or 10 of 10 is reassuring; 6 is considered equivocal; 4 or less is abnormal. Oligohydramnios should always be evaluated further.[20]

BPP measures both chronic and acute hypoxia and asphyxia.[21] Amniotic fluid volume is a marker for chronic conditions, whereas the other 4 measure acute events. A distinct pattern exists regarding the development (and disappearance) of these parameters. The fetal tone center located in the cortex begins to function between 7.5 and 8.5 weeks. The fetal movement center in the cortex-nuclei begins to function at 9 weeks. The fetal breathing movement center located in the ventral surface of the fourth ventricle begins to function between 20 and 21 weeks. The FHR center in the posterior hypothalamus and medulla becomes functional at the end of the second or early third trimester. The biophysical activities that are present earliest in development are the last to disappear with fetal hypoxia.[22]

The stillbirth rate among those with reassuring BPPs is 0.8 per 1000, giving a negative predictive value of greater than 99.9%.[18]

Modified BPP

The modified BPP consists of the NST and amniotic fluid index to assess for fetal well-being. This combines a short-term marker with the chronic marker of amniotic fluid. Amniotic fluid index is measured by summing the measurements of deepest cord-free amniotic fluid pocket in each of the abdominal quadrants. A sum of 5 or greater is considered reassuring. The negative predictive value for this test is similar to the full BPP.[23]

Contraction Stress Test

The contraction stress test (CST) evaluates the FHR response to uterine contractions. It presumes that in the suboptimally oxygenated fetus, transient worsening in oxygen status (contractions) will lead to predictable FHR changes (late decelerations). For the CST, the patient is placed in the recumbent tilted position; FHR and uterine activity are monitored externally. Three contractions of 40 seconds' duration or longer in a 10-minute period are needed. If this does not occur spontaneously, nipple stimulation or intravenous oxytocin administration is used. The CST is interpreted according to the presence or absence of late decelerations.[24] Categories are as follows:

Negative: no late or significant variable decelerations
Positive: late decelerations following 50% or greater of contractions (even if the contraction frequency is less than 3 in 10 minutes)
Equivocal—suspicious: intermittent late decelerations or significant variable decelerations
Equivocal—hyperstimulatory: FHR decelerations that occur in the presence of contractions more frequent than every 2 minutes or lasting longer than 90 seconds
Unsatisfactory—fewer than 3 contractions in 10 minutes or an uninterpretable tracing

The stillbirth rate in the setting of negative CST is 0.3 per 1000, giving a negative predictive value of greater than 99.9%.[18] Relative contraindications to CST include those conditions for which labor would be undesirable.[25] These include preterm labor, preterm rupture of membranes, history of extensive uterine surgery, and placenta previa.

Doppler Velocimetry

Doppler velocimetry is a now well-described technique used to assess fetal status. Several vessels have been interrogated including the (maternal) uterine artery, fetal middle cerebral artery, umbilical artery, umbilical vein, and ductus venosus. The most commonly examined and clinically useful vessel is the fetal umbilical artery. Doppler measurements of flow through this vessel directly reflect the status of fetoplacental circulation. The waveform in normally growing fetuses is characterized by high-velocity diastolic flow and the commonly measured indices include systolic/diastolic ratio, resistance index, and pulsatility index.[26] Marked abnormality in the waveform is characterized by absent or reversed diastolic flow. These waveforms correlate histopathologically with small artery obliteration in placental tertiary villi, and functionally with fetal hypoxia, acidosis, and prenatal morbidity and mortality.[27]

Umbilical artery Doppler velocimetry has not been found to be beneficial in the low-risk population. However, in pregnancies with suspected growth restriction, Doppler velocimetry can follow a predictable pattern and thus be useful in management and intervention in this high-risk population. The Society for Maternal Fetal Medicine recently published a clinical guideline as pertains to Doppler assessment in intrauterine growth restriction (IUGR).[28] Recommendations are as follows:

1. Doppler examination of any vessel is not recommended as a screening tool for identifying pregnancies that will subsequently be complicated by IUGR.
2. Antepartum surveillance of a viable fetus with suspected intrauterine IUGR should include Doppler examination of the umbilical artery, as its use is associated with a significant decrease in perinatal mortality.
3. Once IUGR is suspected, umbilical artery Doppler studies should be performed usually every 1 to 2 weeks to assess for deterioration; if normal, they can be extended to less frequent intervals.
4. Doppler assessment of additional fetal vessels has not been sufficiently evaluated in randomized trials to recommend its routine use in clinical practice in fetuses with suspected IUGR.
5. Antenatal corticosteroids should be administered if absent or reversed end-diastolic flow is noted before 34 weeks in a pregnancy with suspected IUGR.
6. As long as fetal surveillance remains reassuring, women with suspected IUGR and absent umbilical artery end-diastolic flow may be managed expectantly until delivery at 34 weeks.
7. As long as fetal surveillance remains reassuring, women with suspected IUGR and reversed umbilical artery end-diastolic flow may be managed expectantly until delivery at 32 weeks.

Clinical Considerations/Interpreting Test Results

As stated previously, nonreassuring or abnormal results in any of the mentioned tests should prompt further evaluation. The overall clinical scenario should be taken into account because some acute maternal conditions can result in abnormal results. In the absence of worsening maternal status, a stepwise approach can be used.

Maternal reports of decreased fetal movement can be evaluated a number of ways—NST, CST, BPP, modified BPP. A normal result is reassuring and typically enough to exclude imminent fetal distress. A nonreactive NST or abnormal modified BPP should be followed by additional testing (CST or BPP). A positive CST heightens concern for hypoxemia induced acidosis. Usually a nonreactive NST and positive CST is an indication for delivery. However, this combination is also frequently associated with fetal malformation and prompts complete sonographic evaluation.[29] A negative

CST implies that the nonreactive NST is the result of prematurity, sleep cycle, preexisting neurologic damage, or another cause.

As stated previously, a BPP score of 6 is considered equivocal and should prompt delivery in the term fetus. In the preterm fetus, repeat evaluation should be performed in 24 hours and corticosteroid administration can be considered in the interim for gestation less than 34 weeks.[20] Continued equivocal testing should result in delivery or continued surveillance. BPP score of 4 usually indicates delivery. BPP score of less than 4 should prompt expeditious delivery. Delivery of the fetus with an abnormal test result can be attempted via induction of labor unless obstetrically contraindicated (placenta pervia, classical uterine incision, etc).

If the clinical scenario is stable, reassuring tests are considered reliable for 1 week, and testing can be performed on a weekly basis. If the indication for testing is not persistent or recurrent (decreased fetal movement), then the test should not be repeated. Alternatively, in some high-risk populations (eg, diabetes mellitus), testing may be performed more often than on a weekly basis.[30]

Often, clinical situations unrelated to fetal well-being can temporarily affect the interpretation of surveillance techniques. Several maternal behaviors (eg, tobacco and alcohol use) decrease fetal movement, breathing, and heart rate reactivity.[31] Corticosteroids also decrease movement, breathing, and heart rate reactivity but do not compromise neonatal outcome.[32] Finally, several serious maternal medical conditions often result in nonreassuring fetal surveillance: diabetic ketoacidosis and acute asthma exacerbation. Delivery of the infant in this precarious setting is often ill advised and dangerous. Usually, if maternal status can be stabilized and optimized, the fetal status is also improved, avoiding the unnecessary preterm birth.

Ideally, resuscitative efforts can be used in the antepartum period so that pregnancy can be safely prolonged. In an acute, short-lived event such as deceleration on NST, techniques such as maternal repositioning, intravenous fluid bolus, and oxygen administration can be used. Continued monitoring is also warranted. Although technically not resuscitative, antenatal corticosteroid administration for worsening fetal status (declining BPP, abnormal Doppler results) is beneficial for optimizing neonatal outcomes.

As stated previously, antenatal testing is commonly used for pregnancies complicated by chronic conditions. Because techniques for fetal resuscitation are beneficial for common reversible indications, these generally are not effective when trying to resuscitate the growth restricted fetus of a mother with worsening hypertensive disease, for instance. For these particular scenarios, frequent testing with prompt recognition of worsening status to determine need for delivery is indicated.

THE COMPROMISED INTRAPARTUM FETUS

Continuous electronic FHR monitoring is the primary diagnostic tool used to detect the compromised fetus in labor. The previously described 3-tiered system aids in diagnosing and managing FHR tracings. Category I tracings are normal and not associated with fetal acidemia.[9] These can be managed in a routine manner with continuous or intermittent monitoring. Category I tracings should be periodically evaluated and documented during active labor. Management changes should be made if the tracing changes from category I to category II or III.

Category II tracings include all FHR patterns that are not category I or III. These require evaluation and continued surveillance. Several scenarios are described here. Intermittent variable decelerations (occur with <50% of contractions) are a common FHR abnormality in labor and typically do not require treatment.[33] However, recurrent variable decelerations that progress to greater depth and longer duration are more likely to represent acidemia. Thus, resuscitative efforts are directed at relieving umbilical cord compression.[34] This can be accomplished by maternal repositioning and amnioinfusion (**Table 1**).

Recurrent late decelerations reflect transient or chronic uteroplacental insufficiency. The causes are varied and include maternal hypotension from epidural, uterine tachysystole, and maternal hypoxia. Resuscitative techniques involve maneuvers to promote uteroplacental perfusion including maternal lateral positioning, intravenous fluid bolus, and maternal oxygen administration (see **Table 1**).[34] After appropriate resuscitation, reevaluation is necessary. The presence of FHR accelerations or moderate variability greatly reduces the risk for fetal acidemia. However, if recurrent late decelerations persist and moderate variability and accelerations are not present, fetal acidemia must be considered and need for delivery evaluated.

Fetal tachycardia often has an identifiable underlying cause such as infection, maternal medications, maternal medical disorders, obstetric conditions (bleeding), and, less often, fetal tachyarrhythmia. Management should be directed to the underlying cause (ie, administering antibiotics and antipyretics if intra-amniotic infection is diagnosed). Alternatively, it is also important to identify maternal disorders or identify bleeding. Tachycardia is poorly predictive of fetal acidemia unless accompanied by decreased variability or recurrent decelerations.

Fetal bradycardia and prolonged decelerations are initially managed in a similar manner. Evaluation for identifiable causes should be performed promptly. Maternal hypotension, umbilical cord prolapse, rapid fetal descent, tachysystole, abruption, and uterine rupture all can be causes of bradycardic episodes. Less commonly, fetuses with congenital heart defects will present with bradycardia. Again, resuscitative efforts are directed at the underlying cause (see **Table 1**). If prolapsed umbilical cord is identified, a hand can be used to elevate the presenting part until delivery can be accomplished. This is performed by a practitioner placing one hand in the vagina, through the cervix, and physically elevating the presenting part to relieve pressure on the umbilical cord. Hypotension can be corrected by administering

Table 1
Intrauterine resuscitative techniques

Technique	FHR Abnormality	Objective
Maternal repositioning	Bradycardia, prolonged deceleration, minimal variability	Restore blood flow and oxygenation
IV fluid bolus	Recurrent late decelerations, bradycardia, prolonged deceleration, minimal variability	Relieve hypotension, increase blood flow
Sympathomimetic drug administration	Bradycardia, prolonged deceleration	Relieve hypotension, increase blood flow
Oxygen administration	Minimal variability, late decelerations	Promote oxygenation
Amnioinfusion	Recurrent variable decelerations	Alleviate cord compression
Decrease/discontinue oxytocin; administer tocolytic	Tachysystole with category II or III tracing	Decrease contractions
Cervical examination	Bradycardia, prolonged deceleration	Identify cord prolapse or rapid cervical change

intravenous fluids or sympathomimetics. Bradycardia with minimal or absent variability or a prolonged deceleration that does not resolve prompts expeditious delivery.

FHR variability often changes during the course of labor. Minimal variability can indicate acidemia; however, other causes can include maternal opioid administration, other medications such as magnesium sulfate, and fetal sleep cycles.[35,36] Maternal repositioning, maternal oxygen administration, and intravenous fluid bolus can be considered if decreased variability is thought to be the result of decreased fetal oxygenation. Scalp stimulation or vibroacoustic stimulation can be performed if variability does not improve and there are no FHR accelerations. Continued minimal variability that is unexplained and does not resolve should be considered to potentially indicate acidemia and managed accordingly.

Tachysystole can be associated with or without FHR changes. Specific management depends on the category of fetal tracing. Category I tracings can be managed with close observation. Category II or III tracings require resuscitative measures depending on the characterization of the heart rate abnormality. Recurrent FHR decelerations always prompt further evaluation. Specific treatment such as decreasing or discontinuing oxytocin or use of tocolytics may be warranted.[37]

Resuscitative measures or interventions ideally specifically address the abnormal FHR. Several nonsurgical interventions can be used. Even though there is no conclusive evidence that oxygen administration to the mother improves fetal oxygenation, a common technique is to administer oxygen via face mask when the FHR has characteristics suggestive of hypoxia (late decelerations). Repositioning the patient to the lateral recumbent position is another technique. This type of positioning allows for the least amount of blood flow to other muscles and maximizes cardiac return and output. Increasing hydration by extraintravenous fluid administration potentially maximizes intravascular volume and uterine perfusion. Decreasing or discontinuing oxytocin allows for more time between contractions, and therefore more time to perfuse the placenta and deliver oxygen. Administering tocolytics can be used in the patient having excessive spontaneous contractions and associated nonreassuring FHR.

Several other techniques have been used to evaluate nonreassuring FHR. Assessing the fetal scalp pH is a well-tested method for determining fetal acidosis. To perform this, a plastic cone is inserted transvaginally against the fetal vertex. The cervix needs to be at least 4 cm dilated. A lubricant is applied to the scalp to aid in beading of fetal blood. The scalp is then pricked and the blood collected. A scalp pH less than 7.2 typically correlates with fetal acidosis. A pH of 7.2 to 7.25 is borderline and should be repeated immediately. A pH of greater than 7.25 is reassuring, but this measure should be repeated every 30 minutes to ensure well-being.[38] The cartridges required to assess pH are not available in the United States, thus rendering this technique nearly obsolete in this country.

Pulse oximetry has been found to be of great value in assessing the condition of adult and pediatric patients, but technical challenges created barriers to use of this technology for a great period. A device was developed and marketed in the United States with which preliminary data seemed to show significant fetal academia when fetal oximetry readings decreased to less than 30%. The device involved sliding a transducer through the cervix after rupture of membranes, with the transducer sitting adjacent to the fetal cheek. However, a large randomized trial in more than 5000 subjects that compared use of this device with routine electronic fetal monitoring versus routine monitoring only failed to show a benefit in either neonatal outcomes or reduced obstetric interventions.[39]

Category III tracings are abnormal and place the fetus at increased risk for fetal acidemia.[9] They are associated with increased risk for encephalopathy, cerebral palsy, and neonatal acidosis. They have poor predictive value for overall abnormal neurologic outcome. Category III tracings require expeditious delivery if they do not resolve. The same resuscitative measures are used (ie, positioning, fluid bolus, tocolysis if tachysystole is noted, amnioinfusion).[34] Although an optimal time frame in which to accomplish delivery has not been established, in general, a 30-minute decision to incision time is used.[40] Delivery can be accomplished via operative vaginal delivery (vacuum or forceps assisted) if the clinical scenario is appropriate. Often, the patient is remote from vaginal delivery and cesarean delivery is necessary.

Many studies have demonstrated the lack of association of increased adverse outcomes if delivery is accomplished later than 30 minutes after the decision to deliver was made. In a study of 2808 women who had emergent cesarean deliveries, 30% began after greater than 30 minutes from the time of the decision to operate but adverse neonatal outcomes were not increased.[41] When the decision is made, delivery should be accomplished as expeditiously but also as safely as possible. There are logistic issues to consider when preparing for delivery in the setting of a category III tracing, including obtaining informed consent, assembling the necessary personnel (surgical team, anesthesia, neonatal resuscitation team), and ensuring maternal stability.

The initiation of electronic FHR monitoring was expected to reduce the number of cases of intrapartum asphyxia leading to death, neurologic damage, or cerebral palsy. Although intrapartum deaths have significantly declined, the rates of cerebral palsy have remained steady for the past 30 years.[42] In the same time frame, the rate of cesarean delivery has significantly increased to 33% in 2009.[43] It is recognized that intrapartum events are rarely responsible for cerebral palsy. Despite minimal evidence to support long-term benefit from the use of electronic FHR monitoring, it will likely remain as the most common form of intrapartum surveillance for the near future.

SUMMARY

Antepartum and intrapartum surveillance techniques provide an opportunity to monitor fetal well-being. Our gold standard—continuous FHR monitoring—allows for identification of the compromised fetus. It is hoped that the prompt assessment and judicious use of resuscitative techniques can identify the fetus in need of delivery or further evaluation. Further research is still needed to develop new monitoring techniques and resuscitative therapies. One such monitoring technique is currently being researched via a large multicenter trial sponsored by Eunice Kennedy Shriver National Institute of Child Health and Human Development.[44] This randomized trial of fetal electrocardiographic ST segment and T wave ANalysis (STAN) as an adjunct to electronic FHR monitoring seeks to determine whether fetal STAN reduces the risk of perinatal hypoxic-ischemic morbidity and mortality. Conceptually, it is thought that pathologic fetal cardiac hypoxia leading to ST- or T-segment alterations detected by computer analysis can alert physicians in an objective way before overt acidemia occurs. This study is still in the recruiting phase, but its results and outcomes are eagerly awaited.

REFERENCES

1. Manning FA, Platt LD. Maternal hypoxemia and fetal breathing movements. Obstet Gynecol 1979;53(6):758–60.
2. Murata Y, Martin CB Jr, Ikenoue T, et al. Fetal heart rate accelerations and late decelerations during the course of intrauterine death in chronically catheterized rhesus monkeys. Am J Obstet Gynecol 1982;144(2):218–23.

3. Weiner CP, Sipes SL, Wenstrom K. The effect of fetal age upon normal fetal laboratory values and venous pressure. Obstet Gynecol 1992;79(5): 713–8.

4. Manning FA, Snijders R, Harman CR, et al. Fetal biophysical profile score. VI. Correlation with antepartum umbilical venous fetal pH. Am J Obstet Gynecol 1993;169(4):755–63.

5. Kennedy E. Observation on obstetrics auscultation. Dublin (Ireland): Hodges and Smith; 1833. p. 1.

6. Hillis DS. Attachment for the stethoscope. JAMA 1917;68:910.

7. Hon EH. Observations on pathologic fetal bradycardia. Am J Obstet Gynecol 1959;77(5):1084–99.

8. Martin JA, Hamilton BE, Sutton PD, et al. Births: final data for 2002. Natl Vital Stat Rep 2003;52(10):1–113.

9. Macones GA, Hankins GD, Spong CY, et al. The 2008 National Institute of Child Health and Human Development workshop report on electronic fetal monitoring: update on definitions, interpretation, and research guidelines. Obstet Gynecol 2008;112(3):661–6.

10. Parer JT, King T, Flanders S, et al. Fetal acidemia and electronic fetal heart rate patterns: is there evidence of an association? J Matern Fetal Neonatal Med 2006; 19(5):289–94.

11. MacDorman MF, Kirmeyer S. Fetal and perinatal mortality, United States, 2005. Natl Vital Stat Rep 2009;57(8):1–19.

12. Moore TR, Piacquadio K. A prospective evaluation of fetal movement screening to reduce the incidence of antepartum fetal death. Am J Obstet Gynecol 1989; 160(5 Pt 1):1075–80.

13. Neldam S. Fetal movements as an indicator of fetal well-being. Dan Med Bull 1983;30(4):274–8.

14. Lee CY, Di Loreto PC, O'Lane JM. A study of fetal heart rate acceleration patterns. Obstet Gynecol 1975;45(2):141–6.

15. Bishop EH. Fetal acceleration test. Am J Obstet Gynecol 1981;141(8):905–9.

16. Lavin JP Jr, Miodovnik M, Barden TP. Relationship of nonstress test reactivity and gestational age. Obstet Gynecol 1984;63(3):338–44.

17. Zimmer EZ, Divon MY. Fetal vibroacoustic stimulation. Obstet Gynecol 1993;81: 451–7.

18. Manning FA, Morrison I, Harman CR, et al. Fetal assessment based on fetal biophysical profile scoring: experience in 19,221 referred high-risk pregnancies. II. An analysis of false-negative fetal deaths. Am J Obstet Gynecol 1987;157(4 Pt 1):880–4.

19. Manning FA, Platt LD, Sipos L. Antepartum fetal evaluation: development of a fetal biophysical profile. Am J Obstet Gynecol 1980;136(6):787–95.

20. Manning FA, Harman CR, Morrison I, et al. Fetal assessment based on fetal biophysical profile scoring. IV. An analysis of perinatal morbidity and mortality. Am J Obstet Gynecol 1990;162(3):703–9.

21. Hanley M, Vintzileos AM. Biophysical testing in premature rupture of the membranes. Semin Perinatol 1996;20(5):418–25.

22. Vintzileos AM, Knuppel RA. Fetal biophysical assessment in premature rupture of the membranes. Clin Obstet Gynecol 1995;38(1):45–58.

23. Miler DA, Rabello YA, Paul RH. The modified biophysical profile: antepartum testing in the 1990s. Am J Obstet Gynecol 1996;174(3):812–7.

24. Freeman RK, Anderson G, Dorchester W. A prospective multi-institutional study of antepartum fetal heart rate monitoring. I. Risk of perinatal mortality and morbidity

according to antepartum fetal heart rate test results. Am J Obstet Gynecol 1982; 143(7):771–7.

25. Freeman RK. The use of the oxytocin challenge test for antepartum clinical evaluation of uteroplacental respiratory function. Am J Obstet Gynecol 1975;121(4): 481–9.

26. Erkskine RL, Ritchie JW. Umbilical artery blood flow characteristics in normal and growth-retarded fetuses. Br J Obstet Gynaecol 1985;92(6):605–10.

27. Karsdorp VH, van Vugt JM, van Geijn HP, et al. Clinical significance of absent or reversed end diastolic velocity waveforms in umbilical artery. Lancet 1994; 344(8938):1664–8.

28. Society for Maternal-Fetal Medicine Publications Committee, Berkley E, Chauhan SP, et al. Doppler assessment of the fetus with intrauterine growth restriction. Am J Obstet Gynecol 2012;206(4):300–8.

29. Garite TJ, Linzey EM, Freeman RK, et al. Fetal heart rate patterns and fetal distress in fetuses with congenital anomalies. Obstet Gynecol 1979;53(6): 716–20.

30. Boehm FH, Salyer S, Shah DM, et al. Improved outcome of twice weekly nonstress testing. Obstet Gynecol 1986;67(4):566–8.

31. Fox HE, Steinbrecher M, Pessel D, et al. Maternal ethanol ingestion and the occurrence of human fetal breathing movements. Am J Obstet Gynecol 1978; 132(4):354–8.

32. Mulder EJ, Derks JB, Visser GH. Antenatal corticosteroid therapy and fetal behaviour: a randomised study of the effects of betamethasone and dexamethasone. Br J Obstet Gynaecol 1997;104(11):1239–47.

33. Garite TJ, Dildy GA, McNamara H, et al. A multicenter controlled trial of fetal pulse oximetry in the intrapartum management of nonreassuring fetal heart rate patterns. Am J Obstet Gynecol 2000;183(5):1049–58.

34. Simpson KR. Intrauterine resuscitation during labor: review of current methods and supportive evidence. J Midwifery Womens Health 2007;52(3):229–37.

35. Giannina G, Guzman ER, Lai YL, et al. Comparison of the effects of meperidine and nalbuphine on intrapartum fetal heart rate tracings. Obstet Gynecol 1995; 86(3):441–5.

36. Hallak M, Martinez-Poyer J, Kruger ML, et al. The effect of magnesium sulfate on fetal heart rate parameters: a randomized placebo-controlled trial. Am J Obstet Gynecol 1999;181(5 Pt 1):1122–7.

37. Kulier R, Hofmeyr GJ. Tocolytics for suspected intrapartum fetal distress. Cochrane Database Syst Rev 2000;(2):CD000035.

38. Clark SL, Paul RH. Intrapartum fetal surveillance: the role of fetal scalp blood sampling. Am J Obstet Gynecol 1985;153(7):717–20.

39. Bloom SL, Spong CY, Thom E, et al. Fetal pulse oximetry and cesarean delivery. National Institute of Child Health and Human Development Maternal-Fetal Medicine Units Network. N Engl J Med 2006;355(21):2195–202.

40. American Academy of Pediatrics, American College of Obstetricians and Gynecologists. Fetal heart rate monitoring. In: Guidelines for perinatal care. 6th edition. Elk Grove Village (IL); Washington, DC: AAP; ACOG; 2007. p. 146–7.

41. Bloom SL, Leveno KJ, Spong CY, et al. Decision-to-incision times and maternal and infant outcomes. National Institute of Child Health and Human Development Maternal-Fetal Medicine Units Network. Obstet Gynecol 2006;108(1): 6–11.

42. Clark SL, Hankins GD. Temporal and demographic trends in cerebral palsy – fact and fiction. Am J Obstet Gynecol 2003;188(3):628–33.

43. Martin JA, Hamilton BE, Ventura SJ, et al. Births: final data for 2009. Natl Vital Stat Rep 2011;60(1):1–70.
44. Eunice Kennedy Shriver National Institute of Child Health and Human Development (NICHD). A randomized trial of fetal ECG ST Segment and T Wave Analysis as an adjunct to electronic fetal heart rate monitoring (STAN). Available at: Clinicaltrials.gov. identifier NCT01131260.

Physiology of Transition from Intrauterine to Extrauterine Life

Noah H. Hillman, MD, Suhas G. Kallapur, MD,
Alan H. Jobe, MD, PhD*

KEYWORDS

- Corticosteroids • Catecholamines • Lung function • Cardiovascular
- Cesarean section

KEY POINTS

- The transition from fetal to extrauterine life is the summation of multiple rapid organ adaptations that often have redundant mediators.
- The primary mediators that both prepare the fetus for birth and support the multiorgan transitions are cortisol and catecholamines.
- Lung adaptation requires the coordinated clearance of fetal lung fluid, surfactant secretion, and the onset of consistent breathing.
- Cardiovascular transition requires striking changes in blood flow, pressures, and pulmonary vasodilation.
- Abnormalities in adaptation are frequent following preterm birth or delivery by cesarean section at term.

OVERVIEW

The transition from a fetus to a newborn is the most complex physiologic adaptation that occurs in human experience. Before medicalization of delivery, the transition had to occur quickly for survival of the newborn. All organ systems are involved at some level, but the major immediate adaptations are the establishment of air breathing concurrently with changes in pressures and flows within the cardiovascular system. Other essential adaptations are striking changes in endocrine function, substrate metabolism, and thermogenesis (**Box 1**). Hospital-based deliveries increase the difficulties for transition for many fetuses because of the frequent use of cesarean sections, deliveries before the onset of labor, rapid clamping of the cord, and the anesthetics and analgesics associated with these hospital deliveries. The net result is the

Support: NIH R01-HD072842 (PI-Jobe), K08-HL097085 (Hillman-PI).
Conflict of interest: The authors have no conflicts of interest with this article.
Division of Pulmonary Biology, Cincinnati Children's Hospital Medical Center, University of Cincinnati, 3333 Burnet Avenue, ML#7029, Cincinnati, OH 45229-3039, USA
* Corresponding author. Division of Pulmonary Biology, Cincinnati Children's Hospital, 3333 Burnet Avenue, ML#7029, Cincinnati, OH 45229-3039.
E-mail address: alan.jobe@cchmc.org

Clin Perinatol 39 (2012) 769–783
http://dx.doi.org/10.1016/j.clp.2012.09.009
0095-5108/12/$ – see front matter © 2012 Elsevier Inc. All rights reserved.

Box 1

Essential components for a normal neonatal transition

- Clearance of fetal lung fluid
- Surfactant secretion and breathing
- Transition of fetal to neonatal circulation
- Decrease in pulmonary vascular resistance and increased pulmonary blood flow
- Endocrine support of the transition

---

frequent need to assist the newborn with the birth transition. Preterm deliveries cause particular difficulties for transition and expose the preterm infant to lung injury from mechanical ventilation. These components of the fetal to neonatal transition are reviewed for preterm and term deliveries.

ENDOCRINE ADAPTATIONS TO BIRTH
Cortisol

Cortisol is the major regulatory hormone for terminal maturation of the fetus and for neonatal adaption at birth.[1] The "cortisol surge" is initiated with the switch from maternal-transplacental–derived corticosteroids to the ability of the fetal adrenal to synthesize and release cortisol under fetal hypothalamic control. Fetal cortisol levels in the human are low (5–10 µg/mL) relative to normal cortisol levels until about 30 weeks' gestation. Cortisol levels progressively increase to about 20 µg/mL by about 36 weeks' gestation and increase further to about 45 µg/mL before labor at term. Cortisol increases further during labor to peak at high levels of about 200 µg/mL several hours after term delivery. The increase in fetal cortisol throughout late gestation supports multiple physiologic changes that facilitate normal neonatal adaption. For example, over the final weeks of gestation, the conversion of T_4 to T_3 increases, catecholamine release by the adrenal and other chromaffin tissues increases, glucose metabolic pathways in the liver mature, gut digestive capacity increases (enzyme induction), β-adrenergic receptor density increases in many tissues, including the heart and the lungs, and the surfactant system in the lungs is induced to mature.[2] Cortisol, in association with increasing thyroid hormones, activates the sodium pump that clears fetal lung fluid at birth. These cortisol-modulated changes are normally a progressive process of preparation for birth as the cortisol levels rise before birth then peak soon after delivery. This normal increase in cortisol supports an integrated transition following birth (**Box 2**). Cesarean section without labor at term blunts

---

Box 2

Some effects of cortisol on factors contributing to a normal fetal-to-newborn transition

- Lung maturation: anatomy and surfactant
- Clearance of fetal lung fluid
- Increased β receptor density
- Gut functional maturation
- Maturation of thyroid axis
- Regulate catecholamine release
- Control energy substrate metabolism

the postnatal rise in cortisol, and the cortisol responses to preterm birth also are attenuated because of unresponsiveness and immaturity of the adrenal gland.[3] A particularly stressful delivery can uncover a "functional" adrenal insufficiency if the adrenal gland cannot respond to the increased stress. The very preterm infant may have low cortisol levels around birth with symptoms, such as low blood pressure, that are responsive to cortisol treatment. In contrast, antenatal exposure to chorioamnionitis may increase fetal cortisol levels before delivery.[4]

Catecholamines

Despite the enthusiasm of clinicians to use catecholamine infusions to increase the blood pressure of very preterm infants following birth, the normal physiology of endogenous catecholamines during and after birth are not reviewed in recent neonatology textbooks. The term human fetus can release catecholamines (norepinephrine, epinephrine, and dopamine) from adrenal medullary and other sympathetic tissues in response to fetal stresses of various sorts, as evaluated by catecholamine values in cord blood.[5] The preterm fetus has higher cord catecholamine levels than the term fetus, and cesarean delivery is associated with lower cord catecholamine levels. The details of the catecholamine responses to term and preterm labor and delivery were characterized elegantly by Padbury and colleagues[6] in a series of reports beginning in the 1980s. Using catheterized fetal sheep that were transitioned through delivery, they demonstrated that norepinephrine and epinephrine increase to high levels within minutes of term delivery and cord clamping. In contrast, the catecholamines increased more slowly following preterm delivery but to levels that were about threefold higher for norepinephrine and fivefold higher for epinephrine than after term delivery (**Fig. 1**). The lower increases in catecholamines in the term newborn were associated with larger increases in plasma glucose and free fatty acids than in the preterm. Careful measurement of thresholds for responses of fetal sheep to epinephrine and norepinephrine infusion demonstrated that the term fetus had lower thresholds and greater responses for blood pressure, glucose, and free fatty acid increases than did the preterm fetuses.[7] The catecholamine increases at delivery resulted primarily from adrenal release as adrenalectomy ablated the increase in epinephrine and norepinephrine and blunted blood pressure, glucose, and fatty acid increases and pulmonary adaption.[8] The fetus is in part protected from the cardiovascular and metabolic effects of stress-mediated catecholamine release because the placenta increases catecholamine clearance.[9]

These studies demonstrate the importance of a large catecholamine release as a normal response to the birth process for fetal adaption. The catecholamine surge is primarily responsible for the increase in blood pressure following birth, adaption of energy metabolism with support of the primary substrates for metabolism after birth (glucose and fatty acids), and for initiating thermogenesis from brown fat. The preterm secretes more catecholamines because the organ systems are less responsive: higher concentration thresholds for response and lower responses. Cesarean section of the unlabored fetus depresses catecholamine release. Catecholamine release at birth can be viewed as the "gas" that drives the adaptive responses. However, fetal exposure to cortisol is the "carburetor" that is the potent regulator of the responses of the newborn to catecholamines. Antenatal corticosteroid treatments decrease catecholamine levels in preterm infants compared with unexposed infants.[10] Cortisol treatments of fetal sheep also greatly decrease the postnatal increase in both norepinephrine and epinephrine (**Fig. 2**).[11] Nevertheless, the animals had better cardiovascular and metabolic adaptation to preterm birth. These studies demonstrate the importance of both cortisol and catecholamines to adaptations to birth.

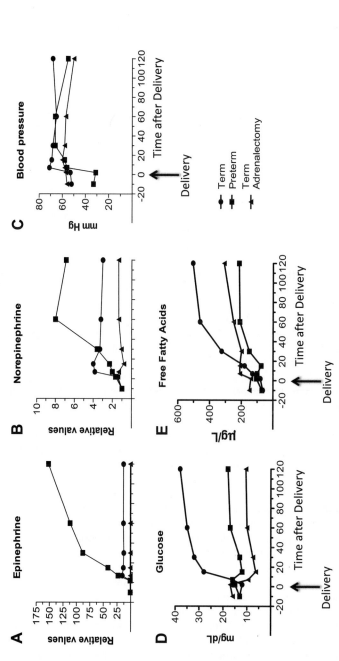

Fig. 1. Catecholamine response to delivery of term lambs, preterm lambs, and term lambs following adrenalectomy. Fetal term (145 ± 2 day gestation) and preterm (130 ± 1 day gestation) lambs were delivered at 0 time following fetal catheter placement. The adrenalectomy lambs had adrenal glands removed at 138 ± 1 days and received continuous cortisol supplemental until delivery at 142 days' gestation. Epinephrine and norepinephrine values are expressed relative to the values measured 10 minutes before delivery. (A) Epinephrine increased about 12-fold over the –10-minute value for the term lambs, and this increase was ablated by adrenalectomy. The increase in epinephrine was much larger for the preterm lambs. (B) There was a similar pattern for the norepinephrine responses. (C) Blood pressure increased in term and preterm animals but not in term adrenalectomized animals. (D, E) Glucose and free fatty acids in blood increased more for term than preterm lambs with minimal increases following adrenalectomy. (Data from Padbury JF, Polk DH, Newnham JP, et al. Neonatal adaptation: greater sympathoadrenal response in preterm than full-term fetal sheep at birth. Am J Physiol 1985;248:E443–9; and Padbury J, Agata Y, Ludlow J, et al. Effect of fetal adrenalectomy on catecholamine release and physiologic adaptation at birth in sheep. J Clin Invest 1987;80:1096-103.)

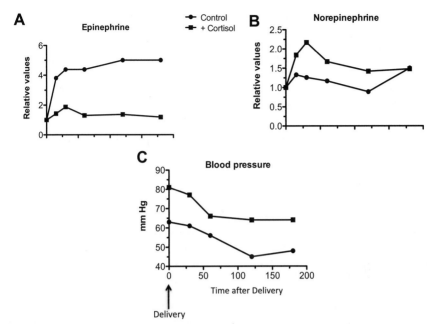

Fig. 2. Antenatal cortisol alters postnatal catecholamine secretion and blood pressure responses to delivery in preterm lambs. Fetal sheep had vascular catheters placed at 122–125 days' gestation, and the fetuses were randomized to a 60-hour cortisol or vehicle infusion at 128 days' gestation. The fetuses were delivered and supported on mechanical ventilation. During transition, epinephrine (*A*) and norepinephrine (*B*) increased more in control lambs than in cortisol-exposed lambs. Nevertheless, blood pressure (*C*) was higher in the cortisol-exposed newborns than the control animals. (*Data from* Stein HM, Martinez A, Oyama K, et al. Effect of corticosteroids on free and sulfoconjugated catecholamines at birth in premature newborn sheep. Am J Physiol 1995;268:E28–32.)

Other vasoactive substances, such as angiotensin II and rennin, also increase greatly at birth in association with increases in blood pressure.[12] The net effect is the normal exposure of the newborn to very high levels of multiple vasoactive substances to support adaption. The basic physiology of these agents was described more than 20 years ago in animal models, with confirmation in term and moderately preterm infants. Much of this work could be profitably repeated for extremely low birth weight infants to better understand how their catecholamine responses to preterm birth may be dysregulated and to better target therapies. For example, Ezaki and colleagues[13] recently reported that very low birth weight infants with severe hypotension had a decreased conversion of dopamine to norepinephrine.

Thyroid Hormones

The thyroid axis matures in late gestation in parallel to the increase in cortisol with increased thyroid simulating hormone (TSH), T_3 and T_4 levels, and decreased rT3 levels as term approaches.[14] Following term birth, TSH quickly peaks and decreases, and T_3 and T_4 increase in response primarily to the increased cortisol, to cord clamping, and to the cold stimulus of birth. Acute ablation of thyroid function at birth did not greatly alter thermogenesis or cardiovascular adaptation in experimental animals. However, inhibition of thyroid function more chronically before birth did interfere with postnatal cardiovascular adaptation and thermogenesis in newborn lambs.[15]

These results demonstrate a supportive and preparative role for thyroid hormones for birth rather than as acute modulators of endocrine adaptation to birth. For example, fetal infusions of T_3 and cortisol can activate the Na^+, K^+, ATPase that helps clear fetal lung fluid after birth.[16] Term infants with congenital hypothyroidism generally do not have abnormalities of early neonatal adaptation that are evident in the controlled environment of hospital deliveries. Very preterm infants have a blunted thyroid functional transition from fetal to newborn life with very low levels of plasma T_3 and T_4 relative to term infants. The effects of the depressed thyroid function on the early postnatal transition in the preterm are unclear but probably contribute to the depressed adaptive behavior of the preterm.

METABOLIC ADAPTATIONS
Energy Metabolism

Fetal energy needs are supported primarily by the transplacental transfer of glucose to the fetus.[17] Although the fetal liver is capable of gluconeogenesis from early gestation, gluconeogenesis is minimal during normal fetal homeostasis. Rather, as term approaches, glucose and other substrates are being stored as glycogen and fat in anticipation of birth in the high insulin and low glycogen fetal environment. With delivery and cord clamping, the maternal glucose supply is removed, and plasma glucose levels normally fall over the early hours after birth. The glucose and free fatty acid levels are accompanied by a fall in insulin, and increase in glycogen, the normal glucose homeostatic hormones. However, the large catecholamine release and increase in cortisol are probably the major acute regulators of plasma glucose and free fatty acid levels in the immediate newborn period. For example, adrenalectomy of the fetal sheep who received cortisol replacement blunts and delays the postdelivery increase in plasma free fatty acids and results in persistent hypoglycemia (see **Fig. 1**).[8] Fetal treatments with cortisol decrease the catecholamine surge at birth, but increase both plasma glucose, and free fatty acids relative to control animals (see **Fig. 2**).[11] Therefore, the metabolic adaptations to birth are regulated by acute changes in insulin and glucogen, but also by catecholamines and cortisol in term infants.

Cortisol and catecholamine responses to preterm birth are dysregulated with less cortisol and more catecholamine release. The preterm also has minimal glycogen and fat stores.[17] Therefore, the availability of energy substrates during the birth transition will be severely challenging for the preterm. This aspect of adaptation in the immediate newborn period is treated routinely with glucose infusion to prevent hypoglycemia; however, the integrated effects of the endocrine abnormalities and responses to glucose infusions have not been well described in extremely low birth weight infants.

Thermoregulation

Fetal body temperature is about $0.5°C$ above the maternal temperature. Although the fetus produces heat from metabolism, that heat is effectively dissipated across the placenta and fetal membranes. At birth, the sympathetic release resulting from the redundant stimuli of increased oxygenation, ventilation, cord occlusion, and a cold stimulus to the skin activates thermogenesis by brown adipose tissue.[18] This thermogenic response potential has developed during late gestation by an increase in brown adipose tissue around the kidney and in the intrascapular areas of the back to become about 1% of fetal weight at term.[19] Brown adipose tissue generates heat by uncoupling oxidative metabolism from ATP synthesis in the mitochondria, with the release of heat.[18] This uncoupling is mediated by the mitochondrial membrane protein uncoupling protein 1 (UCP1), which is activated by norepinephrine released by the sympathetic innervation of brown adipose tissue. UCP1 levels increase in the brown adipose tissue during late gestation in response to a local conversion of T_4 to T_3 and to induction of UCP1 synthesis in response to the increasing cortisol levels in the fetal plasma as term approaches. Thus, the same hormones that modulate the fetal preparation for birth and the transition period are central to thermogenesis by brown adipose tissue. The term infant also can generate some heat by shivering thermogenesis, which is an increase in nonpurposeful skeletal muscle activity signaled by cutaneous nerve endings via central motor neurons. Shivering thermogenesis seems to be of secondary importance to the newborn human. The preterm human is at a major disadvantage for thermoregulation following birth, as brown adipose tissue has not developed in quantity or response potential for a cold stress.

CARDIOVASCULAR ADAPTATIONS

Profound changes in the cardiovascular system occur after delivery in response to removal of the low resistance placenta as the source of fetal gas exchange and nutrition. Much of our knowledge regarding cardiovascular adaptation after birth is based on studies in animals, particularly sheep. The major changes are an increase in the cardiac output and transition of fetal circulation to an adult-type of circulation. Increased cardiac output is required to provide for increases in basal metabolism, work of breathing, and thermogenesis. In the close-to-term fetus, the combined ventricular output is about 450 mL/kg/min, with the right ventricular output accounting for two-thirds of the cardiac output and the left ventricle ejecting one-third of the cardiac output.[20] Soon after birth, the circulation changes from "parallel" to "series," where the right ventricular output equals the left ventricular output. The cardiac output nearly doubles after birth to about 400 mL/kg/min (for the right and the left ventricle). This marked increase in cardiac output parallels closely the rise in oxygen consumption. The organs experiencing increased blood flow after birth are the lungs, heart, and kidney, and the gastrointestinal tract.[21] Although the precise mechanisms mediating increased cardiac output after birth are not known, the increase in cortisol and vasoactive hormones, which include catecholamines, the rennin-angiotensin system, vasopressin, and thyroid hormone, contribute to support of blood pressure and cardiovascular function.[20]

In the fetus, the relatively well-oxygenated blood from the placenta is delivered via the umbilical cord and ductus venous. This ductus venous blood enters the right atrium from the inferior vena cava and is directed preferentially to the left atrium by the foramen ovule and subsequently delivered preferentially to the brain and the coronary circulation by the fetal left ventricle. The right ventricle is the predominant ventricle in the fetus, and most of the right ventricular output goes to the descending aorta via the ductus arteriosus because very little blood enters the pulmonary circulation. With birth and removal of the low resistance placenta, blood flow increases to the pulmonary circulation. Shortly after birth, functional closure of the ductus arteriosus begins. The mechanisms contributing to the high pulmonary vascular resistance in the fetal lung are primarily the low oxygen tension and low pulmonary blood flow, which suppresses the synthesis and release of nitric oxide (NO) and prostaglandin I2 from the pulmonary endothelium.[22] Fetal exposure to hypoxia will increase the already high pulmonary vascular resistance and hyperoxia will decrease pulmonary vascular resistance and increase fetal pulmonary blood flow.[23] Experimentally, ventilation of the fetal lung without changing oxygenation will decrease pulmonary vascular resistance and increase pulmonary blood flow by 400%. With delivery, ventilation, and oxygenation, NO and PGI2 increase with a rapid fall in pulmonary vascular resistance.

The use of supplemental oxygen for the initiation of ventilation will cause pulmonary vascular resistance to decrease more rapidly with the resultant more rapid increase in pulmonary blood flow.[24] There is no benefit in systemic oxygenation, however, and the pulmonary vessels subsequently become more refractory to dilation by NO or acetylcholine.

The cardiovascular transition at birth also is modulated by corticosteroids. Exposure of fetal sheep to betamethasone increased fetal pulmonary blood flow but did not alter postnatal pulmonary vasodilation in preterm sheep.[25] Heart function after preterm birth is improved by antenatal exposure to corticosteroids.[7] The fetal and newborn blood pressures increase, as does cardiac output and left ventricular contractility. These effects are partially explained by an increase in beta-receptor signaling to an increase in cyclic AMP. Similarly, adrenalectomy ablates the increase in blood pressure that normally occurs at birth (see **Fig. 2**).[8] Thus, although there are specific mediators such as NO and PGI2 that facilitate cardiovascular transition, the consistent theme is that the same mediators, corticosteroids and catecholamines, also facilitate this transition.

The normal oxygen saturation of fetal blood in the left atrium is about 65%.[26] During labor, the human fetus tolerates oxygen saturations as low as 30% without developing acidosis.[27] After birth, the preductal saturation in healthy term infants gradually increases to about 90% at 5 minutes of age.[28] This knowledge is important to avoid unnecessary administration of supplemental oxygen during resuscitation.

LUNG ADAPTATIONS
Fetal Lung Fluid

The most essential adaptation to birth is the initiation of breathing, but the airspaces of the fetal lung are filled with fetal lung fluid. What is fetal lung fluid and how is it cleared from the airspaces? Fetal lung fluid is secreted by the airway epithelium as a filtrate of the interstitial fluid of the lung by the active transport of chloride.[29] Consequently, the chloride content of fetal lung fluid is high and protein content is very low. The production rate is high, although direct measurements are not available for the human fetus. The volume of lung fluid of the fetal sheep increases from mid gestation and the secretion rate increases to about 4 mL/kg per hour by late gestation.[30] Production and maintenance of the normal volume of fetal lung fluid is essential for normal lung growth. The electrochemical gradient for the production of fetal lung fluid is substantial and can overdistend the airspaces. This behavior of the production of fetal lung fluid is used to advantage to obstruct the trachea, which will distend the hypoplastic lungs of fetuses with diaphragmatic hernia.

In experiments with fetal rabbits and sheep, Bland and colleagues[31] demonstrated that fetal lung fluid production decreased before the onset of labor, and the volume of lung fluid in the airspaces decreased from about 25 mL/kg to 18 mL/kg. The fetal lung fluid volume decreased further with labor such that the airways contained about 10 mL/kg at delivery. Harding and Hooper[30] measured an airspace fluid volume of about 50 mL/kg in fetal sheep at term and without labor, which is about twice the functional residual capacity of the newborn term lamb after adaptation to air breathing.

The endocrine adaptations that begin before delivery are critical to fluid clearance. Cortisol, thyroid hormones, and catecholamines all increase and shut down the active chloride-mediated secretion of fetal lung fluid and activate the basal Na^+, K^+, ATPase of type II cells on the airway epithelium. Sodium in fetal lung fluid enters the apical surfaces of type II cells and is pumped into the interstitium with water and other electrolytes following passively, thus removing fluid from the airways. In preterm fetal sheep, infusion of cortisol and T_3 will activate the sodium pump, which normally occurs at term.[16] The components of fetal lung fluid then are cleared directly into the vasculature or via lymphatics from the lung interstitium over many hours.

This clearance of a large volume of airspace fluid is remarkably efficient normally. The essential contribution of activation of Na^+ transport was demonstrated by respiratory distress in animals from amiloride inhibition of the Na^+, K^+, and ATPase. Mice with defective Na^+ transporters will die following delivery because of failure to clear fetal lung fluid.[32] The frequent clinical scenario in which retained lung fluid contributes to poor respiratory adaptation is the operative delivery of infants who were not in labor. These infants do not increase their oxygen saturations as quickly as vaginally delivered term infants,[28] and there is an increased incidence of transient tachypnea of the newborn and other respiratory morbidities (**Table 1**).[29] In experimental studies in sheep, the increased volume of fetal lung fluid interferes with respiratory adaptation, and vaginal delivery facilitates adaptation relative to operative delivery at equivalent volumes of fetal lung fluid.[33]

Transient tachypnea of the newborn is most frequent in late preterm infants. This syndrome is thought to directly result from ineffective clearance of fetal lung fluid because of inadequate Na^+ transport, either because of decreased numbers of transporters or lack of activation.[34] Preterm infants also have decreased Na^+ transport, and late preterm infants with transient tachypnea of the newborn have low amounts of surfactant.[35] Thus, the infant with transient tachypnea of the newborn has immaturity of Na^+ transport and a tendency for surfactant deficiency, whereas the infant with respiratory distress syndrome (RDS) has more severe surfactant deficiency that also includes immature Na^+ transport. These 2 diseases probably are, in fact, a continuum of these 2 abnormalities from mild to severe.

A hypothetical calculation may help the clinician to understand why lung fluid can compromise neonatal adaptation. If the 3-kg term infant has about 30 mL/kg of fetal lung fluid in the airspaces at cesarean delivery without labor and that infant is intubated, then no fluid can passively drain from the lungs. Assuming that the blood volume of this infant is 80 mL/kg and the hematocrit is 50%, then the plasma volume is 40 mL/kg. The fetal lung fluid will move from the airspace to the lung interstitium, initially interfering with lung mechanics and gas exchange. This fluid then will be transferred to the plasma, which if this occurred acutely would expand plasma volume from 40 mL/kg to 70 mL/kg. This transfer occurs over hours in reality. Nevertheless, the fetal lung fluid volume that must be accommodated during neonatal adaptation is added stress for the newborn.

Table 1
Respiratory morbidities are increased by Cesarean section deliveries without labor relative to vaginal births after a previous Cesarean section

	Cesarean Section	Vaginal Birth
Number	15,212	8336
Respiratory distress syndrome	2.1%	1.4%[a]
Transient tachypnea	4.1%	1.9%[a]
Oxygen therapy	4.4%	2.5%[a]
Mechanical ventilation	1.3%	0.8%[a]

[a] $P < .001$ versus cesarean section.
   Data from Jain L, Eaton DC. Physiology of fetal lung fluid clearance and the effect of labor. Semin Perinatol 2006;30:34–43.

Breathing at Birth

The essential component to neonatal adaptation to birth is the maintenance of adequate respiratory effort. The stimuli changing the fetal breathing pattern virtually instantaneously to continuous breathing remain incompletely defined and probably are redundant, as are the stimuli for other adaptations to birth. Most of the information about fetal breathing and its transition after birth is from quite old studies using fetal sheep models, with some verification in the human fetus.[36] The fetal state in utero can be classified into rapid eye movement (REM) sleep and quiet sleep with no clear periods of wakefulness. During REM sleep, the fetus has irregular breathing activity characterized by long inspiratory and expiratory times with movement of variable volumes of fetal lung fluid (mixed with amniotic fluid) into and out of the lung. Fetal breathing, swallowing, and licking activities are confined to REM sleep, with minimal movements during quiet sleep. Fetal hypoxia abolishes fetal breathing, whereas high fetal Po_2 values stimulate fetal breathing. With birth, the fetal sheep will not breathe consistently until the cord is clamped. This observation has generated the hypothesis that breathing is suppressed by a placentally derived substance except in the REM state. Fetal sheep given prostaglandin E2 infusions stop breathing, and treatment with prostaglandin synthetase inhibitors, such as indomethacin, cause continuous fetal breathing.[37] The net effect is that the normal fetal-to-neonatal transition results in the rapid onset of vigorous breathing because of the combined stimuli of cord clamping (and the probable removal of rapidly catabolized prostaglandins that suppress breathing), diffuse tactile and cold stimuli that act centrally, and changes in Pco_2 and Po_2 levels in the blood. The newborn will not initiate breathing if hypoxia is severe. Remarkably, in the absence of hypoxia, virtually all term infants will effectively initiate breathing. Most very preterm infants also will successfully initiate breathing if given the opportunity.[38]

Surfactant and Lung Adaptation

The adequate development of the fetal lung to support gas exchange is the essential adaptation in preparation for birth. During the last third of gestation, the fetal lung septates into about 4 million distal saccules (respiratory bronchioles and alveolar ducts) derived from the 17 generations of airways by about 32 weeks and then further separates to form alveoli.[39] In parallel, the lung parenchymal tissue mass decreases relative to body weight such that the potential gas volume of the airways and alveoli increase greatly. Concurrently, from about 22 weeks' gestational age, surfactant lipid and the lipophilic proteins SP-B and SP-C begin to be synthesized and aggregated into lamellar bodies in the maturing type II cells.[40] The lamellar bodies are the storage and secretory packets for the essential biophysically active components of surfactant. As the lung matures, more and more of the lamellar bodies are released into fetal lung fluid and subsequently mix with amniotic fluid or are swallowed. By term, type II cells in the fetal lung contain much more surfactant than does the adult lung, and this large pool of surfactant is poised for release before and at delivery.

As delivery approaches, fetal lung fluid secretion ceases (see earlier in this article) and fetal lung fluid volume may decrease. Simultaneously, surfactant is secreted into the fetal lung fluid with labor, which will increase the surfactant concentration in the fetal lung fluid.[41] The presumed mediators of this secretion are the increases in catecholamines that stimulate Beta-receptors. Purinergic agonists, such as ATP, may also promote this predelivery secretion. Subsequently, the initiation of ventilation following birth causes alveolar stretch and therefore deformations of type II cells, another secretion signal. The large increase in catecholamines following delivery probably further stimulates surfactant secretion. In term animals shortly after birth, the alveolar pool size of surfactant is about 100 mg/kg. This value is 5-fold to 20-fold higher than the amount of surfactant in the alveoli of healthy adult animals or humans. Although no measurements are available for the term human, a similar value is likely based on the amount of surfactant present in amniotic fluid at term. Thus, the term fetus is ensured of having adequate surfactant for the transition to air breathing.[42] The high surfactant pool size decreases to adult levels over the first week of life in animal models. Following operative delivery of preterm lambs, a stable surfactant pool of alveolar surfactant is achieved in about 3 hours despite no labor.[43] Although there has been no surfactant secretion before delivery, the endocrine and lung stretch effects allow the unlabored fetal lung to quickly adapt to air breathing. The secretory events concurrent with birth do not appreciably deplete surfactant stores in type II cells because surfactant synthesis and packaging into lamellar bodies continues and the surfactant that has been secreted also is recycled back into type II cells for secretion as needed.[44]

The preterm lung has several disadvantages for transition to air breathing. The structurally immature lung has less potential lung gas volume relative to body weight and metabolic needs, and secretion of fetal lung fluid may not cease before and after delivery, which will delay clearance of fetal lung fluid. Further, the amount of surfactant stored in type II cells is low, and, thus, less surfactant can be secreted in response to birth. The result is a lower concentration of surfactant to form a surface film and stabilize the lung. Surprisingly, many preterm lungs can adapt, perhaps with a bit of help from continuous positive airway pressure. The small alveolar surfactant pool size need not be more than about 5 mg/kg for the preterm lamb supported by continuous positive airway pressure.[45] This result illustrates that the term infant has large excesses of surfactant to ensure a successful transition to air breathing.

Injury of the Preterm Lung

The transition from a fetus to a newborn requires the initiation of breathing, clearance of fluid from airways, and ventilation of the distal airspaces. Healthy newborns inflate their lungs at birth by generating large negative pressure breaths, which pull the lung fluid from the airways into the distal airspaces. The infant continues to clear lung fluid with subsequent inflations.[46,47] Spontaneously breathing newborn rabbits quickly move fluid from their airways to the alveoli and subsequently into the interstitium at birth, with 50% of lung aeration occurring with the first 3 breaths. They use an increased inspiratory volume–to–expiratory volume ratio to achieve functional residual capacity (FRC).[47] Most of the clearance of fetal lung fluid occurs during inspiration, with a return of lung fluid into airways during expiration when positive end-expiratory pressure (PEEP) is not used.[47] In newborn preterm rabbits, the use of PEEP during initiation of ventilation facilitates the development of FRC and surfactant treatment creates more uniformed distribution of FRC.[48,49]

Many preterm or asphyxiated term infants do not have adequate spontaneous respirations at birth and require positive pressure ventilation. Premature infants have immature lungs that are more difficult to ventilate because of inadequate surfactant to decrease surface tension and maintain FRC. The airways in the preterm lung stretch with positive pressure ventilation and the decreased surfactant pools contribute to nonuniform expansion of the lung with areas of focal overdistension and atelectasis.[50,51] The initial ventilation of the preterm lung will occur before much of the endogenous surfactant is secreted and surfactant therapy cannot practically be given before the initiation of ventilation. The movement of fluid at the air interface across epithelial cells generates high surface forces that distort the cells and injure the epithelium of the small airways, a feature prominent in the lungs of infants who have died of RDS.[52,53] Continuous positive airway pressure or PEEP should minimize the movement of fluid in the airways, and surfactant will lower the pressure required to move fluid into the small airways and decrease the injury from fluid movement.[48,54] As few as 6 large tidal volume breaths at birth can eliminate the surfactant treatment responses of preterm sheep because of acute lung injury.[55] In preterm sheep models, we demonstrated that airway stretch occurs during initiation of ventilation and initial injury is localized primarily to the bronchi and bronchioles.[53] Acute phase response genes involved in inflammation, angiogenesis, vascular remodeling, and apoptosis were activated within the lung, and immunologically active proteins (HSP70, HSP60) were released by the airway epithelium into the airspace fluid.[56]

As with preterm sheep, ventilated very low birth weight infants have increased proinflammatory cytokines (interleukin [IL]-8, IL-1β, IL-6, and monocyte chemotactic protein 1) in tracheal aspirates soon after birth, which correlate with an increased risk of bronchopulmonary dysplasia.[57] Ventilation of preterm infants with respiratory distress increased plasma levels of IL-1β, IL-8, and tumor necrosis factor α, and decreased levels of the anti-inflammatory cytokine IL-10.[58] We previously demonstrated that regardless of the tidal volume or PEEP used, initiation of ventilation in fluid-filled, surfactant-deficient preterm lambs is injurious.[56,59] Small increases in the endogenous surfactant pool size can increase the uniformity of lung expansion and thus decrease focal injury.[60] The preterm lung is likely at risk for small and large airway injury from initiation of ventilation during resuscitation.

REFERENCES

1. Liggins GC. The role of cortisol in preparing the fetus for birth. Reprod Fertil Dev 1994;6:141–50.
2. Padbury JF, Ervin MG, Polk DH. Extrapulmonary effects of antenatally administered steroids. J Pediatr 1996;128:167–72.
3. Watterberg K. Fetal and neonatal adrenalcortical physiology. In: Polin R, Fox W, Abman S, editors. Fetal and neonatal physiology. 4th edition. Philadelphia: Elsevier; 2011. p. 1995–2004.
4. Watterberg KL, Scott SM, Naeye RL. Chorioamnionitis, cortisol, and acute lung disease in very low birth weight infants. Pediatrics 1996;97:210–5.
5. Newnham JP, Marshall CL, Padbury JF, et al. Fetal catecholamine release with preterm delivery. Am J Obstet Gynecol 1984;149:888–93.
6. Padbury JF, Polk DH, Newnham JP, et al. Neonatal adaptation: greater sympathoadrenal response in preterm than full-term fetal sheep at birth. Am J Physiol 1985;248:E443–9.
7. Padbury JF, Ludlow JK, Ervin MG, et al. Thresholds for physiological effects of plasma catecholamines in fetal sheep. Am J Phys 1987;252:E530–7.
8. Padbury J, Agata Y, Ludlow J, et al. Effect of fetal adrenalectomy on catecholamine release and physiologic adaptation at birth in sheep. J Clin Invest 1987; 80:1096–103.
9. Stein H, Oyama K, Martinez A, et al. Plasma epinephrine appearance and clearance rates in fetal and newborn sheep. Am J Physiol 1993;265:R756–60.
10. Kallio J, Karlsson R, Toppari J, et al. Antenatal dexamethasone treatment decreases plasma catecholamine levels in preterm infants. Pediatr Res 1998;43:801–7.
11. Stein HM, Martinez A, Oyama K, et al. Effect of corticosteroids on free and sulfoconjugated catecholamines at birth in premature newborn sheep. Am J Physiol 1995;268:E28–32.

12. Davidson D. Circulating vasoactive substances and hemodynamic adjustments at birth in lambs. J Appl Physiol 1987;63:676–84.
13. Ezaki S, Suzuki K, Kurishima C, et al. Levels of catecholamines, arginine vasopressin and atrial natriuretic peptide in hypotensive extremely low birth weight infants in the first 24 hours after birth. Neonatology 2009;95:248–55.
14. Fisher DA. Thyroid system immaturities in very low birth weight premature infants. Semin Perinatol 2008;32:387–97.
15. Breall JA, Rudolph AM, Heymann MA. Role of thyroid hormone in postnatal circulatory and metabolic adjustments. J Clin Invest 1984;73:1418–24.
16. Olver RE. Fluid secretion and adsorption in the fetus. In: Effros RM, Chang HK, editors. Fluid and solute transport in the airspaces of the lungs. New York: Marcel Dekker, Inc; 1994. p. 281.
17. Ward Platt M, Deshpande S. Metabolic adaptation at birth. Semin Fetal Neonatal Med 2005;10:341–50.
18. Power G, Blood A. Fetal and neonatal physiology. In: Polin R, Fox W, Abman S, editors. Thermoregulation. Philadelphia: Elsevier; 2011. p. 615–24.
19. Merklin RJ. Growth and distribution of human fetal brown fat. Anat Rec 1974;178: 637–45.
20. Heymann MA, Iwamoto HS, Rudolph AM. Factors affecting changes in the neonatal systemic circulation. Annu Rev Physiol 1981;43:371–83.
21. Behrman RE, Lees MH. Organ blood flows of the fetal, newborn and adult rhesus monkey: a comparative study. Biol Neonate 1971;18:330–40.
22. Gao Y, Raj JU. Regulation of the pulmonary circulation in the fetus and newborn. Physiol Rev 2010;90:1291–335.
23. Teitel DF, Iwamoto HS, Rudolph AM. Changes in the pulmonary circulation during birth-related events. Pediatr Res 1990;27:372–8.
24. Lakshminrusimha S, Steinhorn RH, Wedgwood S, et al. Pulmonary hemodynamics and vascular reactivity in asphyxiated term lambs resuscitated with 21 and 100% oxygen. J Appl Physiol 2011;111:1441–7.
25. Crossley KJ, Morley CJ, Allison BJ, et al. Antenatal corticosteroids increase fetal, but not postnatal, pulmonary blood flow in sheep. Pediatr Res 2009;66:283–8.
26. Dawes GS, Mott JC, Widdicombe JG. The foetal circulation in the lamb. J Physiol 1954;126:563–87.
27. Garite TJ, Dildy GA, McNamara H, et al. A multicenter controlled trial of fetal pulse oximetry in the intrapartum management of nonreassuring fetal heart rate patterns. Am J Obstet Gynecol 2000;183:1049–58.
28. Dawson JA, Kamlin CO, Vento M, et al. Defining the reference range for oxygen saturation for infants after birth. Pediatrics 2010;125:e1340–7.
29. Jain L, Eaton DC. Physiology of fetal lung fluid clearance and the effect of labor. Semin Perinatol 2006;30:34–43.
30. Harding R, Hooper SB. Regulation of lung expansion and lung growth before birth. J Appl Physiol 1996;81:209–24.
31. Bland RD, Hansen TN, Haberkern CM, et al. Lung fluid balance in lambs before and after birth. J Appl Physiol 1982;53:992–1004.
32. Grotberg JB. Respiratory fluid mechanics and transport processes. Annu Rev Biomed Eng 2001;3:421–57.
33. Berger PJ, Smolich JJ, Ramsden CA, et al. Effect of lung liquid volume on respiratory performance after caesarean delivery in the lamb. J Physiol 1996;492(Pt 3): 905–12.
34. Gowen CW Jr, Lawson EE, Gingras J, et al. Electrical potential difference and ion transport across nasal epithelium of term neonates: correlation with mode of

delivery, transient tachypnea of the newborn, and respiratory rate. J Pediatr 1988; 113:121–7.

35. Machado LU, Fiori HH, Baldisserotto M, et al. Surfactant deficiency in transient tachypnea of the newborn. J Pediatr 2011;159:750–4.
36. Alvaro R, Rigatt H. Breathing in fetal life and onset and control of breathing in the neonate. In: Polin R, Fox W, Abman S, editors. Fetal and neonatal physiology. 4th edition. Philadelphia: Elsevier; 2011. p. 980–92.
37. Kitterman JA. Arachidonic acid metabolites and control of breathing in the fetus and newborn. Semin Perinatol 1987;11:43–52.
38. O'Donnell CP, Kamlin CO, Davis PG, et al. Crying and breathing by extremely preterm infants immediately after birth. J Pediatr 2010;156:846–7.
39. Burri PH. Structural aspects of postnatal lung development—alveolar formation and growth. Biol Neonate 2006;89:313–22.
40. Clements JA. Lung surfactant: a personal perspective. Annu Rev Physiol 1997; 59:1–21.
41. Faridy EE, Thliveris JA. Rate of secretion of lung surfactant before and after birth. Respir Physiol 1987;68:269–77.
42. Rebello CM, Jobe AH, Eisele JW, et al. Alveolar and tissue surfactant pool sizes in humans. Am J Respir Crit Care Med 1996;154:625–8.
43. Jacobs H, Jobe A, Ikegami M, et al. Accumulation of alveolar surfactant following delivery and ventilation of premature lambs. Exp Lung Res 1985;8:125–40.
44. Jobe AH. Why surfactant works for respiratory distress syndrome. NeoReviews 2006;7:e95–105.
45. Mulrooney N, Champion Z, Moss TJ, et al. Surfactant and physiological responses of preterm lambs to continuous positive airway pressure. Am J Respir Crit Care Med 2005;171:1–6.
46. Vyas H, Milner AD, Hopkins IE. Intrathoracic pressure and volume changes during the spontaneous onset of respiration in babies born by cesarean section and by vaginal delivery. J Pediatr 1981;99:787–91.
47. Siew ML, Wallace MJ, Kitchen MJ, et al. Inspiration regulates the rate and temporal pattern of lung liquid clearance and lung aeration at birth. J Appl Physiol 2009;106: 1888–95.
48. Siew ML, Te Pas AB, Wallace MJ, et al. Positive end-expiratory pressure enhances development of a functional residual capacity in preterm rabbits ventilated from birth. J Appl Physiol 2009;106:1487–93.
49. Siew ML, Te Pas AB, Wallace MJ, et al. Surfactant increases the uniformity of lung aeration at birth in ventilated preterm rabbits. Pediatr Res 2011;70: 50–5.
50. Jobe AH, Hillman NH, Polglase G, et al. Injury and inflammation from resuscitation of the preterm infant. Neonatology 2008;94:190–6.
51. Shaffer TH, Bhutani VK, Wolfson MR, et al. In vivo mechanical properties of the developing airway. Pediatr Res 1989;25:143–6.
52. Robertson D. Pathology and pathophysiology of neonatal surfactant deficiency. In: Robertson B, Van Golde L, Batenburg JJ, editors. Pulmonary surfactant. Amsterdam: Elsevier Science Publishers; 1984. p. 383–418.
53. Hillman NH, Kallapur SG, Pillow JJ, et al. Airway injury from initiating ventilation in preterm sheep. Pediatr Res 2010;67:60–5.
54. Ikegami M, Jobe AH, Yamada T, et al. Relationship between alveolar saturated phosphatidylcholine pool sizes and compliance of preterm rabbit lungs. The effect of maternal corticosteroid treatment. Am Rev Respir Dis 1989;139: 367–9.

55. Bjorklund LL, Ingimarsson J, Curstedt T, et al. Manual ventilation with a few large breaths at birth compromises the therapeutic effect of subsequent surfactant replacement in immature lambs. Pediatr Res 1997;42:348–55.
56. Hillman NH, Nitsos I, Berry C, et al. Positive end-expiratory pressure and surfactant decrease lung injury during initiation of ventilation in fetal sheep. Am J Physiol Lung Cell Mol Physiol 2011;301:L712–20.
57. Tullus K, Noack GW, Burman LG, et al. Elevated cytokine levels in tracheobronchial aspirate fluids from ventilator treated neonates with bronchopulmonary dysplasia. Eur J Pediatr 1996;155:112–6.
58. Bohrer B, Silveira RC, Neto EC, et al. Mechanical ventilation of newborn infant changes in plasma pro- and anti-inflammatory cytokines. J Pediatr 2010;156:16–9.
59. Polglase G, Hillman NH, Pillow JJ, et al. Positive end-expiratory pressure and tidal volume during ventilation of preterm lambs. Pediatr Res 2008;64:517–22.
60. Hillman NH, Kallapur SG, Pillow JJ, et al. Inhibitors of inflammation and endogenous surfactant pool size as modulators of lung injury with initiation of ventilation in preterm sheep. Respir Res 2010;11:151.

Cellular Biology of End Organ Injury and Strategies for Prevention of Injury

Jeffrey M. Perlman, MB, ChB

KEYWORDS

- Asphyxia • Interruption of placental blood flow • Hypoxia-ischemia • Brain injury
- Renal injury • Hepatic injury • Resuscitation

KEY POINTS

- The interruption of placental blood flow induces circulatory responses to maintain cerebral, cardiac, and adrenal blood flow with reduced renal, hepatic, intestinal, and skin blood flow.
- If placental compromise is prolonged and/or severe, circulatory collapse is likely with resultant hypoxic ischemic cerebral injury and accompanying renal, hepatic and intestinal compromise.
- Secondary or reperfusion injury may exacerbate the extent of the primary insult and is likely secondary to extended reactions from the primary insult, including excess in oxygen free radicals, intracellular calcium accumulation, microvascular endothelial dysfunction and nitric oxide formation.
- Treatment strategies should include the judicious use of supplemental oxygen, avoidance of hypoglycemia and elevated temperature in the delivery room, and the early initiation of therapeutic hypothermia to infants at highest risk for evolving encephalopathy.

INTRODUCTION

The process of labor increases the fetal risk for cerebral and systemic end organ damage as a consequence of interruption of placental blood flow with reduction in oxygen delivery. Fetal adaptive mechanisms in part involve circulatory responses with redistribution of cardiac output, to preserve cerebral perfusion and maintain cellular integrity. When the interruption of blood flow is severe or prolonged, these mechanisms fail, increasing the potential for cerebral and systemic end organ injury. After the restoration of blood flow either in utero or, more commonly, in the delivery room, there is the potential for secondary or reperfusion injury. This article concerns the initial circulatory changes that accompany a reduction in placental blood flow

Disclosure: There are no conflicts of interest to disclose.
Division of Newborn Medicine, Department of Pediatrics, Weill Cornell Medical College, 525 East 68th Street, Suite N-506, New York, NY 10065, USA
E-mail address: Jmp2007@med.cornell.edu

Clin Perinatol 39 (2012) 785–802
http://dx.doi.org/10.1016/j.clp.2012.09.002
0095-5108/12/$ – see front matter © 2012 Elsevier Inc. All rights reserved.

perinatology.theclinics.com

and oxygen delivery to the fetus, the fetal adaptive responses, the mechanisms that contribute to ongoing end organ injury after resuscitation, the clinical consequences, and potential strategies to reduce ongoing injury.

CIRCULATORY CHANGES ACCOMPANYING INTERRUPTION OF PLACENTAL BLOOD FLOW

The important circulatory responses to interruption of placental blood flow have been well categorized in experimental studies.[1–4] These include (1) redistribution of cardiac output to preserve blood flow to the more vital organs (ie, brain, myocardium, adrenal gland) with reduced flow to less vital organs (ie, kidney, intestine, muscle); (2) redistribution of umbilical venous blood flow including bypassing the liver through the ductus venosus and preferential streaming of umbilical venous blood across the foramen ovale via the left ventricle toward the upper body circulation to maintain oxygen delivery to the heart and brain[5–7]; and (3) loss of cerebral vascular autoregulation resulting in a pressure passive circulation and eventual diminution in cardiac output with resultant hypotension, and ultimately a critical decrease in cerebral perfusion and oxygen delivery (**Fig. 1**).[1–3,8] The mechanisms involved in the redistribution of blood flow include peripheral vasoconstriction, which is triggered by a carotid chemoreflex, and endocrine factors and then maintained or subsequently modified by endocrine and local components.[9,10] The critical relationship between blood pressure and cerebral blood flow (CBF) has been categorized in the experimental model. Thus, with initial arterial hypoxemia, fetal vascular resistance can decrease by at least 50% to maintain CBF with a minimal decrease in oxygen delivery.[11–13] Critical to this state is a normal or elevated mean arterial blood pressure. However, with persistent hypoxemia, and eventual hypotension, cerebral vascular resistance cannot decrease further, resulting in a marked reduction in CBF.[5,14]

The impact on systemic organ blood flow will vary, also determined in part by both the duration and severity of the insult. Experimental studies in fetal lambs demonstrate that partial occlusion of the umbilical cord causes a prompt reduction in urinary output and in glomerular filtration rate.[15] However, the renal response to experimental hypoxia seems to vary according to levels of CO_2 with a sharp reduction in renal blood flow during hypercapnia but not hypocapnia.[16] If the decrease in renal perfusion is marked, necrosis of the tubular epithelium may occur, resulting in the clinical

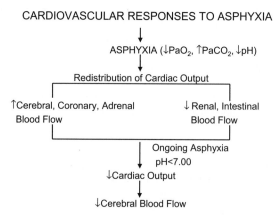

CARDIOVASCULAR RESPONSES TO ASPHYXIA

ASPHYXIA ($\downarrow$PaO$_2$, $\uparrow$PaCO$_2$, $\downarrow$pH)

Redistribution of Cardiac Output

$\uparrow$Cerebral, Coronary, Adrenal Blood Flow $\downarrow$ Renal, Intestinal Blood Flow

Ongoing Asphyxia
pH<7.00
$\downarrow$Cardiac Output

$\downarrow$Cerebral Blood Flow

Fig. 1. Cardiovascular responses to interruption of placental blood flow (asphyxia) with preservation of cerebral, coronary and adrenal blood flow at the expense of flow to other organs.

syndrome of acute tubular necrosis with oliguria and azotemia.[17] Other organs that may be adversely affected by reduced blood flow include the heart with the potential for failure, liver, gastrointestinal tract with an increased risk for necrotizing enterocolitis, the pulmonary circulation with an increased risk for pulmonary hypertension, and muscle with an increased risk for cellular injury and rhabdomyolysis (**Fig. 2**).[18,19]

NONCIRCULATORY FACTORS CONTRIBUTING TO NEURONAL PRESERVATION WITH REDUCED CEREBRAL PERFUSION

Potential mechanisms in preserving neuronal viability with asphyxia include biologic alterations that are maturation dependent. Some examples include (1) a lower rate of brain metabolism during early development resulting in a slower depletion of high-energy compounds during hypoxia–ischemia in the fetus compared with a term infant or adult,[20,21] (2) the use of alternate energy substrate during increased need (ie, the neonatal brain has the capacity to use lactate and ketone bodies for energy production),[22,23] (3) the relative resistance of the fetal and neonatal

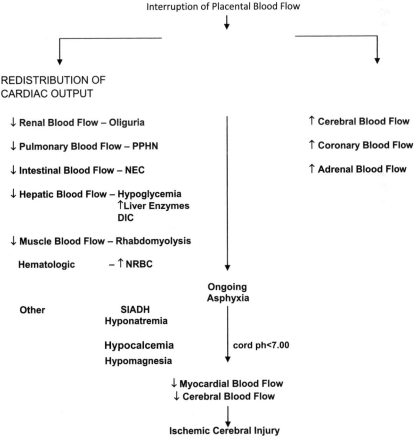

Fig. 2. Consequences of hypoxic–ischemic insult in fetus. DIC, disseminated intravascular coagulation; NEC, necrotizing enterocolitis; NRBC, nucleated red blood cells; PPHN, persistent pulmonary hypertension of the newborn; SIADH, syndrome of inappropriate antidiuretic hormone release.

myocardium to hypoxia–ischemia (see later),[24,25] and (4) the potential protective role of fetal hemoglobin. That is, it has been calculated that if the fetal arterial P_{O_2} were to decrease to a value of less than approximately 3 mm Hg and the fetal venous P_{O_2} were to decrease to approximately 10 mm Hg (a value that may be found in cerebral venous blood with asphyxia), the infant would have more oxygen available for brain uptake with a fetal instead of an adult dissociation curve.[26]

MECHANISMS OF CELL DEATH AFTER HYPOXIA–ISCHEMIA

The mechanisms of cell death after hypoxia–ischemia have been well categorized in the newborn brain and include necrosis and apoptosis.[27] Necrosis is a passive process of cell swelling, with disruption of cytoplasmic organelles, loss of membrane integrity, eventual lysis of cells, and activation of an inflammatory process. In contrast, apoptosis is an active process distinguished from necrosis by the presence of cell shrinkage, nuclear pyknosis, chromatin condensation, and genomic fragmentation, events that occur in the absence of an inflammatory response.[28] Two parallel pathways lead to chromatin processing during apoptosis. One is an intrinsic pathway that involves activation of caspase-3, the most abundant effector caspase in the developing brain.[29] It has been shown that there is a direct correlation between caspase-3 activation and the degree of injury after hypoxia–ischemia.[30] The second pathway involves apoptosis inducible factor (AIF), which is caspase independent and results in DNA fragmentation and chromatin condensation.[31]

Several factors seem to be important in determining the mode of cell death. The first relates to the intensity of the initial insult, with severe injury resulting in necrosis and milder insults resulting in apoptosis.[28] The second relates to the impact of age on cell death mechanisms.[32] Thus, there is a developmental down-regulation of caspase-3 and other elements involved in caspase-3 activation such as Bcl-2–associated X protein that occurs in tandem with a reduction in physiologic programmed cell death seen in the mature brain. Cytochrome c, a critical component of the respiratory chain that generates ATP in the inner mitochondrial membrane, increases during brain development.[32,33] In addition, there is a relative down-regulation of AIF with maturation.[32] Calpains, which are cysteine proteases located within the cytoplasm, are activated by intracellular calcium elevation and have been implicated in excitotoxic neuronal injury.[34] Again, there is a maturational difference with caspain activity peaking 3 hours after hypoxia–ischemia in immature brain, whereas in the mature brain it peaks later at 72 hours and later.[33]

Clearly, because the mechanisms of cell death (ie, necrosis versus apoptosis) differ, strategies to minimize brain damage in an affected infant after hypoxia–ischemia will likely have to include interventions that target both processes.

IMPORTANCE OF THE MITOCHONDRIA TO THE PROCESSES OF CELL DEATH

Mitochondria seem to play a central role in determining the fate of cells subjected to hypoxia–ischemia.[35] Mitochondria are major buffers of intracellular calcium ions and can become overloaded by cytoplasmic Ca^{2+} flooding secondary to opening of N-methyl-D-asparate and voltage-sensitive Ca^{2+} channels (as in the brain) or the opening of the nonspecific pore in the inner mitochondrial membrane (ie, the mitochondrial permeability transition pore [notably in heart and liver] with loss of function).[36] Diminished mitochondrial function can lead to decreased energy production to maintain membrane ion gradients, potentially perpetuating a vicious cycle of membrane depolarization.[37] In addition, mitochondria handle multiple oxidation reactions that can yield highly toxic oxygen free radicals under conditions of oxidative stress.

Mitochondria are key regulators in the process of cell death via release of the numerous proapoptotic proteins such as cytochrome *c*, caspase-2 and -9, and AIF from the intermembrane space.[38–40] Caspase inhibition reduces brain injury after neonatal hypoxia–ischemia, supporting a critical role in hypoxia–ischemia injury and a potential avenue for neuroprotection.[41] AIF, which acts independently of caspases, translocates to the nucleus and induces chromatin condensation and DNA fragmentation.[39,40] AIF levels do not change during development, which is in contrast to the increase in the apoptosis-related intermembrane mitochondrial proteins, cytochrome *c*, and caspase. AIF is released earlier from mitochondria shortly after hypoxia–ischemia and precedes that of cytochrome *c*.[40]

MECHANISMS CONTRIBUTING TO ORGAN INJURY AFTER HYPOXIA–ISCHEMIA
Brain

In the neonate, most of the acute cellular changes result from a reduction in blood flow and include a reduction in oxygen delivery, a switch to anaerobic glycolysis, a progressive decrease in high-energy phosphate compounds (ie, adenosine triphosphate [ATP] and phosphocreatine), intracellular acidosis, and the intracellular accumulation of sodium and calcium. Secondary consequences of these alterations include free radical formation, an increase in extracellular glutamate, intracellular calcium accumulation, and nitric oxide production with eventual mitochondrial cell death. After resuscitation, cerebral perfusion and oxygenation are restored, and there is an initial recovery of the high-energy phosphate compounds. However, there is a subsequent secondary progressive decrease in the high-energy phosphate compounds noted 24 to 48 hours later; this secondary decrease occurs despite the presence of a normal intracellular pH.[42] This may result in further mitochondrial injury with neuronal death during this phase often attributed to apoptosis. In general. the reperfusion injury is likely secondary to extended reactions from the primary insult, including excess in oxygen free radicals, intracellular calcium accumulation, microvascular endothelial dysfunction, nitric oxide formation, and activation of apoptotic pathways.[43]

Myocardium

The newborn myocardium akin to the brain seems to be more tolerant to hypoxia–ischemia. This is in part related to a greater capacity to tolerate near total oxygen deprivation, likely caused by a greater anaerobic glycolytic capacity.[44] In the newborn heart, lactate production increases significantly during near total oxygen deprivation and is greater than in the adult heart. Moreover, there is preservation of ATP in these hearts that is consistent with increased ATP formation from anaerobic glycolysis.[45] Conversely, the newborn myocardium has been shown to be particularly vulnerable to apoptosis. This may reflect that apoptosis and its regulatory factors are closely involved in the morphogenesis of the ventricular wall of the mammalian heart.[46] The generation of reactive oxygen species during reperfusion–reoxygenation seems to be important in the genesis of apoptotic or necrotic cardiac cell death. The reactive oxygen species may overwhelm the immature endogenous antioxidant defense mechanism in the newborn heart, leading to oxidative cellular damage. Mitochondrial permeability transition is a key event in cell death after ischemia–reperfusion.[36] Thus, in the early minutes of reperfusion, there is intracellular calcium accumulation, excessive production of reactive oxygen species, and abrupt restoration of pH that trigger the opening of the nonspecific pore in the inner mitochondrial membrane, known as the mitochondrial permeability transition pore (MPTP). This causes mitochondria uncoupling with breakdown of ATP, which will lead to the loss of ionic homeostasis and promote apoptotic or necrotic cell death. Furthermore, it has been shown that MPTP formation occurs during reperfusion instead of during ischemia.[47] Inhibition of the MPTP has been suggested as a method to limit ischemia–reperfusion injury to the heart or at least prevent the transition of reversible to irreversible myocardial damage.[48] Furthermore, using radioactive tracers, Halestrap and colleagues[47] correlated MPTP closure with cardiac recovery after ischemia–reperfusion injury.

Hepatic

There is a paucity of experimental data related to the mechanisms contributing to hepatic ischemia–reperfusion injury in the developing liver. In the mature system, several key elements seem to predominate. Thus, the generation of reactive oxygen species after reoxygenation inflicts tissue damage and initiates a cascade of deleterious cellular responses leading to inflammation, cell death, and ultimate organ failure. The prime sources of oxygen free radical production include cytosolic xanthine oxidase, Kupffer cells, and adherent polymorphonuclear neutrophils. Increased experimental evidence has suggested that Kupffer cells (resident macrophage located in the sinusoids) and T cells mediate the activation of neutrophil inflammatory responses. Activated neutrophils infiltrate the injured liver in parallel with increased expression of adhesion molecules on endothelial cells, eventually leading to injury.[49,50]

Kidney

The neonatal renal responses to hypoxia–ischemia are less clear. In one study, several differences from the adult were noted. Thus, in response to hypoxia, Na^+-K^+, ATPase redistribution from the plasma membrane was almost 2-fold increased in cells isolated from mature compared with immature kidneys.[51] Reoxygenation resulted in a complete reestablishment of Na^+-K^+, ATPase in the plasma membrane in the immature but not in the mature cells. The expression of μ-calpain, a factor shown to induce ischemic injury to proximal tubular cells, was significantly lower in the immature compared with the mature kidney, whereas the expression of heme oxygenase-1, a factor shown to protect from renal ischemic injury, was significantly higher in the immature kidney. These latter 2 observations suggest that the proximal tubules may be less vulnerable to ischemia–reperfusion injury related to reactive oxygen species.[51]

SYSTEMIC ORGAN INJURY AFTER INTERRUPTION OF PLACENTAL BLOOD FLOW

The extent of systemic organ involvement after interruption of blood flow has been studied in several prospective and retrospective studies. Findings vary in part based on the entry criteria and on the methodology used to determine organ injury.

There are 4 studies with a total of 283 infants available for review (**Table 1**). The first study, by Perlman and colleagues,[52] prospectively evaluated 35 term infants with a 5-minute Apgar score of less than 5 (nonintubated) or less than 6 (intubated) and an umbilical arterial cord pH less than 7.20. Abnormal outcomes included central nervous system (CNS) (moderate to severe encephalopathy [using the Sarnat Staging[53]] with or without an abnormal cranial ultrasound scan), renal (oliguria defined as a urine output <1 mL/kg/h and was further categorized as transient if present for 24 hours only and persistent if for the first 36 hours; azotemia defined as a blood urea nitrogen >25 mg/dL and a creatinine >0.9 mg/dL after the third day), cardiac (abnormal electrocardiograms [ECGs] and/or 2-dimensional echocardiograms), and pulmonary effects (intubation for >48 hours).

Twelve (35%) infants had no evidence of organ injury, 13 (37%) had CNS injury, 14 (40%) had renal injury, 10 (29%) had cardiac injury, and 12 (34%) had pulmonary injury

Table 1
Organ involvement in infants with interruption of placental blood flow

Study	No Organ	CNS	Renal	Cardiac	Pulmonary	Hepatic	Single Organ	Multiple Organs
Perlman et al,[52] 1989 (n = 35) Term infants 5-min Apgar ≤6 Cord I arterial pH <7.20	12/35 (34%)	13/35 (37%)	14/35 (40%)	10/35 (23%)	12/35 (34%)	NA	8/35 (35%)	15/35 (42%)
Martin Ancel et al,[55] 1995 (n = 72) Term infants 5-min Apgar <7 Cord arterial pH <7.20	13/72 (18%)	52/72 (72%)	30/72 (42%)	21/72 (29%)	19/72 (26%)	NA	19/72 (26%)	40/72 (55%)
Shah et al,[56] 2004 (n = 130) Term infants 5-min Apgar <5 Mechanical ventilation Encephalopathy	NA	100%	91/130 (70%)	80/130 (62%)	112/130 (86%)	110/130 (85%)	130/130 (100%)	124/130 (95%)
Hankins et al,[57] 2002 (n = 46) Gestational age >32 wk Acute intrapartum asphyxia Encephalopathy	NA	32/46 (70%)	33/46 (72%)	36/46 (78%)	NA	37/46 (80%)	NA	33/46 (72%)

Abbreviations: FMV, face mask ventilation; NA, not available.

(see **Table 1**), Single organ involvement was noted in 8 (23%) infants (CNS, n = 3; renal, n = 5). Fifteen (42%) had multiple organ involvement. Severe CNS injury almost always occurred with the involvement of other organs. Renal injury was the best systemic marker of potential brain injury. Thus, the presence of altered renal function and specifically oliguria when associated with an abnormal neurologic examination was related to poor long-term neurologic outcome.[54] The odds ratio estimates of poor neurologic outcome in neonates with transient oliguria was 2.8 (95% confidence interval, 0.96–8), and with persistent oliguria was 5.1 (95% confidence interval, 1.95–13.3).

The second study by Martin Ancel and colleagues[55] involved 72 term infants with the following entry criteria: 5 minute Apgar score less than 7, scalp pH less than 7.20, arterial pH less than 7.20, Apgar score less than 7 at 5 minutes, and the requirement of positive pressure ventilation for more than 1 minute before the establishment of sustained respirations. Abnormal outcome included CNS, moderate to severe encephalopathy; renal, oliguria defined as a urine output less than 1 mL/kg/h that persisted for at least 24 hours and a blood urea nitrogen greater than 20 mg/dL; pulmonary, FIO_2 greater than 40% for longer than 4 hours and/or the need for mechanical ventilation; cardiac, ECG abnormalities suggestive of ischemia or signs of heart failure; and gastrointestinal, persistent bloody aspirates or frank necrotizing enterocolitis. Thirteen (18%) of the infants had no organ involvement. CNS involvement occurred in 52 infants (35%), which included 22 (31%) with stage 2/3 encephalopathy and 14 (19%) with seizures; renal involvement was moderate to severe in 30 (42%) including azotemia in 18 infants (25%). Pulmonary abnormalities were noted in 19 (26%) including 14 (19%) who required intubation for at least 24 hours. Cardiac abnormalities in 21 infants (29%) including an abnormal ECG in 14 (19%) and hypotension in 3 infants (4%). Gastrointestinal abnormalities occurred in 21 (29%) including 16 with repeated bloody aspirates. There were 19 (26%) with 1 organ involved and 40 (55%) infants with at least 2 organs involved. When organ involvement was severe and multiple, it was invariably present in the same infants.

There are 2 retrospective studies that have evaluated the extent of organ injury in the context of asphyxia. The first, by Shah and colleagues,[56] enrolled term infants with a 5-minute Apgar score less than 5, metabolic acidosis (ie, base deficit >16 mmol/L), the need for mechanical ventilation, and evidence of encephalopathy. Abnormalities were defined as follows: renal, anuria or oliguria (ie, urine output <1 mL/kg/h ≥24 hours and a serum creatinine concentration >1 mg/dL or any serum creatinine 1.2 mg/dL); cardiovascular, hypotension treated with an inotrope for longer than 24 hours to maintain blood pressure within the normal range or ECG evidence of transient myocardial ischemia; pulmonary, need for ventilator support with oxygen requirement greater than 40% for at least the first 4 hours after birth; and hepatic, aspartate aminotransferase greater than 100 IU/L or alanine aminotransferase greater than 100 IU/L at any time during the first week after birth. Adverse outcomes included death attributable to hypoxic–ischemic encephalopathy or cerebral palsy. Organ abnormalities included renal (n = 91, 70%), cardiac (n = 80, 62%), pulmonary (n = 112, 86%), and hepatic (n = 110, 85%). Multiple organ involvement was noted in 124 (95%) of infants. In the second retrospective study, Hankins and colleagues[57] enrolled 46 infants who met the criteria for an acute intrapartum hypoxic event that included a gestational age greater than 32 weeks, evidence of a sentinel event, an abnormal and sustained intrapartum fetal heart rate abnormality, and evidence of early encephalopathy. Neonatal encephalopathy was defined clinically as a syndrome of disturbed neurologic function in the infant at or near term during the first week after birth, manifested by difficulty with initiating and maintaining respirations, depression of time and reflexes, altered level of consciousness, and often seizures. Hepatic injury was diagnosed based on elevation of aspartate transaminase, alanine transaminase, or lactic dehydrogenase. Cardiac injury was diagnosed on the need for pressor agents beyond 2 hours. Elevation of the creatinine kinase MB isoenzyme was also considered evidence of cardiac injury. Hematologic injury was defined as the development of early thrombocytopenia (<100,000). Renal injury was defined as an elevation in the serum creatinine to greater than 1.0 mg/dL with subsequent return to normal values. Oliguria was defined by the neonatologist as that persisting for longer than 24 hours. Organ involvement included CNS (n = 32, 70%), renal (n = 33, 72%), cardiac (n = 36, 78%), and hepatic (n = 37, 80%). Multiple organ involvement was noted in 33 (72%) of the infants.

In a single-center study, the dynamics of hepatic enzyme activity after birth asphyxia was evaluated in 26 infants and 56 healthy newborns. In 17 of the 26 asphyxiated infants, a serum alanine aminotransferase pattern compatible with hypoxic hepatitis was found. Elevated serum alanine aminotransferase concentrations in the first 72 hours after birth correlated significantly with severity of hypoxic–ischemic encephalopathy.[58]

ORGAN DAMAGE AFTER ASPHYXIA: PATHOLOGIC OBSERVATIONS
Experimental Observations

Eight chronically instrumented near-term fetal lambs were asphyxiated by partial umbilical cord occlusion for approximately 60 minutes until the fetal arterial pH reached less than 6.9 and the base excess reached less than –20 mEq/L.[59] An additional 6 fetuses were used as sham-asphyxiated controls. The brain, heart, kidney, and liver were collected 72 hours after asphyxia. Fetal brain histologic features were classified into 5 grades, with 5 being the most severe damage (4 of the 8 animals were noted to have the more severe injury ie, a grade ≥ 4). Each organ was assayed for tissue concentrations of thiobarbituric acid-reactive substances, superoxide dismutase, glutathione, lactate, and glucose. Myocardial changes of necrosis, phagocytosis, and contraction bands occurred in 2 of the 3 most severely (grade 5) brain-damaged fetuses. The histologic changes in the myocardium and liver were seen only with the most severe brain damage. Infarction of the endocardial muscles, especially sporadic necrosis in papillary muscles, has been previously reported in newborns.[60] The kidney in all cases showed tubular necrosis, but glomeruli were generally spared. There was variable brain damage in these cases. Similar renal findings were reported previously in autopsies of asphyxiated infants.[61] Of the measures of oxidative stress, only liver tissue levels of thiobarbituric acid–reactive substances and superoxide dismutase were significantly higher in the asphyxiated group than in the control group, but there was no correlation with the degree of damage. Thus, it seems that oxidative stress plays a role in the pathogenesis of the liver damage. Lactate levels were higher only in the heart consistent with other experimental observations.[44,45]

Human Autopsy Data

There is one report of 35 infants of gestational age greater than 37 weeks who met the diagnosis of multisystem dysfunction as a result of perinatal asphyxia and underwent autopsy.[62] Entry criteria included 1 or more of the following: 5-minute Apgar score of 3 or less, metabolic acidosis (serum bicarbonate ≤ 12 mmol/L) in cord blood or in the first hour after birth, or onset of spontaneous respiration at 5 minutes; (2) need for positive pressure ventilation after birth; (3) evidence of severe hypoxic–ischemic encephalopathy (intractable seizures starting at age <24 hours or burst suppression pattern on electroencephalogram); (4) clinical evidence of involvement of at least one of the following organs: heart, lungs, kidneys, liver, or intestine, and (5) cause of death stated as perinatal asphyxia or hypoxic–ischemic encephalopathy on autopsy report. The clinical criteria for severe involvement included cardiac, ECG evidence of myocardial ischemia; renal, anuria/oliguria (urine output <1 mL/kg/h) for 24 hours or longer after birth and a rising serum creatinine level after birth; pulmonary, respiratory support at 24 hours of age; hepatic, peak aspartate aminotransferase and alanine aminotransferase values of 200 U/L or higher in the first 48 hours after birth; and gastrointestinal, evidence of intramural air present on plain abdominal radiography. The median age of death was 2 days. Of the 35 patients, 33 had one or more organ involvement. The relationship between clinical and autopsy findings indicated the following. On electrocardiography, 16 of 22 infants (73%) had evidence of myocardial ischemia; 12 of these 16 (75%) had myocardial necrosis at autopsy. Severe renal pathologic conditions were found in 9 of 15 cases (60%) with severe clinical abnormalities versus none of the 9 infants with mild clinical symptoms. There were 15 cases with severe liver dysfunction; severe pathologic conditions were was found in 3 (20%) cases and in none of the 9 cases without severe clinical findings. Three of 35 patients (8.5%) had documented clinical evidence of necrotizing enterocolitis, with autopsy confirming the diagnosis in 2 cases. To summarize, major pathologic involvement was noted in the following proportion of cases: cardiac (62%), pulmonary (33%), renal (28%), hepatic (22%), and intestine (6%). In 9 of 35 autopsies (25%), severe involvement of 2 or more organs was found; 2 infants had severe involvement of 4 organs. The proportions of organs with no pathologic changes were heart (17%), kidneys (14%), and liver (14%). Of the organs studied (excluding the intestine), 38% had either mild or no pathologic change at autopsy.

Long-term Consequences of Organ Injury

The overwhelming long-term data are almost exclusively related to neurocognitive outcome. This outcome is related to the severity of the encephalopathy in the neonatal period. Thus, data before the use of therapeutic hypothermia indicated that approximately 25% of infants who presented with moderate encephalopathy have an abnormal outcome, and with severe encephalopathy, the outcome was invariably abnormal.[63] Long-term consequences of systemic organ injury have not been systematically evaluated but are rare.

Implications

Systemic organ injury reflects the circulatory adaptive responses to interruption of placental blood flow and is modulated by duration and severity. Combining the clinical and pathologic data, it is apparent that renal, cardiac, and hepatic abnormalities predominate and are more pronounced in those cases with severe brain injury. In the one autopsy series with entry criteria consistent with moderate to severe interruption of placental blood flow, approximately 40% of the cases had either mild or no changes noted at autopsy.

Based on these cumulative observations, management strategies should focus on interventions to preserve cerebral perfusion and maintain cerebral energy substrates, avoid hyperoxia and the generation of oxygen free radicals, and contain the inflammatory response.

MANAGEMENT OF INFANTS AT RISK FOR ORGAN INJURY WITH ASPHYXIA
Identification of Infants at Risk for Organ Injury in the Delivery Room

Identification of a high-risk infant begins during labor and extends through the delivery process. Key markers of risk include a history of a sentinel event (fetal bradycardia), low extended Apgar score, the need for delivery room resuscitation (intubation, chest compression, medications), and a cord umbilical arterial pH less than 7.00. Individually, these markers are not related to either brain injury or systemic organ injury in any consistent manner. However, the cumulative data clearly indicate that a combination of these markers is most useful in the early identification (within the first postnatal hour) of infants who are at highest risk for progressing to hypoxic–ischemic encephalopathy.[64]

Management and Stabilization in the Delivery Room

To avoid and/or reduce the long-term morbidity, resuscitative and postresuscitative management should focus on restoring and optimizing supportive care that will facilitate adequate perfusion and supply of nutrients to the brain and to other organs. Resuscitation should include, when indicated, the establishment of functional residual capacity (strategies may include mask ventilation, intubation, and positive pressure ventilation), immediate restoration of spontaneous circulation (strategies may include the need for chest compressions, intravenous epinephrine, and volume replacement),[64] judicious oxygen use,[65] and avoidance of hyperthermia[66] and hypoglycemia.[67] After resuscitation and stabilization, the subsequent care and management of the infant must continue to be coordinated and delivered in a timely manner. The neonate should be cared in an environment where systemic and cerebral function can be closely monitored. Further management includes maintaining cerebral and systemic perfusion, avoidance of hyperoxia, and careful monitoring of fluid and renal homeostasis and of metabolic function, including calcium, magnesium, and glucose.[63,68]

THE ROLE OF SUPPLEMENTAL OXYGEN USE DURING RESUSCITATION

Resuscitation of the depressed neonate is aimed at restoring blood flow and oxygen delivery to the tissues. In the past, it was recommended to initiate resuscitation with 100% oxygen at the time of delivery. However, the most recent international guidelines now recommend beginning resuscitation with room air.[65] The critical clinical indicator of whether to initiate supplemental oxygen during resuscitation is the response in heart rate to ventilation. Under circumstances of profound bradycardia unresponsive to ventilation, blood flow and oxygen delivery to brain and other organs are compromised.[5,8] In experimental studies mirroring this state, resuscitation with 100% oxygen is associated with significantly more rapid restoration of hypoxia-depressed CBF, improved cerebral perfusion, and significantly lower levels of excitatory amino acid levels in striatum and with more favorable short- and long-term outcomes in surviving adult mice.[69,70] Additionally, in mice exposed to hypoxia–ischemia associated with circulatory arrest, resuscitation with 100% oxygen compared with room air resulted in significantly greater rates of return of spontaneous circulation.[71] A crucial role for optimizing oxygen delivery was also observed in an experimental paradigm in newborn piglet animals resuscitated with 18% oxygen as opposed to room air or 100% oxygen after a period of hypoxia. Higher pulmonary arterial pressure at 1 hour was observed in the 18% oxygen group compared with control animals or the room air resuscitated group.[72] Conversely, with a rapid increase in heart rate, after the initiation of positive pressure ventilation, the continued use of room air is appropriate.[73–77]

SUPPORTIVE CARE
Ventilation

Assessment of adequate respiratory function is critical in the infant at risk for evolving encephalopathy. In particular, changes in Pa_{CO_2} can affect CBF such that hypercarbia increases and hypocarbia decreases blood flow.[78] Thus, careful monitoring of arterial blood gases and level of $Paco_2$ is of particular importance. Some experimental studies suggest that modest elevation in Pco_2 (50–55 mm Hg) at the time of hypoxia–ischemia is associated with better outcome than when the $Paco_2$ is within the normal (mid 30s) range.[79] However, this is a complex issue in that progressive hypercarbia in ventilated premature infants is associated with loss of autoregulation.[80] Moreover, when hyperventilation with associated hypocarbia has been used for the treatment of term infants with pulmonary hypertension, there has been associated hearing loss. In a study of term infants diagnosed with intrapartum asphyxia, severe hypocapnia (defined as $Paco_2$ <20 mm Hg) led to increased risk of adverse outcome defined as death or severe neurodevelopmental disability at 12 months of age.[81] Because of the divergent experimental and clinical data, it is recommended that the $Paco_2$ be maintained in the normal range in mechanically ventilated infants at risk for hypoxic-ischemic encephalopathy (HIE). This is more complicated in clinical practice, because these infants often compensate for the underlying metabolic acidosis present via hyperventilation with resultant hypocarbia. In a recent study assessing carbon dioxide levels and adverse outcomes in infants with HIE, only 11.5% of infants demonstrated normocapnia through the first 3 days of life, moderate hypocapnia was seen in 29% of infants, and severe hypocapnia was seen in 5.8%.[81] These observations illustrate the difficulty in maintaining carbon dioxide levels within a target range.

MAINTENANCE OF ADEQUATE PERFUSION

Cardiac injury, as noted previously, is not uncommon, and infants often exhibit hypotension. The hypotension may be related to myocardial dysfunction, endothelial cell damage, or, rarely, volume loss. The treatment should be directed toward the cause (ie, inotropic support for myocardial dysfunction, or volume replacement for intravascular depletion).[82] However, there is no evidence from randomized trials to support the routine use of dopamine in infants with suspected perinatal asphyxia with or without cardiovascular compromise as a therapy for improving mortality and neurodevelopmental outcome.[83]

FLUID STATUS

Infants with organ injury secondary to interruption of placental blood flow often progress to a fluid-overload state. Delivery room management may contribute to this problem, because many infants may receive volume as part of the resuscitation process. Animal studies have suggested that volume infusion at time of resuscitation may be detrimental in some cases. Thus, in the asphyxiated neonatal piglet model, animals who received volume infusion during resuscitation demonstrated increased pulmonary edema and decreased lung compliance 2 hours after resuscitation.[84] The fluid overload seen after delivery may be related to renal failure secondary to acute tubular necrosis or to inappropriate antidiuretic hormone release. Clinically, such infants present with an increase in weight, low urine output, and hyponatremia. The management is fluid restriction. Others have taken a different approach to treat the oliguria based on the following presumed mechanism. After hypoxia–ischemia, adenosine acts as a vasoconstrictive metabolite that contributes to a decreased glomerular filtration rate. This vasoconstriction can be blocked with theophylline. In 2 randomized controlled studies, "asphyxiated" infants received a single dose of theophylline (8 mg/kg) within the first hour. Theophylline was associated with a decrease in serum creatinine and urinary β_2-microglobulin and enhanced creatinine clearance.[85,86] The clinical relevance of these findings in terms of long-term benefit remains unclear.

CONTROL OF BLOOD GLUCOSE CONCENTRATION

In the context of cerebral hypoxia–ischemia, experimental studies suggest that both hyperglycemia and hypoglycemia may accentuate brain damage. In immature animals subjected to cerebral hypoxia–ischemia, hyperglycemia to a blood glucose concentration of 600 mg/dL entirely prevents the occurrence of brain damage.[87] Conversely, the effects of hypoglycemia in experimental neonatal models vary, as do the mechanisms of the hypoglycemia. Thus, insulin-induced hypoglycemia is detrimental to immature rat brain subjected to hypoxia–ischemia. However, if fasting induces hypoglycemia, a high degree of protection is noted.[88] This protective effect is thought to be secondary to the increased concentrations of ketone bodies, which presumably serve as alternative substrates to the immature brain (see earlier discussion of protective mechanisms). In the clinical setting, hypoglycemia that is associated with hypoxia–ischemia is detrimental to the brain. Thus, term infants delivered in the presence of severe fetal acidemia (umbilical arterial pH <7.0) and who presented with an initial blood sugar less than 40 mg/dL were 18 times more likely to progress to moderate to severe encephalopathy than were infants with a blood sugar level greater than 40 mg/dL.[67] In the ongoing management of hypoxia–ischemia, a glucose level should be screened shortly after birth and monitored closely. If the blood glucose is low, it should be promptly corrected.

TARGETED THERAPY

Modest therapeutic hypothermia has been shown to ameliorate the course of infants who present with early hypoxic–ischemic encephalopathy if implemented within 6 hours[89–91] (see the article by Seetha Shankaran for a more detailed review of the topic). Other potential strategies are to limit the production of reactive oxygen species, thereby ameliorating the pathways leading to apoptosis. For example, in a study of neonatal piglets subjected to hypoxia–reperfusion, it was shown that postresuscitation administration of N-acetylcysteine reduces myocardial oxidative stress and caused a prolonged improvement in cardiac function and in newborn piglets with hypoxia–reoxygenation insults.[92] These experimental observations offer the potential opportunity for carefully designed clinical studies, particularly in the infant with early cardiac compromise.

SUMMARY

The consequences of placental blood flow interruption on end organ injury and function depend on the extent and duration of the insult. In practical terms, the long-term consequences are invariably driven by the extent of cerebral injury. In the absence of severe brain injury, there is recovery of systemic organ function in almost all cases. Therapeutic strategies should be targeted at maintaining cerebral perfusion and oxygen delivery. Strategies to minimize the extent of cerebral and systemic organ injury include the judicious use of supplemental oxygen and early treatment of high-risk infants with therapeutic hypothermia.

REFERENCES

1. Behrman RE, Lees MH, Petersen EN, et al. Distribution of circulation in the normal and asphyxiated fetal primate. Am J Obstet Gynecol 1970;108:956–69.
2. Cohn EH, Sacks EJ, Heymann MA, et al. Cardiovascular responses to hypoxemia and acidemia in fetal lambs. Am J Obstet Gynecol 1974;120:817–24.

3. Peeters L, Sheldon R, Jones MD Jr, et al. Blood flow to fetal organs as a function of arterial oxygen content. Am J Obstet Gynecol 1979;135:637–46.

4. Jensen A, Garnier Y, Berger R. Dynamics of fetal circulatory responses to hypoxia and asphyxia. Eur J Obstet Gynecol Reprod Biol 1999;84:155–72.

5. Block BS, Schlafer DH, Wentworth RA, et al. Intrauterine asphyxia and the breakdown of physiologic circulatory compensation in fetal sheep. Am J Obstet Gynecol 1990;162(5):1325–31.

6. Reuss ML, Rudolph AM. Distribution and recirculation of umbilical and systemic venous blood flow in fetal lambs during hypoxia. J Dev Physiol 1980;2:71–84.

7. Edelstone DI, Rudolph AM, Heymann MA. Effects of hypoxemia and decreasing umbilical flow on liver and ductus venosus blood flows in fetal lambs. Am J Physiol 1980;7:H656–63.

8. Dawes G. Foetal and neonatal physiology. Chicago: Year Book Medical Publishers, Inc; 1968. p. 111.

9. Giussani DA, Spencer JA, Moore PJ, et al. Afferent and efferent components of the cardiovascular responses to acute hypoxia in term fetal sheep. J Physiol 1993;461:431–9.

10. Morrison S, Gardner DS, Fletcher AJ, et al. Enhanced nitric oxide activity offsets peripheral vasoconstriction during acute hypoxemia via chemoreflex and adrenomedullary actions in the fetus. J Physiol 2003;547:283–91.

11. Jones MD Jr, Sheldon RE, Peeters LL, et al. Regulation of cerebral blood flow in the ovine fetus. Am J Physiol 1978;235:H162–6.

12. Koehler RC, Jones MD Jr, Traystman RJ. Cerebral circulation response to carbon monoxide and hypoxic hypoxia in the lamb. Am J Physiol 1982;243:H27–32.

13. Ashwal S, Dale PS, Longo ID. Regional cerebral blood flow: studies in the fetal lamb during hypoxia, hypercapnia, acidosis and hypotension. Pediatr Res 1984;18:1309–16.

14. Johnson EW, Palahniwk RJ, Tween WA, et al. Regional cerebral blood flow changes during severe fetal asphyxia produced by slow partial umbilical cord compression. Am J Obstet Gynecol 1979;135:48–52.

15. Dauber IM, Krauss AN, Symchych PS, et al. Renal failure following perinatal anoxia. J Pediatr 1976;88:851–5.

16. Begwin F, Dunnihood DB, Quilligan EJ. Effect of carbon dioxide elevation on renal blood flow in the fetal lamb in utero. Am J Obstet Gynecol 1974;199:630–5.

17. Stork H, Geiger R. Renal tubular dysfunction following vascular accidents of the kidneys in the newborn period. J Pediatr 1973;83:933–7.

18. Perlman JM. Intrapartum asphyxia and cerebral palsy: is there a link? Clin Perinatol 2006;33:335–53.

19. Kasik JW, Leuschen MP, Bolam DL, et al. Rhabdomyolysis and myoglobinemia in neonates. Pediatrics 1985;76:255–8.

20. Duffy TE, Kohle SJ, Vannucci RC. Carbohydrate and energy metabolism in perinatal rat brain: relation to survival in anoxia. J Neurochem 1975;24:271–6.

21. Holowach-Thurston J, McDougal DB Jr. Effects of ischemia on metabolism of the brain of the newborn mouse. Am J Physiol 1964;216:348–52.

22. Cremer JE. Substrate utilization and brain development. J Cereb Blood Flow Metab 1982;2:394–407.

23. Yager J, Heitjan DF, Towfighi J, et al. Effect of insulin-induced and fasting hypoglycemia on perinatal hypoxic ischemic brain damage. Pediatr Res 1992;31:138–42.

24. Dawes GS, Mott JC, Shelley HJ. The importance of cardiac glycogen for the maintenance of life in foetal lambs and newborn animals during anoxia. J Physiol 1959;146:519–38.

25. Wells RJ, Friedman WF, Sobel BE. Increased oxidative metabolism in the fetal and newborn lamb heart. Am J Physiol 1972;222:1488–93.
26. Wimberley PD. A review of oxygen and delivery in the neonate. Scand J Clin Lab Invest Suppl 1982;160:114–8.
27. Northington FJ, Ferriero DM, Graham EM, et al. Early neurodegeneration after hypoxia-ischemia in neonatal rat is necrosis while delayed neuronal death is apoptosis. Neurobiol Dis 2001;8:207–19.
28. Bonfoco E, Krainc D, Ankarcrona M, et al. Apoptosis and necrosis: two distinct events, induced respectively by mild and intense insults with N methyl – dospartate or nitric oxide/superoxide in cortical cell cultures. Proc Natl Acad Sci U S A 1995;92:7162–6.
29. Enari M, Sakahira H, Nagata S. Cleavage of CAD inhibitor in CAD activation and DNA degradation during apoptosis. Nature 1998;391:43–50.
30. Zhu C, Wang X, Hagberg H, et al. Correlation between caspase-3 activation and three different markers of DNA damage in neonatal cerebral hypoxia-ischemia. J Neurochem 2000;75:819–29.
31. Susin SA, Daugas E, Ravagnan L, et al. Two distinct pathways leading to nuclear apoptosis. J Exp Med 2000;192:571–80.
32. Zhu C, Wang X, Bahr BA, et al. The influence of age on apoptotic and other mechanisms of cell death after cerebral hypoxia-ischemia. Cell Death Differ 2005;12:162–76.
33. Kalou M, Rauchova H, Drahota Z. Postnatal development of energy metabolism in the rat brain. Physiol Res 2001;50:315–9.
34. Siman R, Noszek JC. Excitatory amino acids activate calpain I and induce structural protein breakdown in vivo. Neuron 1988;1:279–87.
35. Gilland E, Puka-Sundvall M, Hillered L, et al. Mitochondrial function and energy metabolism after hypoxia-ischemia in the immature brain: involvement of NMDA-receptors. J Cereb Blood Flow Metab 1998;18:297–304.
36. Crompton M. Mitochondrial intermembrane junctional complexes and their role in cell death. J Physiol 2000;529:11–21.
37. Johnston MV, Trescher WH, Ischida A, et al. Neurobiology of hypoxic-ischemic injury in developing brain. Pediatr Res 2001;49:735–41.
38. Kroemer G, Dallaporta B, Resche-Rigon M. The mitochondrial death/life regulator in apoptosis and necrosis. Annu Rev Physiol 1998;60:619–64.
39. Susin SA, Loernzo HK, Zamzami N, et al. Molecular characterization of the mitochondrial apoptosis-inducing factor. Nature 1999;397:441–6.
40. Zhu C, Qiu L, Wang X, et al. Involvement of apoptosis-inducing factor in neuronal death after hypoxia-ischemia in the neonatal rat brain. J Neurochem 2003;86:306–17.
41. Cheng Y, Deshmukh M, D'Costa A, et al. Caspase inhibitor affords neuroprotection with delayed administration in a rat model of hypoxic-ischemic brain injury. J Clin Invest 1998;101:1992–8.
42. Lorek A, Takei Y, Cady EB, et al. Delayed secondary cerebral energy failure after acute hypoxia-ischemia in the newborn piglet: continues 48-hour studies by phosphorus magnetic resonance spectroscopy. Pediatr Res 1994;36:699–706.
43. Shalak L, Perlman JM. Hypoxic-ischemic brain injury in the term infant- current concepts. Early Hum Dev 2004;80:125–41.
44. Lopaschuk GD, Collins-Nakai RL, Itoi T. Developmental changes in energy substrate use by the heart. Cardiovasc Res 1992;26:1172–80.
45. Jarmakani JM, Nakazawa M, Nagatomo T, et al. Effect of hypoxia on myocardial high-energy phosphates in the neonatal mammalian heart. Am J Physiol 1978;235:H475–81.

46. Abdelwahid E, Pelliniemi LJ, Niinikoski H, et al. Apoptosis in the pattern formation of the ventricular wall during mouse heart organogenesis. Anat Rec 1999;256:208–17.
47. Halestrap AP, Clarke SJ, Javadov SA. Mitochondrial permeability transition pore opening during myocardial reperfusion - a target for cardioprotection. Cardiovasc Res 2004;61:372–85.
48. Cour M, Loufouat J, Paillard M, et al. Inhibition of mitochondrial permeability transition to prevent the post cardiac arrest syndrome: a preclinical study. Eur Heart J 2011;32:226–35.
49. Farmer DG, Amersi F, Kupiec-Weglinski JW, et al. Current status of ischemia and reperfusion injury in the liver. Transplant Rev 2000;14:106–26.
50. Fondevila C, Busuttil RW, Kupiec-Weglinski JW. Hepatic ischemia/reperfusion injury—a fresh look. Exp Mol Pathol 2003;74:86–93.
51. Adachi S, Zelenin S, Matsuo Y, et al. Cellular response to renal hypoxia is different in adolescent and infant rats. Pediatr Res 2004;55:485–91.
52. Perlman JM, Tack ED, Martin T, et al. Acute systemic organ injury in term infants following asphyxia. Am J Dis Child 1989;143:617–62.
53. Sarnat HB, Sarnat MS. Neonatal encephalopathy following fetal distress. A clinical and electroencephalographic study. Arch Neurol 1976;33:696–705.
54. Perlman JM, Tack ED. Renal injury in the asphyxiated newborn infant: relationship to neurological outcome. J Pediatr 1988;113:875–9.
55. Martin-Ancel A, Garcia-Alix A, Caba Ã, et al. Multiple organ involvement in perinatal asphyxia. J Pediatr 1995;127:786–93.
56. Shah P, Riphagen S, Beyene J, et al. Multiorgan dysfunction in infants with post-asphyxial hypoxic-ischaemic encephalopathy. Arch Dis Child 2004;89:F152–5.
57. Hankins GD, Koen S, Gei AF, et al. Neonatal organ system injury in acute birth asphyxia sufficient to result in neonatal encephalopathy. Obstet Gynecol 2002; 99:688–91.
58. Karlsson M, Blennow M, Nemeth A, et al. Dynamics of hepatic enzyme activity following birth asphyxia. Acta Paediatr 2006;95:1405–11.
59. Ikeda T, Murata Y, Quilligan EJ, et al. Histologic and biochemical study of the brain, heart, kidney, and liver in asphyxia caused by occlusion of the umbilical cord in near-term fetal lambs. Am J Obstet Gynecol 2000;182:449–57.
60. Setzer E, Ermocilla R, Tonkin I, et al. Papillary muscle necrosis in a neonatal autopsy population: incidence and associated clinical manifestations. J Pediatr 1980;96:289–94.
61. Anand SK, Northway JD, Crussi FG. Acute renal failure in newborn infants. J Pediatr 1978;92:985–8.
62. Barnett CP, Perlman M, Ekert PG. Clinicopathological correlations in postasphyxial organ damage: a donor organ perspective. Pediatrics 1997;99:797–9.
63. Volpe JJ. Neurology of the newborn. 5th edition. Philadelphia: WB Saunders; 2008.
64. Stola A, Perlman JM. Post resuscitation strategies to avoid ongoing injury following intra-partum hypoxia-ischemia. Semin Fetal Neonatal Med 2008;13: 424–31.
65. Perlman JM, Wyllie J, Kattwinkel J, et al. Neonatal resuscitation: 2010 International consensus on cardiopulmonary resuscitation and emergency cardiovascular care science with treatment recommendations. Pediatrics 2010;126(5): e1319–44.
66. Petrova A, Demissie K, Rhoads GG, et al. Association of maternal fever during labor with neonatal and infant morbidity and mortality. Obstet Gynecol 2001;98: 20–7.

67. Salhab WA, Wyckoff MH, Laptook AR, et al. Initial hypoglycemia and neonatal brain injury in term infants with severe fetal acidemia. Pediatrics 2004;114:361–6.
68. Kasdorf E, Perlman JM. Management of the term infant with neonatal encephalopathy following intrapartum hypoxia-ischemia. In: Perlman JM, editor. Neonatology: questions and controversies: neurology. 2nd edition. Philadelphia: Saunders/Elsevier; 2012. p. 77–90.
69. Solas AB, Kutzsche S, Vinje M, et al. Cerebral hypoxemia-ischemia and reoxygenation with 21% or 100% oxygen in newborn piglets: effects on extracellular levels of excitatory amino acids and microcirculation. Pediatr Crit Care Med 2001;2:340–5.
70. Presti AL, Kishkurno SV, Slinko SK, et al. Reoxygenation with 100% oxygen versus room air: late neuroanatomical and neurofunctional outcome in neonatal mice with hypoxic-ischemic brain injury. Pediatr Res 2006;60:55–9.
71. Matsiukevich D, Randis TM, Utkina-Sosunova I, et al. The state of systemic circulation, collapsed or preserved defines the need for hyperoxic or normoxic resuscitation in neonatal mice with hypoxia-ischemia. Resuscitation 2010;81:224–9.
72. Cheung PY, Johnson ST, Obaid L, et al. The systemic, pulmonary and regional hemodynamic recovery of asphyxiated newborn piglets resuscitated with 18%, 21% and 100% oxygen. Resuscitation 2008;76:457–64.
73. Davis PG, Tan A, O'Donnell CP, et al. Resuscitation of newborn infants with 100% oxygen or air: a systematic review and meta-analysis. Lancet 2004;364:1329–33.
74. Tan A, Schulze A, O'Donnell CP, et al. Air versus oxygen for resuscitation of infants at birth. Cochrane Database Syst Rev 2005;(2):CD002273.
75. Rabi Y, Rabi D, Yee W. Room air resuscitation of the depressed newborn: a systematic review and meta-analysis. Resuscitation 2007;72:353–63.
76. Vento M, Asensi M, Sastre J, et al. Resuscitation with room air instead of 100% oxygen prevents oxidative stress in moderately asphyxiated term neonates. Pediatrics 2001;107:642–7.
77. Vento M, Sastre J, Asensi MA, et al. Room-air resuscitation causes less damage to heart and kidney than 100% oxygen. Am J Respir Crit Care Med 2005;172:1393–8.
78. Rosenberg AA, Jones MD Jr, Traystman RJ, et al. Response of cerebral blood flow to changes in PCO2 in fetal, newborn, and adult sheep. Am J Physiol 1982;242(5):H862–6.
79. Vannucci RC, Brucklacher RM, Vannucci SJ. Effect of carbon dioxide on cerebral metabolism during hypoxia-ischemia in the immature rat. Pediatr Res 1997;42(1):24–9.
80. Kaiser JR, Gauss CH, Williams DK. The effects of hypercapnia on cerebral autoregulation in ventilated very low birth weight infants. Pediatr Res 2005;58(5):931–5.
81. Nadeem M, Murray D, Boylan G, et al. Blood carbon dioxide levels and adverse outcome in neonatal hypoxic-ischemic encephalopathy. Am J Perinatol 2010;27:361–5.
82. Wyckoff MH, Perlman JM, Laptook AR. Use of volume expansion during delivery room resuscitation in near-term and term infants. Pediatrics 2005;115(4):950–5.
83. Hunt R, Osborn D. Dopamine for prevention of morbidity and mortality in term newborns with suspected perinatal asphyxia. Cochrane Database Syst Rev 2002;(3):CD003484.
84. Wyckoff M, Garcia D, Margraf L, et al. Randomized trial of volume infusion during resuscitation of asphyxiated neonatal piglets. Pediatr Res 2007;61:415–20.
85. Jenik AG, Ceriani Cernadas JM, Gorenstein A, et al. A randomized, double-blind, placebo-controlled trial of the effects of prophylactic theophylline on renal function in term neonates with perinatal asphyxia. Pediatrics 2000;105:E45.

86. Bhat MA, Shah ZA, Makhdoomi MS, et al. Theophylline for renal function in term neonates with perinatal asphyxia: a randomized, placebo-controlled trial. J Pediatr 2006;149:180–4.

87. Vannucci RC, Mujsce DJ. Effect of glucose on perinatal hypoxic-ischemic brain damage. Biol Neonate 1992;62:215–24.

88. Yager JY. Hypoglycemic injury to the immature brain. Clin Perinatol 2002;29(4): 651–74.

89. Gluckman PD, Wyatt JS, Azzopardi D, et al. Selective head cooling with mild systemic hypothermia after neonatal encephalopathy: multicentre randomised trial. Lancet 2005;365:663–70.

90. Shankaran S, Laptook AR, Ehrenkranz RA, et al. Whole-body hypothermia for neonates with hypoxic-ischemic encephalopathy. N Engl J Med 2005;353: 1574–84.

91. Azzopardi DV, Strohm B, Edwards AD, et al. Moderate hypothermia to treat perinatal asphyxial encephalopathy. N Engl J Med 2009;361:1349–58.

92. Liu JQ, Lee TF, Bigam DL, et al. Effects of post-resuscitation treatment with N acetylcysteine on cardiac recovery in hypoxic newborn piglets. PLoS One 2010;5: e15322.

The Role of Oxygen in the Delivery Room

Jay P. Goldsmith, MD[a],*, John Kattwinkel, MD[b]

KEYWORDS

- Infant • Newborn • Resuscitation • Oxygen

KEY POINTS

- All hospitals should have the capacity to blend oxygen and air in their delivery facilities and have pulse oximetry immediately available for all births.
- Avoid hyperoxia. Starting resuscitation with no supplemental oxygen (ie, air) is probably the best choice for babies born at term.
- It is reasonable to match the oxyhemoglobin saturation increase demonstrated by healthy term newborns, taking approximately 10 minutes to increase the intrauterine saturation of approximately 50% to 60% to the conventional neonatal targets. Long-term exposure of neonates to Spo_2 targets of 85% to 89% versus 91% to 95% has been associated with complications of hypoxemia or hyperoxemia, respectively, so many clinicians have chosen to use an intermediate target range (eg, 88%–92%).
- Blended oxygen permits achievement of term targets faster than when using either 21% or 100%, so if the need for resuscitation can be anticipated (eg, the delivery of a very low birth weight infant), it may be preferable to begin with an oxygen-air blend. A lower starting percentage (eg, 30%) may be preferable to higher (eg, 90%).
- Use of any supplemental oxygen should trigger attachment of an oximeter to the newborn.

All substances are toxic: only the dose makes a thing not a poison.
—Paracelsus, 1524.

....the air which nature has provided for us is as good as we deserve.
—Priestley, 1775.

HISTORICAL BACKGROUND

Although Joseph Priestley is usually credited with the discovery of oxygen in 1774, a Polish alchemist, Michal Sendivogius, recognized its existence as early as 1604.[1] Unlike Priestley, he seems to have acknowledged its full significance. Sendivogius

Conflict of interest statement. Neither of the authors has any conflict of interest.
[a] Department of Pediatrics, Tulane University, 1430 Tulane Avenue, SL37, New Orleans, LA 70112, USA; [b] Department of Pediatrics, University of Virginia, Charlottesville, VA 22908, USA
* Corresponding author.
E-mail address: goldsmith.jay@gmail.com

Clin Perinatol 39 (2012) 803–815
http://dx.doi.org/10.1016/j.clp.2012.09.003
0095-5108/12/$ – see front matter © 2012 Elsevier Inc. All rights reserved.
perinatology.theclinics.com

was perhaps the first person to appreciate that air was not a single entity but that it was a mixture of gases containing "aerial nitre" (oxygen) as an essential ingredient. Sendivogius produced "aerial nitre" by heating saltpeter (also known as nitre, potassium nitrate or KNO_3). He reasoned that this gas made all animal life possible and was a "universal spirit that pervades all matter."

The first concerns regarding the safety of this gas were raised by Priestly in 1775.[2] He wrote: "though pure dephlogisticated air (ie, oxygen) might be very useful as a medicine, it might not be so proper for us in the usual healthy state of the body for, as a candle burns out much faster in dephlogisticated air than in common air, so we might, as may be said, live out too fast and the animal powers be too soon exhausted in this pure kind of air."

However for nearly two centuries the admonitions of Priestly were largely ignored. Many great clinicians recommended the liberal use of oxygen in the treatment of sick and premature newborns. In 1900, Budin recommended oxygen for premature infants during episodes of cyanosis. Hess (1931) advised oxygen for infants with apnea, cyanosis, and perinatal asphyxia. In Detroit, Wilson (1942) observed that the typical form of respiration seen in premature infants while in room air (the regular-irregular pattern, known as "periodic breathing") could be converted to a regular ("normal") rhythm by increasing the fraction of inspired oxygen (Fio_2) to high levels (70%).[3] Other investigators noted that the skin color of small neonates was an unreliable indicator of the state of oxygenation. The skin remained pink in small infants even when blood oxygen levels were relatively low; the term "subcyanotic anoxia" was coined as a label for this unusual circumstance.

These observations were used to rationalize the liberal use of supplemental oxygen in the care of premature infants. Additionally, the availability of newly designed incubators in the late 1940s (built with tightly fitting gaskets, sleeved access ports, and novel float valves in an oxygen-intake plenum) made it possible to maintain high concentrations of oxygen for prolonged intervals. It took several years to recognize the causal connection between these changes in routine management and the appearance of a new form of infantile blindness: retrolental fibroplasia.[4]

It was not until the epidemic of retrolental fibroplasia, now called retinopathy of prematurity, was recognized in premature babies treated with high concentrations of oxygen in the 1940s that physicians began to understand the potential toxicity of this gas. From the early 1950s attempts were made to control the use of oxygen in the management of preterm infants. Initial admonitions to limit exposure of infants to concentrations less than 40% to reduce retinopathy of prematurity were associated with an increase in mortality and in the prevalence of cerebral palsy. Subsequently, attempts to avoid hyperoxia were made by advocating frequent measurement of arterial blood gases and the use of transcutaneous oxygen electrodes in the neonatal intensive care unit. The measurement of oxygen saturation by pulse oximetry was introduced in the 1980s and quickly supplanted transcutaneous electrodes. Although this surrogate for oxygen tension gave a continuous measure of saturation, the imprecise correlation with oxygen tension at saturations greater than 93% was perhaps a step back in the clinical mission to control hyperoxia.[3]

However, until recently, concerns about oxygen use in the neonatal intensive care unit were slow to translate into recommendations for resuscitation of depressed and premature newborns in the delivery room. Throughout this period of increased focus on avoiding hyperoxia, especially in the premature infant, the standard recommendations of the Neonatal Resuscitation Program (NRP) were to provide 100% oxygen for the resuscitation of babies having difficulty making transition at birth. This recommendation was based on the assumption that newborns requiring resuscitation were likely to have experienced a period of anaerobic metabolism with the resulting accumulation of lactic acid, which would require rapid metabolism, and that a high concentration of oxygen would result in faster generation of energy through more efficient creation of ATP, thus perhaps ultimately lessening the likelihood of neurologic or organ sequelae. There was also a presumption that a relatively brief exposure to a high oxygen concentration would not be harmful or carry any long-term consequences.[5]

It had been known since the middle of the last century that the fetus normally develops in a relatively hypoxemic environment (oxygen saturations of 50%–60%),[6] and if hypoxic tissue is abruptly exposed to high concentrations of oxygen during resuscitation, cell and tissue injury are worsened.[7] Subsequent research in the ensuing six decades demonstrated the role of oxygen free radicals, antioxidants, and their link with apoptosis and reperfusion injury.[8] The concepts of oxidative stress and oxygen injury were gradually accepted by the medical community and the International Liaison Committee on Resuscitation (ILCOR) began to change its recommendations concerning the use of oxygen in the delivery room in 2005.[9] The most recent recommendations have swung to an even more restrictive use of supplemental oxygen, to the point of recommending the use of non–oxygen-enriched air (ie, 21% oxygen) when assisting ventilation of the compromised baby born at term.[10]

PHYSIOLOGIC PRINCIPLES

In the at-risk fetus or neonate, conditions of poor cardiac output, decreased oxygen carrying capacity (ie, anemia or abnormal hemoglobin), or inadequate inspired oxygen may result in anaerobic metabolism during which incomplete metabolism results in the production of lactic acid. The creation of ATP is reduced and over time purine derivatives accumulate in the cytoplasm and extracellular spaces.[11] This time period may be relatively short and alleviation of the harmful processes may result in rapid repayment of the "oxygen debt" resulting in no harm. However, prolonged energy failure results in cellular membrane depolarization, followed by cellular injury or death. Moreover, sublethal hypoxic ischemia may result in the later death of less affected cells (apoptosis) and contribute to the down-regulation of gene expression for future cell growth and reproduction. In the context of a hypoxic ischemic event immediately before birth, the rapid establishment of pulmonary gas exchange to replace the failure of placental gas exchange is essential to effective resuscitation. The difficulty encountered by the health care provider is to decide when the effects of excess oxygen administration in a situation of acute asphyxia are overtaken by the concern of continuing anaerobic metabolism. This problem is exacerbated in delivery room resuscitation because the resuscitator does not know how severe and prolonged the anaerobic metabolism has been in the newly born infant before birth. Recent concerns over the potential toxic effects of high concentrations of oxygen and the balancing concerns over the effects of prolonged anaerobic metabolism have led to the administration of blended air and oxygen at concentrations between 21% and 100% as a common practice during delivery room resuscitation. However, when blended oxygen is not available in the delivery room, the provider is often forced to choose to use either 100% oxygen or air. A third choice in this situation would be to use 100% oxygen delivered with a self-inflating resuscitation bag without a reservoir, which would provide approximately 40% inspired oxygen.

ILCOR RECOMMENDATIONS 2010: THE EFFICACY OF AIR

In 2010, ILCOR modified its recommendation on the initial gas to use in resuscitation of term and preterm newborns to achieve the "oxygen saturation value in the interquartile range of preductal saturations measured in healthy term babies following vaginal birth at sea level (Class IIb, LOE B). These targets may be achieved by initiating resuscitation with air or blended oxygen and titrating the oxygen concentration to achieve a SpO2 in the target range... using pulse oximetry."[10] Numerous animal and human studies were considered in making these recommendations. The studies support using room air or blended air and oxygen rather than 100% oxygen as the initial gas in resuscitation of all newborns regardless of gestational age, and also suggest that blended oxygen will permit one to achieve the target Spo_2 range more quickly if one starts with a blend, rather than the extremes of either air or 100% oxygen. Multiple human studies have also demonstrated the feasibility and reliability of using pulse oximetry in the delivery room to guide gas delivery and have confirmed that, with sufficient anticipation and preparation, a pulse oximetry probe can be attached and be operational within 1 to 2 minutes after delivery.[10]

The clinicians' and public's love of oxygen as a life giving and sustaining gas was not easily overcome. In the last two decades researchers have shown that brief exposure to high concentrations of oxygen to an organism that has previously been developing in a relatively hypoxemic environment before the time of birth might be dangerous, and several randomized and pseudorandomized studies of the effectiveness of resuscitation of "asphyxiated" newborn babies with air or 100% oxygen were performed.[12–17] In each of these studies, air was at least as effective as oxygen in the short term, although no study individually showed a statistical advantage to either gas. Several meta-analyses reviewed human trials of 100% oxygen versus air for newborn resuscitation.[18–20] In the most recent of these, Saugstad and colleagues[20] analyzed mortality and hypoxic ischemic encephalopathy in a meta-analysis of 10 randomized and pseudorandomized studies of resuscitation of depressed newborns with air or 100% oxygen published up until 2008. In this meta-analysis, 1082 newborns received air initially and 1051 were allocated to the 100% oxygen group. Results of the meta-analysis revealed a reduced relative risk of death in the newborns receiving air (relative risk [RR] = 0.69; 95% confidence interval [CI], 0.54–0.88). This reduction of risk was accentuated when comparing the truly randomized babies (RR = 0.32; 95% CI, 0.12–0.84) with the pseudorandomized group (RR = 0.74; 95% CI, 0.57–0.95). All of the published meta-analyses were criticized because a substantial number of babies entered into the studies were included from under-resourced countries where the efficacy of resuscitation and equipment available could be questioned. Moreover, a substantial number of babies required crossover to the other gas (similar in both groups) and there was no statistical difference in hypoxic ischemic encephalopathy between the two groups.[21] Finally, there was concern that several of the trials excluded babies most likely to be severely asphyxiated (eg, meconium aspiration, infection, or apparent stillbirths), which might have introduced a type II statistical error bias against the most compromised newborns. Interestingly, the growing medical awareness of the potential harmful effects of oxygen has curtailed human experimentation and may have made it unethical to use 100% oxygen as the initial gas in a future human trial. How ironic, because it was not that long ago that the lack of scientific equipoise made it unethical to not use oxygen to begin resuscitation of newborns in a human trial.

A minority of studies examining resuscitation of newborn term and immature animals have suggested that high concentrations of oxygen during resuscitation might be beneficial. Three studies by Solås and coworkers in a hypoxic ischemic piglet model demonstrated higher levels of brain excitatory amino acids (suggesting a greater degree of cell damage), lower mean arterial pressure, reduced perfusion of the cerebral cortex, and less complete restoration of the microcirculation in the piglets resuscitated with air than the group resuscitated with 100% oxygen.[22–25] Similarly, Matsiukevich and colleagues[26] demonstrated that more asphyxiated mice returned to spontaneous circulation and restored cerebral blood flow faster on reoxygenation with 100% oxygen than with air, depending on the condition of their systemic circulation at initiation of resuscitation. Of the 32 animal studies reviewed for the ILCOR 2010 Consensus on Science and Treatment document, 29 did not demonstrate any distinct advantage to the use of increased concentrations of oxygen for resuscitation.[10] However, all studies were conducted in animals that had already made transition from intrauterine to extrauterine life; researchers also used different combinations of hypoxia, ischemia, or hypercarbia in the animal models of "asphyxia"; and all trials were conducted in nonmammalian species.

THE CASE AGAINST OXYGEN: ANIMAL AND HUMAN STUDIES

Studies in newly born infants and neonatal animals have also demonstrated disadvantages to the use of oxygen as a resuscitation gas. A single breath of 100% oxygen given to babies in the first week of life has resulted in a decrease in minute volume, more so in preterm than in term infants.[27] A similar effect was demonstrated by Lofaso and colleagues[28] who exposed mice to 100% oxygen for 3 minutes followed by air for 12 minutes. The oxygen-exposed mice had reduced minute ventilation, which increased in severity with repeated exposures. Two studies in animals showed significantly delayed initiation of breathing and subsequent hyperoxia when resuscitated with 40% or 100% oxygen than the control groups that were resuscitated with air.[29,30]

Other investigators have shown that hyperoxia in newborn animals also causes histologic changes in the brain and other organ injury. Hoehn and colleagues[31] exposed 7-day-old rats to more than 80% oxygen for 24 hours and demonstrated evidence of apoptotic cell death in the retrosplenial cortex, hippocampus, frontal cortex, and thalamus. There were no such changes in the brains of control animals. The same laboratory further elaborated this concept by exposing rat pups aged 14 days old or less, and 7-day-old synRas-transgenic or wild-type mice to 40%, 60%, or 80% oxygen/air for 2 to 72 hours and then sacrificed the animals at 2, 6, 12, 24, 48, and 72 hours after oxygen exposure. Cell death seemed to be dose dependent, both to the amount of oxygen to which the mice were exposed and the length of time of exposure. The amount and distribution of damage was also age dependent. In the youngest animals (Day 0), the areas most affected were the thalamic nuclei, caudate nucleus, putamen, hypothalamus, and white matter tracts.[32] When 7-day rats were treated with an antioxidant precursor (N-acetylcysteine) before and after 12 hours of exposure to 80% oxygen, less brain injury was seen compared with control animals, suggesting that the effect was mediated by reactive oxygen species. Animals exposed to 60% oxygen had significantly greater apoptotic scores than littermates exposed to 40% oxygen or air.[32]

These experiments suggest that hyperoxia causes apoptotic brain damage in developing rodent brains by interfering with the production of the neurotropins necessary for the continued function of developing neurons. Other studies have suggested that exposing infant rodents to hours of hyperoxia not only causes an increased rate of apoptosis in their brains but also elicits long-term alterations in cell growth and differentiation, synaptic function, neuronal migration, and axonal arborization.[33] In addition, other studies in mice exposed to 100% oxygen in postnatal Days 1 to 4 revealed evidence of pulmonary vascular disease and cardiac failure more than a year later, which led to shortened life spans in the oxygen-exposed group suggesting the loss of bone morphogenetic protein signaling.[34]

In rodents, the period of brain vulnerability to hyperoxia seems to be limited to the first 2 weeks of life, which is comparable in the human to the period from the third trimester of pregnancy to several weeks after birth. High concentration of oxygen exposure does not cause these changes in older rodents. However, compared with delivery room oxygen use for neonates, these are extremely long exposures.

Concerns have also been raised by studies of short-term exposures to high oxygen concentrations resulting in hyperoxia. In a randomized study of preterm infants, Lundstrøm and colleagues[35] stabilized 70 babies with either air or 80% oxygen in the delivery room. After oxygen exposure, global cerebral blood flow was decreased up to 2 hours after birth in the oxygen-exposed group compared with those stabilized with air. A similar decrease in measured cerebral blood flow velocity was found by Niijima and colleagues[36] in preterm and term infants after exposure to oxygen. Neither investigative group could detect any short- or long-term effects of these changes in cerebral blood flow. However, in the study by Niijima and colleagues,[36] the term infants who were not mechanically ventilated experienced a simultaneous fall in Pco_2, which the investigators suggested as the cause of the alterations in blood flow velocity. Bookatz and colleagues[30] found a similar unexplained hypocarbic effect in rats breathing high-concentration oxygen in association with a decrease in bicarbonate and delayed initiation of spontaneous respirations. Two large epidemiologic studies have also suggested that brief exposure to high oxygen concentration for 3 minutes or longer after birth is associated with increased risk of childhood cancer, primarily acute lymphatic leukemia.[37–39]

In newborn animals, several studies have shown that brief exposures to oxygen during resuscitation result in significant oxygen stress detectable in multiple organ systems and metabolic pathways that is not apparent in the control animals resuscitated with air.[40–44] A Canadian laboratory using a piglet model has noted deleterious effects of high oxygen concentration used for resuscitation on mesenteric blood flow and biomarkers in the liver and heart.[43,44] In human newborns, Vento and coworkers[15,16] have demonstrated similar findings of oxidative stress associated with high oxygen administration with measurable effects lasting at least 28 days. A particularly disturbing study by Vento and colleagues[45] reported major implications of a very brief exposure of extremely low birthweight infants to high inspired oxygen concentrations at birth. The babies were randomly assigned to starting resuscitation with 30% or 90% oxygen, but with both groups having their inspired oxygen adjusted to achieve normal Spo_2, term-baby targets within 5 minutes of birth. Despite the saturations and inspired oxygen concentrations being equivalent within 5 minutes from birth, the duration of supplemental oxygen required, number of assisted ventilation days, time on continuous positive airway pressure, and incidence of chronic lung disease were two to nearly four times greater in those babies who received the brief higher oxygen exposure. Such dramatic differences in outcome were not reported from a multicenter trial comparing starting resuscitation with air versus 100% oxygen, also aiming at term-baby saturation targets.[46]

EFFECT OF OXYGEN CONCENTRATION ON PULMONARY VASCULAR RESISTANCE AT BIRTH

A major concern regarding the recommendation to minimize oxygen use in neonatal resuscitation was the possible deleterious effect the inspired gas might have on pulmonary vascular resistance (PVR). Oxygen has long been recognized as a pulmonary vasodilator; and one concern was that the use of air or low concentrations of oxygen to inflate the lungs might result in persistence of the normal intrauterine state of pulmonary vascular constriction. Once the placental source of oxygen is removed, this phenomenon might then lead to a failure of systemic arterial oxygenation and the vicious cycle known as persistent pulmonary hypertension of the newborn (PPHN). Because most of the animal models demonstrating air as equal to oxygen had already made transition from the intrauterine to extrauterine environment, PVR might have been less of a factor in the efficacy of the gas used for resuscitation in those studies. In addition, many of the human studies had excluded newborns with meconium aspiration syndrome, a condition associated with the development of PPHN.[12–17] Moreover, the diagnosis of asphyxia in many of the human studies was questioned because entry criteria varied among studies and most infants included would not meet the accepted criteria of intrapartum asphyxia.[47] Several animal studies have addressed these concerns.[48–52] Using newborn piglets, Medbo and colleagues[48] found that PVR rose significantly with induced hypoxia, but could demonstrate no difference in the fall in PVR when subsequent resuscitation was performed with air or 100% oxygen. A series of studies by the groups at Northwestern and Buffalo under the direction of Lakshminrusimha and Steinhorn has provided some of the most important evidence in this regard. Lakshminrusimha and colleagues[49] studied full-term lambs delivered by caesarean section and then ventilated with 21%, 50%, or 100% oxygen for 30 minutes. Using the decrease in PVR in response to 100% oxygen as indicative of the best response, these studies demonstrated that by 2 minutes of age PVR had achieved 72% and 80% of this optimum reduction in those lambs resuscitated with 21% and 50% oxygen, respectively. By 30 minutes of age, the PVR of the 100% and 50% oxygen groups was identical and by 60 to 90 minutes of age, the decrease in PVR in all three groups was not statistically different. It is interesting to note that Rudolph and Yuan had demonstrated as early as 1966 that PVR can be shown to relax with oxygen tensions as low as 60 mm Hg, which are easily achievable with exposure to the oxygen content in air at sea level.[53]

In the study by Lakshminrusimha and colleagues,[50] the lambs were subsequently ventilated with 10% oxygen or given a thromboxane analog to cause an increase in PVR, resulting in a similar response in all groups. However, treatment with nitric oxide (NO) or acetylcholine was blunted in the groups previously ventilated with additional oxygen. Furthermore, after withdrawal of the pulmonary vasodilators, rebound pulmonary hypertension occurred in the group resuscitated with 100% oxygen to a level higher than that before the initiation of NO/acetylcholine. Both of these findings suggest that the high oxygen exposure might actually increase, rather than decrease, the predilection to PPHN. In a subsequent study, this group demonstrated that a maximal change in PVR was achieved at Pao_2 values less than 60 mm Hg and that oxygen tensions higher than this (ie, hyperoxia) did not confer significant additional pulmonary vasodilation in lambs with induced PPHN.

Potential mechanisms to explain this phenomenon have been explored in subsequent studies by Farrow and colleagues[51] demonstrating that reactive oxygen species produced by exposure to 100% oxygen can react with arachidonic acid leading to the production of isoprotanes, which are potent constrictors of pulmonary arteries. Similarly superoxide radicals react with NO to produce peroxynitrite, a potent oxidant causing vasoconstriction, lipid peroxidation, and damage to surfactant proteins. Lakshminrusimha and colleagues[52] demonstrated in their same lamb model that short hyperoxia exposures produce significant changes in critical cellular signaling pathways in fetal pulmonary artery smooth muscle cells, leading to a degradation of cyclic GMP and inhibition of NO-mediated cGMP-dependent pulmonary vasorelaxation (**Fig. 1**).

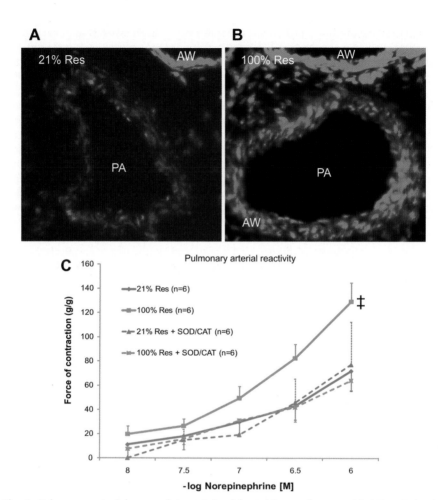

Fig. 1. Pulmonary arteriolar vasculature stained for evidence of superoxide injury in lambs resuscitated with air (*A*) or 100% oxygen (*B*) at birth. Conversion of dihydroethidium to ethidium results in red nuclear florescence. When pulmonary vascular rings were stimulated with norepinephrine (*C*), those that had been dissected from 100% oxygen lungs had significantly greater contraction, but when subjected to antioxidants (superoxide dismutase and catalase) contraction was similar to those resuscitated with air. (*From* Lakshminrusimha S, Steinhorn RH, Wedgwood S, et al. Pulmonary hemodynamics and vascular reactivity in asphyxiated term lambs resuscitated with 21 and 100% oxygen. J Appl Physiol 2011;111(5):1441–7; with permission.)

It seems that resuscitation with air or low concentrations of oxygen decreases PVR if the Pao_2 can be raised to the 60 mm Hg range, which is the approximate level experienced by term babies undergoing cardiopulmonary transition while breathing air at sea level. Moreover, the creation of hyperoxia by the use of higher concentrations of oxygen may have a deleterious effect on signaling pathways and actually inhibit the ability of the pulmonary vasculature to dilate by blunting the endogenous NO response. Is it possible that in the fervor to reverse the effects of intrauterine or peripartum hypoxia, clinicians have unwittingly increased the risk of the phenomenon of persistent pulmonary hypertension?

HOW HAVE THESE NEW FINDINGS BEEN TRANSLATED INTO NEW RECOMMENDATION FOR RESUSCITATING NEWBORNS?

After several years of reviewing and debating the new evidence, the neonatology section of ILCOR and the NRP Steering Committee have been convinced that the traditional recommendation of using high concentrations of supplemental oxygen during resuscitation of the compromised newly born infant was incorrect.[10] Although there is no doubt that oxygen is essential to mammalian survival, and anaerobic metabolism is an inefficient pathway for generating metabolic energy, abrupt exposure to oxygen in excessive quantities can also be toxic, particularly when such tissues have had restricted exposure throughout their ontogeny. All of the evidence suggests that exposure of neonatal tissues to high amount of supplemental oxygen is unnecessary and generally contraindicated, unless measurement of blood oxygen levels can be confirmed to be significantly below those existing in the intrauterine environment. Contemporary oximeters are relatively easy to apply and are capable of accurately estimating tissue oxygenation, particularly when such levels are in the normal range encountered by the uncompromised fetus and newborn (50%–90% oxyhemoglobin saturation). Strategies have been suggested in the NRP Textbook and Instructor's Manual for ensuring the immediate availability of oximeters for every hospital-based delivery where supplemental oxygen may become necessary,[54,55] and multiple studies have demonstrated that obtaining reliable preductal oximeter readings can be achieved within 1 to 2 minutes after birth.[56–59] There is good evidence that using blended oxygen in the 30% to 90% range in premature infants can achieve targeted oximeter readings more rapidly than using either air or 100%,[60] and some evidence that attaching the probe to the baby before attaching to the instrument results in acquisition of a signal more quickly.[61] Until further studies may indicate otherwise, aiming for targets demonstrated by healthy babies born at term is recommended. These interquartile target ranges are displayed in **Fig. 2**, which demonstrates that the average newborn may take longer than 10 minutes after birth to achieve normal extrauterine values.

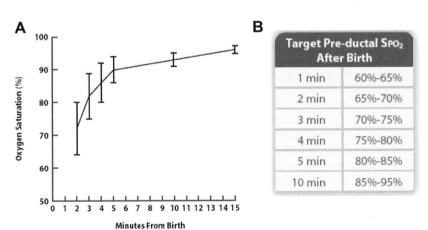

A

Oxygen Saturation (%) / Minutes From Birth

B

Target Pre-ductal SpO_2 After Birth	
1 min	60%-65%
2 min	65%-70%
3 min	70%-75%
4 min	75%-80%
5 min	80%-85%
10 min	85%-95%

Fig. 2. (*A*) Preductal oxygen saturations in healthy babies born at term. In utero SpO_2 during labor is approximately 60%. (*B*) Approximate ranges of interquartile SpO_2 values recommended for targets during resuscitation. ([*A*] *From* Mariani G, Dik PB, Ezquer A, et al. Pre-ductal and post-ductal O2 saturation in healthy term neonates after birth. J Pediatr 2007;150:418, with permission; and [*B*] AAP/AHA Neonatal Resuscitation Program. 6th edition. 2010; with permission.)

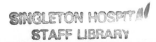

There is no evidence that achieving normal neonatal Spo_2 levels more rapidly than shown in **Fig. 2** is beneficial, and significant evidence that hyperoxygenation can be harmful.

Thus, from the multiple studies that have been conducted as of 2012, the following recommendations can be made about the use of supplemental oxygen to assist the newly born infant who is having difficulty making cardiopulmonary transition at birth:

- All hospitals should have the capacity to blend oxygen and air in their delivery facilities and have pulse oximetry immediately available for all births.
- Avoid hyperoxia. Starting resuscitation with no supplemental oxygen (ie, air) is probably the best choice for babies born at term.
- It is reasonable to match the oxyhemoglobin saturation increase demonstrated by healthy term newborns, taking approximately 10 minutes to increase the intra-uterine saturation of approximately 50% to 60% to the conventional neonatal targets. Long-term exposure of neonates to Spo_2 targets of 85% to 89% versus 91% to 95% have been associated with complications of hypoxemia or hyperox-emia, respectively, so many clinicians have chosen to use an intermediate target range (eg, 88%–92%).
- Blended oxygen permits achievement of term targets faster than when using either 21% or 100%, so if the need for resuscitation can be anticipated (eg, the delivery of an very low birth weight infant), it may be preferable to begin with an oxygen-air blend. A lower starting percentage (eg, 30%) may be preferable to higher (eg, 90%).
- Use of any supplemental oxygen should trigger attachment of an oximeter to the newborn.

WHAT MORE NEEDS TO BE KNOWN ABOUT TRANSITIONAL OXYGEN BEFORE PERHAPS CHANGING THE RECOMMENDATIONS FOR FUTURE NEWBORN RESUSCITATION?

More research will be required in terms of in vitro and animal studies, and new multi-center clinical trials to answer the following questions regarding the optimum oxygen environment for assisting compromised neonates to make the transition from intra-uterine to extrauterine oxygenation:

- Are the interquartile targets extrapolated from uncomplicated term births really the best target for all babies requiring resuscitation?
- Should babies with evidence of severe intrauterine asphyxia or poor cardiac output, and therefore compromised myocardial perfusion, receive efforts to increase oxygenation more rapidly?
- Should the extremely preterm infant, with less innate antioxidant protection, perhaps have oxygenation increased more slowly?
- Are the saturation targets really the best final goal, or are there implications of the inspired oxygen concentrations used to achieve them?
- Should clinicians delay clamping of the umbilical cord in babies requiring resus-citation, so as to make better use of placental oxygenation during transition?

Studies to answer most of these questions are currently underway and will likely result in even more changes in the recommendations regarding the use of supple-mental oxygen in the delivery room over the next few years.

REFERENCES

1. Szydlo Z. Water which does not wet hands: the alchemy of Michael Sendivogius. Warsaw (Poland): Polish Academy of Sciences; 1994.

2. Priestley J. Experiments and observations on different kinds of air. Birmingham (England): 1775.
3. Silverman WA. A cautionary tale about supplemental oxygen: the albatross of neonatal medicine. Pediatr 2002;113:394–6.
4. Silverman WA. Retrolental fibroplasia: a modern parable. New York, NY: Grune & Stratton, Inc.; 1980.
5. Niermeyer S, Kattwinkel J, Van Reempts P, et al. International guidelines for neonatal resuscitation. Pediatrics 2000;106:29.
6. Barcroft, Joseph Sir. Researches on prenatal life. Oxford (United Kingdom): Blackwell; 1946.
7. Latham F. The oxygen paradox. Experiments on the effects of oxygen in human anoxia. Lancet 1951;1:77–81.
8. Paneth N. The evidence mounts against use of pure oxygen in newborn resuscitation. J Pediatr 2005;147:4–6.
9. Kattwinkel J, Perlman J, Boyle D, et al. 2005 American Heart Association (AHA) guidelines for Cardiopulmonary Resuscitation (CPR) and Emergency Cardiovascular Care (ECC) of pediatric and neonatal patients: Neonatal resuscitation guidelines. Pediatrics 117:e1–10;2006.
10. Perlman JM, Wyllie J, Kattwinkel J, et al. Part 11: neonatal resuscitation: 2010 international consensus on cardiopulmonary resuscitation and emergency cardiovascular care science with treatment recommendations. Circulation 2010; 122:S516–38.
11. Saugstad OD. Hypoxanthine as an indicator of hypoxia: its role in health and disease through free radical production. Pediatr Res 1988;23:143–50.
12. Ramji S, Ahuja S, Thirupuram S, et al. Resuscitation of asphyxic newborn infants with room air or 100% oxygen. Pediatr Res 1993;34:809–12.
13. Saugstad OD, Rootwelt T, Aalen O. Resuscitation of asphyxiated newborn infants with room air or oxygen: an international controlled trial: the Resair 2 Study. Pediatrics 1998;102:1–7.
14. Ramji S, Rasaily R, Mishra PK, et al. Resuscitation of asphyxiated newborns with room air or 100% oxygen at birth: a multicentric trial. Indian Pediatr 2003;40:510–7.
15. Vento M, Asensi M, Sastre J, et al. Resuscitation with room air instead of 100% oxygen prevents oxidative stress in moderately asphyxiated term neonates. Pediatrics 2001;107:642–7.
16. Vento M, Asensi M, Sastre J, et al. Oxidative stress in asphyxiated term infants resuscitated with 100% oxygen. J Pediatr 2003;142:240–6.
17. Bajaj N, Udani RH, Nanavati RN. Room air vs 100 per cent oxygen for neonatal resuscitation: a controlled clinical trial. J Trop Pediatr 2005;51:206–11.
18. Tan A, Schulze A, O'Donnell CP, et al. Air versus oxygen for resuscitation of infants at birth. Cochrane Database Syst Rev 2005:CD002273.
19. Rabi Y, Rabi D, Yee W. Room air resuscitation of the depressed newborn: a systematic review and meta-analysis. Resuscitation 2007;72:353.
20. Saugstad OD, Ramji S, Soll R, et al. Resuscitation with room air or pure oxygen: an updated meta-analysis. Neonatology 2008;94:176–82.
21. Richmond S, Goldsmith JP. Refining the role of oxygen administration during delivery room resuscitation: what are our future goals? Semin Fetal Neonatal Med 2008;13:368–74.
22. Solås AB, Kutzsche S, Vinje M, et al. Cerebral hypoxemia-ischemia and reoxygenation with 21% or 100% oxygen in newborn piglets: effects on extracellular levels of excitatory amino acids and microcirculation. Pediatr Crit Care Med 2001;2:340–5.

23. Solås AB, Kalous P, Saugstad OD. Reoxygenation with 100 or 21% oxygen after cerebral hypoxemia-ischemia-hypercapnia in newborn piglets. Biol Neonate 2004;85:105–11.

24. Solås AB, Munkeby BH, Saugstad OD. Comparison of short- and long-duration oxygen treatment after cerebral asphyxia in newborn piglets. Pediatr Res 2004; 56:125–31.

25. De Lee JB. Asphyxia neonatorum: causation and treatment. Medicine (Detroit) 1897;3:643–60.

26. Matsiukevich D, Randis TM, Utkina-Sosunova I, et al. The state of systemic circulation, collapsed or preserved defines the need for hyperoxic or normoxic resuscitation in neonatal mice with hypoxia–ischemia. Resuscitation 2010;81(2):224–9.

27. Aizad T, Bodani J, Coates D, et al. Effect of a single breath of 100% oxygen on respiration in neonates during sleep. J Appl Physiol 1984;57:1531–5.

28. Lofaso F, Dauger S, Matrot B, et al. Inhibitory effects of repeated hyperoxia on breathing in newborn mice. Eur Respir J 2007;29:18–24.

29. Hutchison AA. Recovery from hypopnea in preterm lambs: effects of breathing air or oxygen. Pediatr Pulmonol 1987;3:317–23.

30. Bookatz GB, Mayer CA, Wilson CG, et al. Effect of supplemental oxygen on reinitiation of breathing after neonatal resuscitation in rat pups. Pediatr Res 2007;61: 698–702.

31. Hoehn T, Felderhoff-Mueser U, Maschewski K, et al. Hyperoxia causes inducible nitric oxide synthase-mediated cellular damage to the immature rat brain. Pediatr Res 2003;54:179–84.

32. Felderhoff-Mueser U, Bittigau P, Sifringer M, et al. Oxygen causes cell death in the developing brain. Neurobiol Dis 2004;17:273–82.

33. Kaindl AM, Sifringer M, Zabel C, et al. Acute and long-term proteome changes induced by oxidative stress in the developing brain. Cell Death Differ 2006;13: 1097–109.

34. Yee M, White RJ, Awad HA, et al. Neonatal hyperoxia causes pulmonary vascular disease and shortens life span in ageing mice. Am J Pathol 2011;178(6): 2601–10.

35. Lundstrøm KE, Pryds O, Greisen G. Oxygen at birth and prolonged cerebral vasoconstriction in preterm infants. Arch Dis Child 1995;73:F81–6.

36. Niijima S, Shortland DB, Levene MI, et al. Transient hyperoxia and cerebral blood flow velocity in infants born prematurely and at full term. Arch Dis Child 1988;63: 1126–30.

37. Cnattingius S, Zack M, Exbom A, et al. Prenatal and neonatal risk factors for childhood lymphatic leukaemia. J Natl Cancer Inst 1995;87:908–14.

38. Naumburg E, Bellocco R, Cnattingius S, et al. Supplementary oxygen and risk of childhood lymphatic leukaemia. Acta Paediatr 2002;91:1328–33.

39. Spector LG, Klebanoff MA, Feusner JH, et al. Childhood cancer following neonatal oxygen supplementation. J Pediatr 2005;147:27–31.

40. Goplerud JM, Kim S, Delivoria-Papadopoulos M. The effect of post-asphyxial reoxygenation with 21% vs. 100% oxygen on Na+, K(+)-ATPase activity in striatum of newborn piglets. Brain Res 1995;696:161–4.

41. Huang CC, Yonetani M, Lajevardi N, et al. Comparison of postasphyxial resuscitation with 100% and 21% oxygen on cortical oxygen pressure and striatal dopamine metabolism in newborn piglets. J Neurochem 1995;64:292–8.

42. Kondo M, Itoh S, Isobe K, et al. Chemiluminescence because of the production of reactive oxygen species in the lungs of newborn piglets during resuscitation periods after asphyxiation load. Pediatr Res 2000;47:524–7.

43. Haase E, Bigam DL, Nakonechny QB, et al. Resuscitation with 100% oxygen causes intestinal glutathione oxidation and reoxygenation injury in asphyxiated newborn piglets. Ann Surg 2004;240(2):364–73.
44. Haase E, Bigam DL, Nakonechny QB, et al. Cardiac function, myocardial glutathione, and matrix metalloproteinase-2 levels in hypoxic newborn pigs reoxygenated by 21%, 50% or 100% oxygen. Shock 2005;23(4):383–9.
45. Vento M, Moro M, Escrig R, et al. Preterm resuscitation with low oxygen causes less oxidative stress, inflammation, and chronic lung disease. Pediatrics 2009; 124:e439–49.
46. Rabi Y, Singhal N, Nettel-Aguirre A. Room-air versus oxygen administration for resuscitation of preterm infants: the Roar Study. Pediatrics 2011;128(2):e374–81.
47. American College of Obstetricians and Gynecologists. Neonatal encephalopathy and cerebral palsy: defining the pathogenesis and pathophysiology. Washington: American College of Obstetricians and Gynecologists; 2003.
48. Medbo S, Yu XQ, Asberg A, et al. Pulmonary hemodynamics and plasma endothelin-1 during hypoxemia and reoxygenation with room air or 100% oxygen in a piglet model. Pediatr Res 1998;44:843–9.
49. Lakshminrusimha S, Russell JA, Steinhorn RH, et al. Pulmonary hemodynamics in neonatal lambs resuscitated with 21%, 50% and 100% oxygen. Pediatr Res 2007; 62:313–8.
50. Lakshminrusimha S, Swartz DD, Gugino SF, et al. Oxygen concentration and pulmonary hemodynamics in newborn lambs with pulmonary hypertension. Pediatr Res 2009;66(5):539–44.
51. Farrow KN, Lee KJ, Perez M, et al. Brief hyperoxia increases mitochondrial oxidation and increases phosphodiesterase 5 activity in fetal pulmonary artery smooth muscle cells. Antioxid Redox Signal 2012;17(3):460–70.
52. Lakshminrusimha S, Steinhorn RH, Wedgwood S, et al. Pulmonary hemodynamics and vascular reactivity in asphyxiated term lambs resuscitated with 21 and 100% oxygen. J Appl Physiol 2011;111(5):1441–7.
53. Rudolph AM, Yuan S. Response of the pulmonary vasculature to hypoxia and H+ ion concentration changes. J Clin Invest 1966;45(3):399–411.
54. Kattwinkel J, editor. Neonatal resuscitation textbook. 6th edition. Elk Grove Village (IL): American Academy of Pediatrics; American Heart Association; 2011. p. 52–8.
55. Zaichkin J, editor. Neonatal resuscitation instructor manual. 6th edition. Elk Grove Village (IL): American Academy of Pediatrics; American Heart Association; 2011. p. 73.
56. Mariani G, Brener P, Ezquer A. Pre-ductal and post-ductal O2 saturation in healthy term neonates after birth. J Pediatr 2007;150:418–21.
57. Dawson JA, Kamlin COF, Vento M, et al. Defining the reference range for oxygen saturation for infants after birth. Pediatrics 2010;125(6):e1340–7.
58. Rabi Y, Yee W, Chen SY, et al. Oxygen saturation trends immediately after birth. J Pediatr 2006;148:590–4.
59. Wang CL, Anderson C, Leone TA, et al. Resuscitation of preterm neonates by using room air or 100% oxygen. Pediatrics 2008;121:1083–9.
60. Escrig R, Arruza L, Izquierdo I, et al. Neonates resuscitated with low or high oxygen concentrations: a prospective randomized trial. Pediatrics 2008;121:875–81.
61. O'Donnell CP, Kamlin CO, Davis PG, et al. Feasibility of and delay in obtaining pulse oximetry during neonatal resuscitation. J Pediatr 2005;147:698–9.

Delivery Room Management of Meconium-Stained Infant

Rama Bhat, MD[a],*, Dharmapuri Vidyasagar, MD[b]

KEYWORDS

- MSAF • DR-management • MAS • Neonatal resuscitation

KEY POINTS

- Common risk factors for meconium-stained amniotic fluid (MSAF) include postdate pregnancies, nonreassuring fetal heart rate, African and South Asian ethnicity, maternal smoking/drug abuse, and chorioamnionitis.
- MSAF occurs in 3% to –14% of the pregnancies. Incidence can be as high as 40% in postdate pregnancies. Delivering the infant by 41 weeks can decrease the incidence of MSAF and meconium aspiration syndrome (MAS).
- Meconium aspiration is an in utero phenomenon. Decreasing postmaturity, early diagnosis of high-risk pregnancies, and better intrapartum surveillance can help further to decrease MAS.
- Amnioinfusion for MSAF, routine oropharyngeal suction at the perineum, and intubation of vigorous infants born through MSAF are not recommended based on recent large randomized controlled studies.
- In developed countries the incidence of meconium aspiration has been decreasing steadily over the last 15 years from 5% to around 2% and mortality for infants with MAS has decreased from 40% to less than 5%.

INTRODUCTION

Meconium-stained amniotic fluid (MSAF) has been described several hundred years ago by Aristotle, who coined the term meconium (Greek word: meconiumarion). Obstetric textbooks from the beginning of the last century described the passage of meconium in utero as an impending sign of fetal death.[1] Improved obstetric care both antenatal and intrapartum and better neonatal intensive care unit care, along with improved understanding of the maternal and fetal physiology during the second

Disclosure: Both authors declare no financial or other conflicts of interest.
[a] Department of Pediatrics, Children's Hospital of Wisconsin, Medical College of Wisconsin, Room 410, CCC, 999 North 92 Street, Wauwatosa, WI 53226, USA; [b] Department of Pediatrics, University of Illinois at Medical Center at Chicago, 840 South Wood Street, Chicago, IL 60612, USA
* Corresponding author.
E-mail address: ribhat@mcw.edu

Clin Perinatol 39 (2012) 817–831
http://dx.doi.org/10.1016/j.clp.2012.09.004
0095-5108/12/$ – see front matter © 2012 Elsevier Inc. All rights reserved.

half of the last century, has led to improved survival and decreased morbidity. Management of MSAF and the baby born through MSAF has also undergone similar changes in the last 40 years. In this article the authors discuss the epidemiology, pathophysiology, and significance of MSAF and the changes in intrapartum and delivery room management of the newborn over the last 40 years to the current evidence-based approaches.

EPIDEMIOLOGY OF MSAF

The incidence of MSAF in the United States has ranged from 3% to 14%.[2–5] Meconium aspiration syndrome (MAS), the severest of all the morbidities, occurs in 1.5% to 5% of infants born through MSAF.[6] MSAF can also increase the risk of neonatal infection and pulmonary hypertension. Several investigators have reported the epidemiology of MSAF during the past 2 decades.[7–10] Some of the earlier reports were based on a small number of cases and were limited to regional institutions and selected population.[7,8] These reports, one from United Arab Emirates and the other from the United States, showed that there are ethnic differences in the incidence of MSAF. Sedaghatian and colleagues[7] from UAE analyzed their data prospectively to examine the incidence of MSAF among 7 different ethnic groups. They also analyzed the relationship of confounding factors, such as birth weight, gestational age, and maternal gravidity, on MSAF. The overall incidence of MSAF was 19% (13% thin meconium, 6% thick meconium). The prevalence of MAS was 5% in the thick MSAF group and none in the thin MSAF group. The incidence of MSAF, besides being associated with increasing gestational age (6% at <36 weeks to 46% at 42 weeks) and birth weight (11% at <2500 g to 28% at >5000 g), also differed significantly by ethnicity (14% in South Asians to 30% in East Africans). After controlling for these clinical variables, the African infants had a higher percentage of MSAF at all gestational ages as compared with the other ethnic groups. Although there was a higher incidence of MSAF in African babies, there was no increase in MAS. Authors concluded that compared with other ethnic groups, the higher incidence of MSAF without an increase in MAS in black Africans indicates advanced maturity of the gastrointestinal system for gestational age.

In the United States, Alexander and colleagues[8] also found a 50% higher prevalence of MSAF among non-Hispanic black babies compared with non-Hispanic white babies. Similar findings were reported by Sriram and colleagues,[9] who analyzed US birth and infant death cohorts during the period of 1998 to 2000 to estimate the prevalence of MSAF and MAS between non-Hispanic black and non-Hispanic white babies. They calculated the risk of developing MSAF, the risk of developing MAS, and the rate of case fatality of MAS by race, gestational age (GA), and birth weight among the population studied. Non-Hispanic black babies had an 80% greater risk of being born via MSAF (Odds Ratio [OR]: 1.81; 95% confidence interval [CI] 1.80–1.82), and 67% higher incidence of MAS (OR: 1.67; 95% CI: 1.64–1.70) compared with non-Hispanic whites. There were no differences, however, in rates of case fatality between the groups.

In another recent large epidemiology study from the United Kingdom, Balchin and colleagues[10] analyzed the data of 499,996 singleton live births (Birth weight >500 g, GA >24 weeks) to study the incidence of MSAF. The racial composition of the population studied was as follows: white, 70.5%; South Asian, 13%; black, 6.1%. MSAF was present in 81,405 (16.3%; 95% CI: 16.2–16.4). Incidence of MSAF increased by gestation: preterm 5.1%, term 16.5%, and postterm 27%, respectively. After the exclusion of preterm babies, they found that increasing GA and race were independent predictors of

MSAF. In black babies, the OR of having or being born via MSAF was 8.4 (95% CI: 2.4–28.8), and in South Asian babies, the OR was 3.3 (95% CI:4.2–5.3) compared with whites. At every GA, black babies had a far higher rate of MSAF than white babies. They concluded that these findings support the hypothesis that MSAF was associated more with fetal maturity in black and South Asian babies than hypoxia. They suggested that "consideration should be given to increased monitoring or labor induction earlier than 41 weeks' gestation in South Asian and black women."

Fischer and colleagues[11] reported a population-based retrospective study of MAS from a region in France. They found that among 132,884 term (37- to 43-week GA) newborns, the rate of MSAF was 7.93%. The overall prevalence of MAS was 0.18% and the overall prevalence of severe MAS was 0.067%. The incidence of MAS increased with gestational age: 0.11% at 37 to 38 weeks of GA, 0.20% at 39 to 41 weeks of GA, and 0.49% at 42 to 43 weeks of GA. Thick MSAF, fetal tachycardia, Apgar score ≤3 at 1 minute, and birth in a level I, II facility each independently were associated with severe MAS. The frequency of severe MAS decreased following the adaptation of new international recommendations for the management of babies born with MSAF.[12]

Dargaville and colleagues[13] studied the epidemiology of MAS requiring ventilator support in Australia and New Zealand (ANZNN database) for the period 1995 to 2002. Data of 1061 infants ventilated for MAS were analyzed. There was no information on the incidence of MSAF in their population. Overall incidence of MAS requiring intubation during the 7-year period (1995–2002) was 0.43/1000 live births. During this period, the MAS requiring ventilator support decreased steadily to 0.37/1000 live births. Incidence of MAS was also significantly higher for infants born to Pacific Islander and Aboriginal mothers. Data from Australia also showed that the incidence of MAS increased from 0.4/1000 live births at 36 weeks' gestation to 1.42/1000 live births at 42 weeks' gestation. The overall decrease in MAS during the study period was attributed to a significant reduction in births beyond 41 weeks' gestation (2.8% in 1995 to 1.6% in 2002; P<.001).

A recent Cochrane review, which included 19 trials, showed that a policy of induction of labor at 41 weeks' gestation reduced the risk of perinatal mortality (risk ratio [RR]: 0.30; 95% CI: 0.09-0.99) with no increase in operative delivery. This review also reported that among the 41-weeks group, the incidence of MAS was lower in the induced group than the expectantly managed group (RR: 0.29; 95% CI: 0.12–0.68; N = 1325).[14]

SIGNIFICANCE OF MSAF

Between 1of 5 and 1 of 20 babies born at term or near term is born through MSAF. Of this, 1.5% to 5% develop MAS (7500–25,000 cases/yr in the United States) and another 3.4% to 5.2% develop other respiratory problems, such as transient tachypnea, delayed adaptation after birth, pulmonary hypertension, sepsis/pneumonia, and pneumothorax. Thirty percent to 50% of newborns with MAS require ventilator support and treatment of pulmonary hypertension. The last 4 decades have witnessed a significant decrease in mortality from as high as 40% to less than 5%.[15,16] In resource-poor countries, MAS is still associated with high mortality and morbidity. The respiratory problems can be influenced by many factors, among them type of MSAF, namely thick versus thin, intrapartum fetal distress, the presence of chorioamnionitis, and cesarean versus vaginal delivery.[17] Even though a small percentage of newborns (1.5% to 5%) born through MSAF develop MAS and other respiratory disorders and require neonatal intensive care, the presence of meconium in the amniotic fluid indicates the need for close observation for any signs of fetal compromise. The decision to deliver the infant should be based on fetal well-being rather than the presence of meconium. The presence of meconium also calls for the presence of neonatal rapid response team at the time of delivery.

PATHOPHYSIOLOGY OF MSAF

MSAF is uncommon between 20 and 32 weeks' gestation. **Fig. 1** shows the physiologic and stress-mediated mechanisms in the development of MSAF. Higher levels of motilin and increased cholinergic innervation with advancing gestation can explain the higher incidence in MSAF in term and postterm (>294days) infants.[3] Yoder and colleagues[18] reported that reducing post maturity by 33% in a span of 9 years decreased the MAS from 5.8% to 1.5%. They attributed the decrease in MAS to a reduction in post maturity and better intrapartum surveillance, early diagnosis of nonreassuring fetal heart rate, and higher rate of cesarean section. **Fig. 1** describes the various conditions and the possible mechanisms for MSAF.

Other factors associated with meconium passage are drug abuse,[19] intrauterine infection,[20] use of vaginal misoprostol for labor induction,[21] and gestational cholestasis.[22] In the latter instance, MSAF was attributed to an increased fetal colonic stimulation by higher bile acid accumulation in the maternal serum. Infusion of bile acids to fetal lambs did increase colonic motility.[23] In a recent study, Ahanya and colleagues[24] reported that fetal stress increases corticotrophin-releasing factor (CRF) and CRF-R1 receptor, which increase the colonic contractility. Levels of cortisol and CRF in fetuses with MSAF were higher and administration of glucocorticoid and thyroxin to the fetus showed increased colonic contractility and passage of meconium.[25] MSAF can be thin, thick, and or moderately thick depending on the amount of meconium passed, volume of the amniotic fluid, and its clearance from the amniotic fluid. Understanding the mechanisms of meconium passage in utero can lead to preventive treatments in the future.[26] The low incidence of MSAF in preterm infants may be secondary to low motilin, decreased peristalsis, and a small amount of meconium in the gut.[27]

PERINATAL MANAGEMENT
Amnioinfusion to Reduce MAS

Recognizing the strong association of MSAF and MAS, several investigators have attempted to decrease the effect of meconium using amnioinfusion of saline. The hypothesis behind amnioinfusion was 2-fold: (1) to dilute the thick meconium to prevent obstruction of airways if aspirated; (2) to relieve any cord compression, oligohydramnios, and fetal distress. However, the results from several retrospective and prospective randomized trials were conflicting.[28–30]

In an effort to resolve the controversy, Fraser and colleagues[31] conducted a large multinational, multicenter randomized control study of amnioinfusion in women with

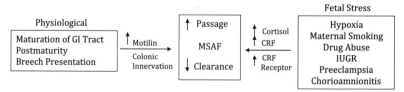

Fig. 1. Pathophysiology of MSAF. CRF, corticotropin releasing factor; CRF-R, CRF receptor; GI, gastrointestinal; MSAF, meconium-stained amniotic fluid; IUGR, intrauterine growth restriction.

thick MSAF. The study included 1998 women in labor and at greater than 36 weeks' gestation from 56 centers with thick MSAF. The study was stratified according to the presence or absence of abnormal fetal heart rate defined as variable decelerations and randomized into an amnioinfusion group or a standard treatment group. Investigators found no difference in the incidence of primary outcome of MAS or in the number of perinatal deaths. MAS or perinatal death or both occurred in 4.5% of infants in the amnioinfusion group compared with 3.5% in the standard treatment group (RR: 1.26; 95% CI: 0.82–1.95). They concluded that amnioinfusion should not be recommended for the prevention of MAS. Other studies have also expressed serious concerns regarding the complications of amnioinfusion, such as uterine rupture and amniotic fluid embolism.[32,33] The American College of Obstetrics and Gynecology (ACOG) subsequently stated that routine prophylactic amnioinfusion for the dilution of MSAF is not recommended.[34]

The most recent Cochrane Review by Hoffmeyr and Xu on amnioinfusion to prevent MAS was published in 2010. Their review included 13 studies with a total of 4143 patients. They found that in settings with standard peripartum surveillance, amnioinfusion showed no significant reduction in primary outcomes, namely MAS, perinatal death, and maternal death or severe morbidity, compared with controls.[35] However, a separate subanalysis of 2 studies from settings with limited perinatal surveillance capabilities showed the following: (1) a reduction in cesarean section for fetal distress and overall reduction in MAS (RR: 0.25; 95% CI: 0.13–0.47); (2) a reduction in need for neonatal ventilation or neonatal intensive care unit admission; and (3) a trend toward reduced perinatal mortality (RR: 0.37; 95% CI: 0.13–1.01). In one of the studies, the presence of meconium below the vocal cords was reduced and, in the other study, neonatal encephalopathy was reduced.[36,37] These findings led to the conclusion that amnioinfusion is associated with substantive improvements in perinatal outcome only in facilities with limited perinatal surveillance. It was not clear whether the benefits were due to dilution of meconium or relief of oligohydramnios.

EVOLUTION OF DELIVERY ROOM MANAGEMENT OF INFANTS BORN THROUGH MSAF

The Neonatal Resuscitation Program (NRP) was launched in the late 1980s in the United States, under the aegis of American Academy of Pediatrics (AAP) and the American Heart Association (AHA). Earlier guidelines were based largely on clinical experience with some supportive experimental evidence. In the 1990s there was an increasing emphasis toward the practice of evidence-based medicine using randomized controlled clinical trials as the gold standard; however, the number of available controlled studies in the 1990s was limited. In 2000, the International Committee on Cardiopulmonary Resuscitation undertook an evidenced-based review of delivery room resuscitation practices. Evidence for several delivery room practices was gathered and analyzed critically by expert committees. The management of infants born through MASF and the prevention of MAS was one of the important topics reviewed by the International Committee on Cardiopulmonary Resuscitation committee. The details of the elaborate process of developing evidence-based recommendations have been described previously.[38] These recommendations were eventually adopted by the NRP committee of AAP and AHA.

The recommendations for the intrapartum and delivery room management of mother and the newborn have gone through significant changes during the last 4 decades based on several observational, randomized controlled trials (RCTs) and systematic reviews regarding intrapartum suctioning, and postdelivery endotracheal suctioning. **Table 1** shows the AAP/ACOG recommendations starting from 1977 until

Table 1
AAP-NRP recommendations for delivery room management of meconium-stained newborn over the years

Guidelines	1977[39]	1983[40]	1992[41]	2002[42]	2006[43]	2011[44]
Oral and nasopharyngeal suction in the perineum	Recommended	Recommended	Recommended	Recommended	Not Recommended	Not Recommended
Intubate and suction all	Yes	Yes[a]	No	No	No	No
Selective intubation and suction	No	No	Yes	Yes	Yes	Yes

[a] In the presence of thick meconium.

2011.[39–44] In 1977 the first set of guidelines were published on the delivery room management of MSAF by the Committee on Fetus and Newborn in the 6th edition of Standards and Recommendations for Hospital Care of Newborn Infants.[39] It is recommended that both oropharyngeal suction at perineum and intubation and suctioning of trachea is performed. These recommendations were based on clinical studies of Gregory and colleagues and Carson and colleagues.[45,46] In the first edition of Guidelines for Perinatal Care in 1983, the recommendations for thick MSAF included direct visualization of the larynx and suction with an endotracheal tube by mouth, covered with a surgical mask. Subsequently, intrapartum oropharyngeal suction with a De Lee trap became routine on delivery of the shoulder. These recommendations continued until the RCT of tracheal intubation in meconium-stained vigorous newborns was published by Linder and colleagues[47] in 1988. In the 3rd edition of Guidelines for Perinatal Care published in 1992, intubation was recommended only if meconium is present in the larynx and the infant is depressed.[41] Evidence for this recommendation, however, was weak, with only one controlled trial in a selective population. In the 5th edition of Guidelines for Perinatal Care (2002), the recommendation was to intubate and suction only depressed infants at birth born through MSAF.[42] Oropharyngeal suction at the perineum was still recommended for all infants born through MSAF. These recommendations were based on the large RCT of intubation of vigorous infants born through MSAF.[17] In 2005 Vain and colleagues[48] reported the results from a large multicenter RCT of oropharyngeal suction at the perineum in meconium-stained infants. The study showed no benefit in preventing MAS. Following its publication both ACOG and AHA/AAP recommended not to suction at the perineum.[49] The sixth edition of the NRP textbook and the current Guidelines for Perinatal Care recommend no oropharyngeal suction at the perineum and no endotracheal suction of vigorous infants after birth.[44]

Obstetric Intervention Before Delivery of the Shoulders

Intrapartum oropharyngeal and nasopharyngeal suctioning became a routine procedure for all newborns born through MSAF since the first report by Carson and colleagues.[46] In this part prospective and part retrospective study they compared the effectiveness of combined obstetric and pediatric suctioning with that of direct tracheal suction alone by the pediatrician. The results showed that the infants (n = 273) who received combined obstetric and selective neonatal tracheal suctioning had the lowest incidence of MAS (0.37%) and 0% mortality. In infants who received only endotracheal suction (n = 947), the incidence of MAS was 1.9% and the addition of lung lavage did not decrease MAS (1.8%). They concluded that deep nasopharyngeal suctioning on the delivery of the head in the perineum rarely requires any further tracheal suction after delivery. Since then, routine oropharyngeal and nasopharyngeal suction with a large-bore 12- to 13-French catheter at the perineum became standard of care. Subsequently, 2 reports by Falciglia in 1988 and Falciglia and colleagues in 1992 showed that oropharyngeal suction at the perineum followed by tracheal suction after birth decreased only the severity of the disease but not the incidence of MAS. He speculated that "aspiration of the meconium is an in utero phenomena and presence of meconium in the trachea is merely a marker of earlier fetal hypoxia."[50,51] Despite these and other similar observational reports showing no benefit, oropharyngeal suctioning before the delivery of the shoulders remained a standard of care until the results of a large RCT published by Vain and colleagues[48] in 2004. This multicenter RCT conducted in 12 centers (1 in USA and 11 in Argentina) enrolled 2514 term newborns born through MSAF irrespective of the consistency of meconium. Infants were randomized to either oropharyngeal suction or no suction before the delivery of the shoulders. Infants randomized to suction received oropharyngeal suction followed by nasopharyngeal suction using 10- to 13-French catheters. The suction was performed in vaginally born and in those born by cesarean section. Management immediately after birth was according to NRP guidelines recommended by AAP and AHA. The primary outcome measure was the incidence of MAS. The secondary outcomes included mortality, need for mechanical ventilation, pneumothorax, and respiratory disorders other than MAS. The incidence of MAS remained the same (4% vs 3.7%) between groups. There were no differences in the need for mechanical ventilation, length of stay, and duration of oxygen between groups (**Table 2**). They concluded that nasopharyngeal suction at the perineum before delivery of the shoulders decreased neither the incidence nor the severity of MAS (Level 1A evidence).

Neonatal Management After Delivery

James first described the technique of tracheal suctioning for infants born through MSAF.[52] Burke-Strickland and Edwards in 1973 first reported the results of aggressive management for infants born through MSAF with intubation and tracheal lavage. Over a 2-year period they encountered 101 infants with MSAF; 84 of these had meconium and 17 had no meconium in oropharynx. Fifty of 84 intubated infants also had meconium in the trachea. Infants who received intubation and suction or intubation and suction and lavage had significant reduction in respiratory distress and shorter hospital stays. Based on these findings, Burke-Strickland and Edwards recommended that all infants born through MSAF should be intubated and suctioned immediately at birth.[53] Two other reports, one by Gregory and colleagues[45,54] and the second by Ting and Brady, showed that tracheal suction was associated with immediate improved outcome. Although the first study was prospective without concurrent controls, the latter study was retrospective, comparing the intubated and suctioned infants to those not suctioned. Since the publication of these studies, intubation and suctioning of all infants born through MSAF became routine practice. In a RCT, the first of its kind in terms of meconium-stained newborns, Linder and colleagues[47] showed that endotracheal suction of vigorous meconium-stained infants provided no benefits compared with controls. The study included 572 meconium-stained vigorous newborns born vaginally who were randomized to either endotracheal suction or no suction. The study excluded infants born by cesarean section and by instrument-assisted delivery. All newborns had their oropharyngeal suction in

Table 2
Major primary and secondary outcomes in the randomized controlled trial oropharyngeal and nasopharyngeal suction at the perineum

Outcome	Intrapartum Suction N = 1263 (%)	No Intrapartum Suction N = 1251 (%)	RR (CI)
N in each group	N = 1263 (%)	N = 1251 (%)	
Need for intubation/suction and Positive Pressure Ventilation (PPV)	106 (8%)	113 (9%)	1.1 (0.8–1.4)
Meconium aspiration syndrome	52 (4%)	47 (3.8%)	0.9 (0.6–1.3)
Ventilatory support	24 (2%)	18 (1%)	0.8 (0.4–1.4)
Respiratory disorders other than MAS	61 (5%)	79 (6%)	1.3 (0.9–1.8)
Mortality	9 (0.7%)	4 (0.32%)	0.4 (0.1–1.5)

Data from Vain NE, Szyld EG, Prudent LM, et al. Oropharyngeal and nasopharyngeal suctioning of meconium stained neonates before the delivery of their shoulders: multicenter randomized controlled trial. Lancet 2004;364:597–602.

perineum before complete delivery. There were no deaths in either group. However, 6 infants in the suctioned group experienced complications, namely, 4 with MAS, and 2 with laryngeal stridor. The control group had no complications. They concluded that endotracheal intubation is not without complications and should be considered unnecessary in vigorous term neonates born through MSAF. Cunningham and colleagues[55] later proposed standard of care, namely, a selective approach of endotracheal intubation and suction.

Intubation of babies born with MSAF, however, remained a controversy until Wiswell and colleagues[17] published the results of the large multicenter RCT. In this multicenter RCT 2094 vigorous newborns born through meconium-stained (including thick and thin) amniotic fluid were randomized to either intubation and suction or no intubation and suction. There were no differences in the incidence of MAS (3.2% vs 2.7%) and other respiratory disorders (3.8% vs 4.5%). The study concluded that intubation and suctioning the trachea of vigorous meconium-stained infants do not confer any benefits over expectant management. Based on this evidence, the 5th edition of Guidelines for Perinatal Care changed its recommendations to no endotracheal suction in vigorous infants born through MSAF.[42] The most recent Cochrane Review analyzed 4 RCTs on intubation at birth for preventing morbidity and mortality in vigorous, meconium-stained infants born at term. The metaanalysis of these trials failed to show any difference in mortality and morbidity between the intubated and control group. It was concluded that routine intubation cannot be recommended for vigorous meconium-stained infants.[56] Kabbur and colleagues[57] in a retrospective study looked at the impact of the above NRP recommendation on delivery room practices in their institution. They looked at the delivery room practices for 3 years immediately before the 2000 NRP to 3 years after its introduction. **Fig. 2** shows the incidence of MSAF and MAS and rate of intubation for the 2 periods. The incidence of MSAF, MAS, and other respiratory disorders did not change significantly during the 2 periods. The rate of intubation in period 1 was 67%, whereas in period 2 it was 41%, a significant decrease ($P<.001$) from 3 years before. The incidence of MAS both before and after introducing NRP guidelines, however, was lower in this report (0.85%–1.3%) compared with the incidence reported in the multicenter

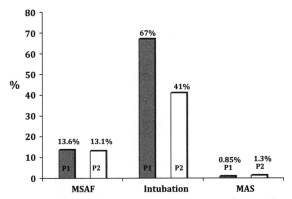

Fig. 2. Impact of Year 2000, NRP Delivery Room Management of Meconium Stained Infants. P1, January 1997–December 1999; P2, January 2000–December 2002. MAS, meconium aspiration syndrome; MSAF, meconium-stained amniotic fluid. (*Data from* Kabbur PM, Herson VC, Zaremba S, et al. Have the year 2000 Neonatal resuscitation program guidelines changed the delivery room management or outcome of meconium stained infants? J Perinatol 2005;25:694–7.)

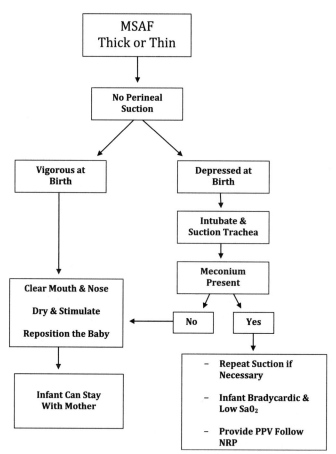

Fig. 3. Algorithm for current management of meconium-stained newborn as recommended in the textbook of "Neonatal Resuscitation" 6th Edition, 2011. NRP, Neonatal Resuscitation Program; PPV, Positive Pressure Ventilation.

randomized control study by Wiswell and colleagues (3.2% vs 2.7%). The results of this study support the NRP recommendations that delivery room intubation and suction are not necessary in vigorous meconium-stained infants.

Despite these evidence-based practice guidelines, it is not clear whether these guidelines are followed by the clinicians in their practice. A recent national survey conducted in Argentina[58] after the publication of 2 large multicenter RCTs[17,48] and subsequent recommendations from AAP/NRP, ACOG, and Argentinian scientific societies reported that 50% of the centers continued the practice of oropharyngeal suction some times and 7% at every birth. Furthermore, 30% of the institutions intubated and suctioned vigorous infants. Surprisingly 31% of the centers did not even suction the depressed meconium-stained infants. Another survey conducted in France by Michel and colleagues reported that the incidence of MSAF was 3% (N = 199/6761) and 26% of these infants were nonvigorous and 74% were vigorous at birth. The survey was conducted 7 years after establishing regional guidelines that recommended intubation of only nonvigorous infants. However immediate intubation and tracheal suction is performed in 42% of nonvigorous and 18% of vigorous newborns despite the regional guidelines.[59] Others have reported variations in delivery room practices between level 3 versus level 2 centers. Continuation of the old guidelines, despite the evidence-based recommendations, is of great concern, underscoring the need for continued educational and quality improvement reviews in each hospital.

UNPROVEN THERAPIES

In the past, several reports have described the methods to prevent meconium aspiration both in utero and at birth. These methods included the following: (1) maternal administration of narcotics like fentanyl (tested in a small number of pregnant baboons) given before the induction of hypoxia was shown to reduce the severity of MAS but did not prevent MAS[60]; (2) cricoid pressure and compression of thorax by the obstetricians at birth have been suggested but never studied. These methods were intended to prevent aspiration of meconium to the trachea. These procedures may increase the risk of injury to the airway and esophagus; and (3) gastric suction in the delivery room less than 5 minutes of age: Liu and Harrington reported a higher incidence of MAS in infants who received gastric suction before 5 minutes of age ($P = .032$; OR 2.81; CI: 1.17–6.74).[61] Another recent report looked at the effect of gastric lavage after birth to prevent subsequent aspiration of meconium from the stomach. In this only observational randomized prospective study, gastric lavage was performed within 1 h of birth in 227 newborns born through thick or thin MSAF. Another 275 newborns born through MSAF served as controls. This study showed no difference in secondary MAS in control versus lavaged group and none had experienced any feeding difficulties.[62] NRP recommends gastric decompression in the presence of gastric distension and if prolonged bag and mask ventilation is needed.

Summary

Intrapartum care and delivery room care of the newborn born through MSAF have gone through significant changes during the last decade primarily because of the large randomized multicenter, multinational controlled studies on amnioinfusion, oropharyngeal suction at perineum, and intubation of vigorous infants born through MSAF. These changes have been incorporated in the most recent guidelines of perinatal care, NRP textbooks, and obstetric textbooks. Although developed countries have seen a steady decline not only in incidence but also in mortality and morbidity from MAS and MAS-related respiratory disorders, it is still a major contributor for neonatal mortality in developing countries. The improvements in the developed countries have been attributed to better intrapartum surveillance, decreasing postmature births, and improved perinatal and neonatal care.

Current NRP recommendations for infants born through MSAF are shown in the algorithm in **Fig. 3**. These recommendations can be summarized as follows:

1. Close intrapartum monitoring of at-risk mother and fetus.
2. Informing the neonatal rapid response team about the impending delivery. Communication before delivery should include relevant antenatal and intrapartum findings, including FHR interpretations, chorioamnionitis, and obstetric interventions if including any cord blood gas results.
3. No oropharyngeal or nasopharyngeal suction at the perineum.
4. After delivery of the newborn, the rapid response team, skilled in neonatal resuscitation, needs to assess the infant quickly to see if the newborn is vigorous or depressed based on heart rate, tone, and respiratory effort.
5. If the newborn is vigorous, the mouth and nose must be cleaned, the infant should be dried, stimulated, and repositioned. The infant can stay with the mother.

6. All depressed infants born through MSAF irrespective of amniotic fluid consistency must be intubated and suctioned. If there is no meconium in the trachea and the infant responds quickly to stimulation, the infant can stay with the mother but may need short-term observation. If meconium is recovered from the trachea, depending on the hemodynamic stability of the infant, suction can be repeated. Endotracheal suction should not take longer than 5 seconds after intubation. This recommendation for depressed newborns is not evidence based at this time.

7. If the infant is bradycardic and has low oxygen saturation, Positive Pressure Ventilation (PPV) must be initiated and further steps taken as recommended in the NRP textbook.

REFERENCES

1. Schultz M. The significance of the passage of meconium during labor. Am J Obstet Gynecol 1925;10:83.
2. Cleary GM, Wiswell TE. Meconium stained amniotic fluid and meconium aspiration syndrome: an update. Pediatr Clin North Am 1998;45:511–29.
3. Poggi SH, Ghidini A. Pathophysiology of meconium passage in to amniotic fluid. Early Hum Dev 2009;85:607–10.
4. Wiswell TE, Bent RC. Meconium staining and meconium aspiration syndrome. Pediatr Clin North Am 1993;40:955–81.
5. Ramin KD, Leveno KJ, Kelly MA, et al. Amniotic fluid meconium: a fetal environmental hazard. Obstet Gynecol 1996;87:181–4.
6. Wiswell TE, Henly MA. Intratracheal suctioning, systemic infection and the meconium aspiration syndrome. Pediatrics 1992;89:203–6.
7. Sedaghatian MR, Othman L, Hossain MM, et al. Risk of meconium stained amniotic fluid in different ethnic groups. J Perinatol 2000;20:257–61.
8. Alexander GR, Hulsey TC, Robillard PY, et al. Determinants of meconium stained amniotic fluid in term pregnancies. J Perinatol 1994;14:259–63.
9. Sriram S, Wall SN, Khoshnood B, et al. Racial disparity in meconium-stained amniotic fluid and meconium aspiration syndrome in the United States, 1998-2000. Obstet Gynecol 2003;102:1262–8.
10. Balchin I, Whitaker JC, Lamont RF, et al. Maternal and fetal characteristics associated with meconium stained amniotic fluid. Obstet Gynecol 2011;117:828–35.
11. Fischer C, Rybakowski C, Ferdynus C, et al. A population based study of meconium aspiration syndrome in neonates born between 37 and 43 weeks gestation. Int J Pediatr 2012;2012:321545.
12. Nolan JP, Soar J, Zideman DA, et al. European resuscitation guidelines for resuscitation 2010: section 1.Executive summary. Resuscitation 2010;81(10):1219–76.
13. Dargaville PA, Copnell B, For the Australian and New Zealand Neonatal Network. The epidemiology of meconium syndrome: incidence, risk factors, therapies and outcome. Pediatrics 2006;117:1712–21.
14. Gulmezoglu AM, Crowther CA, Middleton P. Induction of labor for improving birth outcomes for women at or beyond term. Cochrane database for systematic reviews 2006;(4):CD004945.
15. Vidyasagar D, Harris V, Pildes RS. Assisted ventilation in infants with meconium aspiration syndrome. Pediatrics 1975;56:208–13.
16. Whitfield J, Charsha D, Chiruvolu A. Prevention of meconium aspiration syndrome: an update and the Baylor experience. Proc (Bayl Univ Med Cent) 2009;22:128–31.

17. Wiswell TE, Gannon CM, Jacob J, et al. Delivery room management of apparently vigorous meconium stained neonate. Results of multicenter, international collaborative trial. Pediatrics 2000;105:1–7.
18. Yoder BA, Kirsch EA, Barth WH, et al. Changing obstetric practice associated with decreasing incidence of meconium aspiration syndrome. Obstet Gynecol 2002;126:712–5.
19. Chasnoff IJ, Burns KA, Burns WJ. Cocaine use in pregnancy; perinatal morbidity and mortality. Neurotoxicol Teratol 1987;9:291–3.
20. Mazor M, Froimovich M, Lazer S, et al. Listeria monocytogens. The role of transabdominal amniocentesis in febrile patients with preterm labor. Arch Gynecol Obstet 1992;252:109–12.
21. Vaginal misoprostol for cervical ripening and induction of labor. Cochrane Database Syst Rev 2003;(1):CD000941.
22. Roncaglia N, Arreghini A, Locatelli A, et al. Obstetric cholestasis: outcome with active management. Eur J Obstet Gynecol Reprod Biol 2002;100:167–70.
23. Campos GA, Guerra FA, Israel EJ. Effects of cholic acid infusion in fetal lambs. Acta Obstet Gynecol Scand 1986;65:23–6.
24. Ahanya SN, Lakshmanan J, Morgan BL, et al. Meconium passage in utero: mechanisms, consequences and management. Obstet Gynecol Surv 2005; 60:45–56.
25. Ahanya SN, Lakshmanan J, Babu J, et al. In utero betamethasone administration induces meconium passage in fetal rabbits. J Soc Gynecol Investig 2004;11: 102-A.
26. Lakshmanan J, Ross MG. Mechanisms of in utero meconium passage. J Perinatol 2008;28:S8–13.
27. Tybulewicz AT, Clegg SK, Fonfe GJ, et al. Preterm meconium staining of the amniotic fluid: associated findings risk of adverse clinical outcome. Arch Dis Child Fetal Neonatal Ed 2004;89:F328–30.
28. Macri CJ, Schrimmer DB, Leung A, et al. Prophylactic amnioinfusion improves outcome of pregnancy complicated by thick meconium and oligohydramnios. Am J Obstet Gynecol 1992;167:117–21.
29. Uhing MR, Bhat R, Philobos M, et al. Value of amnioinfusion in reducing meconium aspiration syndrome. Am J Perinatol 1993;10:43–5.
30. Usta IM, Mercer BM, Aswad NJ, et al. The impact of a policy of amnioinfusion for meconium stained fluid. Obstet Gynecol 1995;85:237–41.
31. Fraser WD, Hoffmeyr GJ, Lede R, et al. An international trial for the prevention of meconium aspiration syndrome. N Engl J Med 2005;353:909–17.
32. Maher JE, Wenstrom KD, Hauth JC, et al. Amniotic fluid embolism after saline amnioinfusion: two cases and review of literature. Obstet Gynecol 1994;83:851–4.
33. Dorairajan G, Sundara Raghavan S. Maternal death after intrapartum saline amnioinfusion-report of two cases. Br J Obstet Gynaecol 2005;112:1331–3.
34. ACOG committee opinion number 346 October 2006: amnioinfusion does not prevent meconium aspiration syndrome. Obstet Gynecol 2006;108:1053.
35. Hoffmeyr GJ, Xu H. Amnioinfusion for meconium stained liquor in labour. Cochrane Database Syst Rev 2010;(1):CD000014.
36. Mahomed K, Mulambo T, Woelk G, et al. Collaborative randomized amnioinfusion for meconium project (CRAMP): 2. zimbabwe. Br J Obstet Gynaecol 1998;105:309–13.
37. Rathore AM, Singh R, Ramji S, et al. Randomized trial of amnioinfusion during labour with meconium stained amniotic fluid. BJOG 2002;109:17–20.
38. The International Liaison Committee on Resuscitation. The International Liaison Committee on Resuscitation (ILCOR) consensus on science with treatment

recommendations for pediatric and neonatal patients: neonatal resuscitation. Pediatrics 2006;117:e978–88.

39. Committee on fetus and Newborn. Standards and recommendations for hospital care of newborn infants. 6th edition. Evanston (IL): American Academy of Pediatrics; 1977. p. 54–5.

40. Guidelines for perinatal care/American Academy of Pediatrics and the American College of Obstetricians and Gynecologists. In: Brann AW, Cefalo RC, editors. 1st edition. American Academy of Pediatrics/American College of Obstetricians; 1983. p. 69.

41. Guidelines for Perinatal Care/American College of Obstetricians and Gynecologists. In: Frigoletto FD, Little GA, editors. 3rd edition. American Academy of Pediatrics/American College of Obstetricians; 1988.

42. Guidelines for Perinatal Care/American Academy of Pediatrics/American College of Obstetrics and Gynecologists. In: Gilstrap L, Oh W, editors. 5th edition. American Academy of Pediatrics/American College of Obstetricians & Gynecologists; 2002. p. 190.

43. Text book of neonatal resuscitation. In: Kattwinkel J, editor. 5th edition. American Academy of Pediatrics/American Heart Association; 2006. p. 42–4.

44. Text book of neonatal resuscitation. In: Kattwinkel J, editor. 6th edition. American Academy of Pediatrics/American Heart Association; 2011. p. 176–8.

45. Gregory GA, Gooding CA, Phibbs RH, et al. Meconium aspiration in infants- a prospective study. J Pediatr 1974;85:848–52.

46. Carson BS, Losey RW, Bowes WA, et al. Combined obstetric and pediatric approach to prevent meconium aspiration syndrome. Am J Obstet Gynecol 1976;126:712–5.

47. Linder NJ, Aranda V, Tsur M, et al. Need for endotracheal intubation and suction in meconium stained neonates. J Pediatr 1988;112:613–5.

48. Vain NE, Szyld EG, Prudent LM, et al. Oropharyngeal and nasopharyngeal suctioning of meconium stained neonates before the delivery of their shoulders: multicenter randomized controlled trial. Lancet 2004;364:597–602.

49. Committee on Obstetric Practice, American College of Obstetricians and Gynecologists. ACOG Committee opinion. Management of delivery of a newborn with meconium stained amniotic fluid. Number 379. Obstet Gynecol 2007;110(3):739.

50. Falciglia HS. Failure to prevent meconium aspiration syndrome. Obstet Gynecol 1988;71:349–53.

51. Falciglia HS, Henderschott C, Potter P, et al. Does De Lee suction at the perineum prevent meconium aspiration syndrome? Am J Obstet Gynecol 1992;167:1243–9.

52. James LS. Resuscitation procedures in the delivery room. In: Abramson H, editor. Resuscitation of newborn infant. St Louis (MO): CV Mosby Co.; 1960. p. 141–61.

53. Burke-Strickland M, Edwards NB. Meconium aspiration in the newborn. Minn Med 1973;57:1031–5.

54. Ting P, Brady JP. Tracheal suction in meconium aspiration. Am J Obstet Gynecol 1975;122:767–71.

55. Cunningham AS, Lawson EE, Martin RJ, et al. Tracheal suction and meconium: a proposed standard of care. J Pediatr 1990;116:153–4.

56. Halliday HL, Sweet DG. Endotracheal intubation at birth for preventing morbidity and mortality in vigorous, meconium-stained infants born at term. Cochrane Database Syst Rev 2001;(1):CD000500:

57. Kabbur PM, Herson VC, Zaremba S, et al. Have the year 2000 Neonatal resuscitation program guidelines changed the delivery room management or outcome of meconium stained infants? J Perinatol 2005;25:694–7.

58. Aguilar AM, Satragno DS, Vain NE, et al. Delivery room practices in infants born through meconium stained amniotic fluid: a national survey. Arch Argent Pediatr 2010;108:31–9.
59. Michel F, Nicaise C, Camus T, et al. Management of newborns with meconium stained amniotic fluid: prospective evaluation of practice. Ann Fr Anesth Reanim 2010;29:605–9.
60. Block MF, Kallenberger DA, Kern JD, et al. In utero meconium aspiration by the baboon fetus. Obstet Gynecol 1981;57:37–40.
61. Liu WF, Harrington T. Delivery room risk factors for meconium aspiration syndrome. Am J Perinatol 2002;19:367–77.
62. Narchi H, Kulaylat N. Is gastric lavage needed in neonates with meconium stained amniotic fluid. Eur J Pediatr 1999;158:315–7.

Chest Compressions for Bradycardia or Asystole in Neonates

Vishal Kapadia, MD, Myra H. Wyckoff, MD*

KEYWORDS

- Neonatal • Newborn • Cardiac compressions • Cardiopulmonary resuscitation
- Asphyxia • Resuscitation

KEY POINTS

- When effective ventilation of the newborn fails to establish a heart rate of greater than 60 bpm, cardiac compressions to support the circulation should be initiated in hope of improving perfusion of the coronary arteries and brain. The 2-thumb method is the most effective and least fatiguing technique of newborn cardiac compressions and should be used to compress the lower third of the sternum about one third of the anterioposterior diameter of the chest.
- A compression to ventilation ratio of 3 compressions to 1 breath is recommended to provide adequate ventilation in the face of asphyxia, which is the most common cause of newborn cardiovascular collapse. Interruptions in compressions should be limited to not diminish the perfusion generated by the cardiac compressions.
- One hundred percent oxygen is recommended during cardiac compressions and can be reduced once an adequate heart rate and oxygen saturation is achieved.
- Newborn cardiac compression recommendations are primarily based on physiologic plausibility, data from older patients, and experimental neonatal simulation and animal models because limited clinical data are available.

Most newborns successfully transition from in utero to ex utero life without any help beyond provision of warmth, drying, and stimulation; however, approximately 10% need some form of respiratory support and on rare occasions even cardiovascular support via cardiac compressions and medications at the time of birth.[1] A lack of gas exchange with simultaneous hypoxia and carbon dioxide elevation leading to a mixed metabolic and respiratory acidosis, otherwise known as asphyxia, is the

---

Disclosure: The authors have nothing to disclose.
Division of Neonatal-Perinatal Medicine, Department of Pediatrics, The University of Texas Southwestern Medical Center at Dallas, 5323 Harry Hines Boulevard, Dallas, TX 75390-9063, USA
* Corresponding author.
E-mail address: myra.wyckoff@utsouthwestern.edu

most common reason that newborns fail to successfully transition. Such asphyxia can stem from either failure of placental gas exchange before delivery (eg, abruption, chorioamnionitis) or deficient pulmonary gas exchange after birth (eg, apnea, airway obstruction, hyaline membrane disease). Thus, babies who have an inadequate heart rate despite what would otherwise seem to be effective positive pressure ventilation, are likely to have significant hypoxemia and acidosis, which depresses myocardial function and promotes maximal vasodilation and very low diastolic blood pressures. When the heart is unable to contract strongly enough to pump blood to the lungs to pick up the oxygen delivered by effective positive pressure ventilation, chest compressions can mechanically pump the blood through the heart until the myocardium becomes sufficiently oxygenated to recover spontaneous function.[2]

Although optimized cardiac compressions only achieve approximately 30% of normal perfusion,[3,4] there is preferential perfusion of the heart and brain during cardiac compressions. Thus, myocardial and cerebral blood flow of greater than 50% of normal may well be achieved,[5–7] which is of significant help in recovering oxygen delivery to these vital organs. During cardiac compressions, coronary blood flow occurs exclusively during diastole, presumably because of increased intramyocardial resistance and increased right atrial pressure during chest compressions.[8,9] Therefore, coronary perfusion pressure is determined by the aortic diastolic blood pressure minus the right atrial diastolic blood pressure. Diastolic blood pressure during cardiac compressions is enhanced by repetitive, uninterrupted compressions as well as by a systemic vasoconstrictors such as epinephrine. Concerning morbidity and mortality for both preterm[10,11] and term infants[12,13] who receive cardiac compressions in the delivery room or during neonatal intensive care unit admission[14] suggest the need for continued optimization of neonatal cardiac compression methodology.

CURRENT GUIDELINES

The most recent International Liaison Committee on Resuscitation guidelines for neonatal resuscitation[1] and the American Academy of Pediatrics/American Heart Association Neonatal Resuscitation Program[2] continue to emphasize that it is absolutely critical that effective ventilation be established before initiation of chest compressions. Strategies including checking the mask seal, optimization of the position of the head in the "sniffing" open airway position, suctioning to remove obstructing secretions, opening the newborn's mouth to decrease resistance to ventilation, increasing the peak inspiratory pressure used for ventilation, and even insertion of an advanced airway via endotracheal intubation or laryngeal mask should all be done to enhance ventilation before initiation of cardiac compressions (**Box 1**). This

---

Box 1
MRSOPA: Critical steps to enhance ventilation before initiation of cardiac compression

Mask: Check the mask seal

Reposition: Put the neonate's head in the "sniffing" position

Suction: Remove obstructing secretions

Open the mouth: To decrease resistance to gas flow

Pressure: Increase the peak inflating pressure to see if it will help establish a functional residual capacity

Advanced airway: Intubate or place laryngeal mask device

is because ventilation is the most effective action in neonatal resuscitation and because chest compressions are likely to compete with effective ventilation, ventilation must be optimized first.

Neonatal guidelines continue to recommend cardiac compressions for a newborn infant with a heart rate less than 60 bpm despite at least 30 seconds of adequate ventilation.[1,2] The optimal time interval of ventilation before initiation of cardiac compressions is unknown. Logically, ensuring adequate ventilation in the hope of avoiding compressions altogether must be balanced against the risk of additional hypoxic/ischemic injury if circulation is not assisted in a timely enough manner.[15] A recent experiment in asphyxiated neonatal pigs found that, under conditions of asystole, there was no benefit or harm in delaying initiation of compressions for 1 minute compared with an initial 30 seconds of room air ventilation. When initiation of compressions was delayed for 90 seconds of initial ventilation, fewer animals were successfully resuscitated and those that were resuscitated required more doses of epinephrine to stabilize the heart rate.[16] Whether longer delays in initiation of compressions for bradycardia as opposed to asystole would have the same potential harm is unknown. There are no clinical data to offer guidance.[15] Once chest compressions are initiated, 100% oxygen should be used as the ventilation gas until the heart rate rises above 60 bpm and the pulse oximeter reading is available and reliable so that oxygen concentration can be adjusted to meet the target saturation range per minute of life.

The remainder of the guidelines for neonatal cardiac compressions focus on the optimal neonatal compression technique, thumb position on the sternum, depth of compression, chest compression to ventilation ratio, and the importance of limiting interruptions as much as possible when cardiac compressions are administered (**Box 2**). These recommendations are discussed in greater detail in the sections that follow.

OPTIMAL VENTILATION GAS DURING NEONATAL CARDIAC COMPRESSIONS

Although currently 100% oxygen is still recommended if cardiac compressions are administered, there is concern from animal studies[17,18] as well as some data from newborns with hypoxic-ischemic encephalopathy that hyperoxia during resuscitation and stabilization after asphyxia has the potential to exacerbate brain injury via oxygen free radical damage.[19,20] As soon as an adequate heart rate is restored and pulse oximetry data are available, the oxygen should be titrated to minimize exposure to

---

Box 2
Neonatal cardiac compression guidelines

- Optimize ventilation (including advanced airway placement) before starting cardiac compressions.
- Switch to 100% oxygen when starting compressions.
- Compress to a depth of one third of the anterioposterior diameter of the chest.
- Compress the lower one third of the sternum.
- Use the 2-thumb technique rather than the 2-finger technique.
- Deliver a 3:1 compression to ventilation ratio for asphyxial arrest.
- Coordinate compressions and ventilations.
- Avoid frequent interruptions in compressions.

hyperoxia. A neonatal pig study of asystole after asphyxia reported that cardiac compressions with room air seemed to be as safe and effective as the use of 100% oxygen.[21] However, in the absence of clinical data, the current recommendation is the most logical compromise to limit both hypoxia and hyperoxia.[15]

OPTIMAL DEPTH OF NEONATAL CARDIAC COMPRESSION

Compressions should be administered to a depth of approximately one third of the anterioposterior (AP) diameter of the chest.[1,2] Thus, the depth of compression is determined by the size of the baby. Computed tomography of the chest estimates of the chest dimensions of 20 babies less than 3 months of age suggested that a compression depth of one half of the AP diameter of the chest would likely cause internal structural damage but that one third of the AP diameter should compress the heart enough to pump blood out with less risk of internal damange.[22] Similar conclusions were drawn from computed tomography of the chest of a more recent, larger cohort of 52 neonates less than 28 days of age. Mathematical modeling of the chest dimensions suggest that the recommendations of one third of the AP chest compression depth should be more effective than one quarter of the AP diameter compression depth, and safer than one half of the AP compression depth.[23] A small case series of 6 cardiac surgery infants (2 weeks–7 months of age) who had arterial lines in place at the time cardiac compressions were administered concluded that although a compression depth of one half of the AP diameter of the chest resulted in higher systolic, mean and systemic perfusion pressures, this deeper depth did not improve diastolic blood pressure compared with one third of the AP diameter compressions.[24] Given that the primary goal of cardiac compressions is to perfuse the heart and brain while awaiting definitive restoration of a cardiac rhythm and that diastolic blood pressure is the critical determinant of coronary perfusion, compression depth should favor one third of the AP diameter of the chest rather than deeper compressions.[15] It has also been noted that a compression to relaxation ratio with a slightly shorter compression than relaxation phase offers theoretical advantages for blood flow in the very young infant.[25] The chest should be allowed fully recoil before the next compression to allow the heart to refill with blood.

OPTIMAL THUMB POSITION

Compressions should be centered over the lower third of the sternum rather than the mid sternum to compress most directly over the heart.[26–28] A radiographic study of 55 infants with an age range of 27 weeks' gestation to 13 months post-term demonstrated that the center of the heart was positioned under the lower third of the sternum in 48 cases. In 4 infants, the position was slightly more cephalad, but still below the lower half of the sternum.[27] For 10 children ages 1 month to 3 years who had cardiac compressions administered with an arterial line in place, higher mean arterial pressures were generated when compressions were administered over the lower one third compared with the mid sternum.[26] Positioning the thumbs centrally over the sternum is also critical to decrease risk of rib fracture, which can lead to a flail chest or pneumothorax (both of which inhibit effective ventilation) or dislocating the xiphoid process, which can lead to devastating liver laceration.[15,29]

OPTIMAL COMPRESSION METHOD

The 2-thumb method, in which the hands encircle the newborn chest while the thumbs compress the sternum, should be used for neonatal cardiac compressions.[1,2] The

2-finger technique, a less effective method, uses the tips of the middle and index finger to depress the sternum while the free hand is used to provide a firm support behind the baby's back.[9] Over short, 2-minute intervals, the 2-thumb method produced higher systolic but equivalent diastolic blood pressures compared with the 2-finger method in a newborn pig model of asystole after asphyxia.[30] When the 2 techniques were compared over longer, 10-minute compression intervals using a manikin with a customized artificial fixed volume "arterial system," the 2-thumb method produced higher mean, systolic, and diastolic blood pressures.[15,31] A recent neonatal manikin study demonstrated that over 2-minute intervals of cardiac compressions, the 2-thumb method resulted in improved depth and consistency of compressions, as well as less drift away from correct thumb/finger position.[32] The only available clinical data stems from 2 case reports involving just 3 newborns in which the 2-thumb technique generated improved arterial mean blood pressures and systolic blood pressure.[33,34]

The 2-finger technique is still mentioned as a possible technique to use if umbilical access is needed so that the compressors arms would be out of the way.[1,2] However, once the airway is secured (which should have been done to optimized ventilation before starting compressions), the compressor can move to the head of the bed to continue the 2-thumb technique while providing ample space for another person to access to the umbilical stump (**Fig. 1**). It is critical that compressions from the head of the bed should in no way conflict with adequate ventilation or establishment and maintenance of an advanced airway.

OPTIMAL COMPRESSION TO VENTILATION RATIO

The exact ratio of compressions to ventilations to best enhance both perfusion and ventilation during resuscitation from cardiopulmonary arrest owing to asphyxia

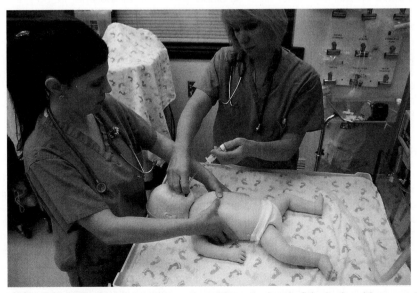

Fig. 1. The 2-thumb technique can be continued from the head of the bed position once the airway is secured, leaving ample access to the umbilical stump for emergent umbilical venous catheter placement. (*From* Wyckoff MH. Respiratory and cardiovascular support in the delivery room. In: Bancalari E, editor. The newborn lung. 2nd edition. Philadelphia: Elsevier; 2012. p. 257; with permission.)

remains unclear. However, it is clear from animal models of asphyxia that a combination of chest compressions and ventilations generates better outcomes and survival than resuscitation with ventilations or compressions alone,[35,36] especially during prolonged resuscitation.[25] This dependence on ventilation as a critical part of the resuscitation process after asphyxia is quite different from resuscitation after cardiac arrest (typically caused by ventricular fibrillation). Immediately after cardiac arrest, the aortic oxygen and carbon dioxide concentrations are close to the pre-arrest state. When compressions are initiated, the blood that will be flowing to the coronaries has adequate oxygenation and a reasonable pH. Thus, the problem in cardiac arrest is more the lack of flow and less the content of the blood. As such, resuscitation algorithms for cardiac arrest (eg, ventricular fibrillation) focus much more on providing continuous, uninterrupted compressions and less on ventilation. Adequate oxygenation and ventilation can continue without rescue breathing for several minutes because of chest compression-induced gas exchange and spontaneous gasping during compressions in victims of sudden cardiac arrest.[9] During asphyxia, blood continues to flow, although with ever-increasing hypoxemia, hypercarbia, and acidemia, until the heart runs out of adenosine triphosphate and stops beating. Thus, it is not surprising that ventilation to reverse the hypercarbia is critical.

A physiologic mathematical modeling study suggests that higher compression to ventilation ratios would result in underventilation of asphyxiated infants.[37] The model predicts that 3 to 5 compressions to 1 ventilation should be most efficient for newborns. A compression to ventilation ratio of 3:1 such that 90 compressions and 30 breaths are achieved per minute is currently recommended to optimize ventilation.[1,2] Recent studies have compared 3:1 to 9:3[38] and 3:1 to 15:2 compression to ventilation ratios[39] in piglet models of asystole owing to asphyxia. Although the 15:2 ratio provided more compressions per minute without compromising $Paco_2$ and generated statistically higher diastolic blood pressures, the diastolic blood pressure was still inadequate until epinephrine was given; thus, there was no difference in time to return of spontaneous circulation.[15,39] A recent simulation model study found that compression rates were least and ventilations breaths were highest for 3:1 as opposed to 15:2 ratios. Providers using a 3:1 versus 15:2 achieve a greater depth of compressions over 2-minute intervals. A more consistent compression depth over time was achieved with 3:1 as opposed to other ratios.[40] Thus, there is no convincing evidence from clinical or experimental studies to justify a change from the current compression to ventilation ratio of 3:1.

WHY AVOID INTERRUPTIONS IN COMPRESSIONS?

There is persuasive evidence from ventricular fibrillation arrest models that frequent or prolonged interruption of chest compressions worsens coronary perfusion pressure,[7,41] increases mortality,[41] and worsens neurologic function in survivors.[42,43] A recent neonatal study suggests that it may take up to 17 seconds for some providers to assess the heart rate during resuscitation.[44] Every time compressions are paused, the diastolic blood pressure (and thus the coronary perfusion pressure) that was being generated via repetitive compressions is transiently diminished and has to be built back up again when compressions are reinitiated. Because of this, the most recent neonatal resuscitation guidelines increased the interval of uninterrupted compressions from 30 seconds to 45 to 60 seconds before pausing for assessment of return of an adequate heart rate during a 6-second auscultation pause.[1,2]

End-tidal CO_2 capnography during cardiac compressions may provide a continuous, noninvasive way to eliminate frequent pauses to auscultate for heart rate. During asystole, changes in end-tidal CO_2 primarily reflect changes in cardiac output.[45] This is because the positive pressure ventilation before intubation may have successfully removed most of the CO_2 present in the lung. With such limited pulmonary blood flow owing to the failing pump action of the heart, little subsequent CO_2 is delivered to the lungs and the $ETCO_2$ detector has negligible CO_2 to detect even if the airway is in the correct position.[45] A piglet model of asphyxia-induced asystole demonstrated that, after positive pressure ventilation, end-tidal CO_2 falls to near zero with loss of pulmonary blood flow and then increases slightly with initiation of cardiac compressions, reflecting blood being pumped through the lungs by effective cardiac compressions. Return of spontaneous circulation correlates with a sudden increase in end-tidal CO_2 as the reestablished perfusion brings CO_2 rich blood back to the lungs. In that model, an end-tidal CO_2 of greater than 14 mm Hg correlated well with return of an audible heart rate greater than 60 bpm.[46] Clinical correlates are needed.[15]

IS COORDINATION OF COMPRESSIONS AND VENTILATIONS IMPORTANT?

Current neonatal resuscitation guidelines continue to recommend that compressions and ventilations be coordinated (synchronized) to avoid simultaneous delivery.[1,2] Thus, the chest compressions and ventilations are given in cycles alternating between the 2 in the specific ratio of 3 compressions to 1 breath. Simultaneous chest compressions and ventilations that are delivered at a specific rate per minute have been examined in neonatal cardiac arrest models.[47–49] In these studies, simultaneous compressions compared with 5:1 synchronized cardiac compressions did not enhance cerebral or myocardial perfusion and resulted in higher arterial P_{CO_2} values, raising concern that this technique might limit ventilation; however, it should be noted that both groups were significantly over-ventilated despite this. These studies have limited applicability because they used a cardiac arrest model, very high peak inspiratory pressures for ventilations, and compressions rate of 60 bpm. Asynchronous chest compressions and ventilations are delivered independently of one another; each has its own target rate per minute. Asynchronous compression and ventilation ratios are recommended during advanced cardiac life support in adults and older children once a secure airway such as an endotracheal tube or laryngeal mask is established. There are no clinical or experimental studies of asynchronus compressions in neonates.

SUMMARY

Fortunately, when effective ventilation is provided, the need for cardiac compressions in newborns is rare; however, the infrequency of cardiac compression use has made it difficult to complete rigorous clinical studies to determine how to best optimize cardiac compressions. The need for better science to inform the cardiac compression recommendations is paramount.

REFERENCES

1. Kattwinkel J, Perlman JM, Aziz K, et al. Part 15: neonatal resuscitation: 2010 American Heart Association Guidelines for Cardiopulmonary Resuscitation and Emergency Cardiovascular Care. Circulation 2010;122:S909–19.
2. Kattwinkel J, editor. Textbook of neonatal resuscitation. Elk Grove (IL): American Academy of Pediatrics AHA; 2011.
3. Delguercio LR, Coomaraswamy RP, State D. Cardiac output and other hemodynamic variables during external cardiac massage in man. N Engl J Med 1963; 269:1398–404.

4. Voorhees WD, Babbs CF, Tacker WA Jr. Regional blood flow during cardiopulmonary resuscitation in dogs. Crit Care Med 1980;8:134–6.

5. Berg RA, Kern KB, Hilwig RW, et al. Assisted ventilation does not improve outcome in a porcine model of single-rescuer bystander cardiopulmonary resuscitation. Circulation 1997;95:1635–41.

6. Berkowitz ID, Gervais H, Schleien CL, et al. Epinephrine dosage effects on cerebral and myocardial blood flow in an infant swine model of cardiopulmonary resuscitation. Anesthesiology 1991;75:1041–50.

7. Berg RA, Sanders AB, Kern KB, et al. Adverse hemodynamic effects of interrupting chest compressions for rescue breathing during cardiopulmonary resuscitation for ventricular fibrillation cardiac arrest. Circulation 2001;104:2465–70.

8. Kern KB, Hilwig R, Ewy GA. Retrograde coronary blood flow during cardiopulmonary resuscitation in swine: intracoronary Doppler evaluation. Am Heart J 1994; 128:490–9.

9. Wyckoff MH, Berg RA. Optimizing chest compressions during delivery-room resuscitation. Semin Fetal Neonatal Med 2008;13:410–5.

10. Wyckoff MH, Salhab WA, Heyne RJ, et al. Outcome of extremely low birth weight infants who received delivery room cardiopulmonary resuscitation. J Pediatr 2012;160:239–44.e2.

11. Shah PS. Extensive cardiopulmonary resuscitation for VLBW and ELBW infants: a systematic review and meta-analyses. J Perinatol 2009;29:655–61.

12. Barber CA, Wyckoff MH. Use and efficacy of endotracheal versus intravenous epinephrine during neonatal cardiopulmonary resuscitation in the delivery room. Pediatrics 2006;118:1028–34.

13. Harrington DJ, Redman CW, Moulden M, et al. The long-term outcome in surviving infants with Apgar zero at 10 minutes: a systematic review of the literature and hospital-based cohort. Am J Obstet Gynecol 2007;196:463.e1–5.

14. Chamnanvanakij S, Perlman JM. Outcome following cardiopulmonary resuscitation in the neonate requiring ventilatory assistance. Resuscitation 2000;45: 173–80.

15. Wyckoff MH. Respiratory and cardiovascular support in the delivery room. In: Bancalari E, editor. The newborn lung. 2nd edition. Philadelphia: Elsevier; 2012. p. 247–62.

16. Dannevig I, Solevag AL, Wyckoff M, et al. Delayed onset of cardiac compressions in cardiopulmonary resuscitation of newborn pigs with asphyctic cardiac arrest. Neonatology 2011;99:153–62.

17. Koch JD, Miles DK, Gilley JA, et al. Brief exposure to hyperoxia depletes the glial progenitor pool and impairs functional recovery after hypoxic-ischemic brain injury. J Cereb Blood Flow Metab 2008;28:1294–306.

18. Solberg R, Andresen JH, Escrig R, et al. Resuscitation of hypoxic newborn piglets with oxygen induces a dose-dependent increase in markers of oxidation. Pediatr Res 2007;62:559–63.

19. Sabir H, Jary S, Tooley J, et al. Increased inspired oxygen in the first hours of life is associated with adverse outcome in newborns treated for perinatal asphyxia with therapeutic hypothermia. J Pediatr 2012;161(3):409–16.

20. Aydemir O, Akar M, Uras N, et al. Total antioxidant capacity and total oxidant status in perinatal asphyxia in relation to neurological outcome. Neuropediatrics 2011;42:222–6.

21. Solevag AL, Dannevig I, Nakstad B, et al. Resuscitation of severely asphyctic newborn pigs with cardiac arrest by using 21% or 100% oxygen. Neonatology 2010;98:64–72.

22. Braga MS, Dominguez TE, Pollock AN, et al. Estimation of optimal CPR chest compression depth in children by using computer tomography. Pediatrics 2009;124:e69–74.
23. Meyer A, Nadkarni V, Pollock A, et al. Evaluation of the Neonatal Resuscitation Program's recommended chest compression depth using computerized tomography imaging. Resuscitation 2010;81:544–8.
24. Maher KO, Berg RA, Lindsey CW, et al. Depth of sternal compression and intra-arterial blood pressure during CPR in infants following cardiac surgery. Resuscitation 2009;80:662–4.
25. Dean JM, Koehler RC, Schleien CL, et al. Age-related effects of compression rate and duration in cardiopulmonary resuscitation. J Appl Physiol 1990;68: 554–60.
26. Orlowski JP. Optimum position for external cardiac compression in infants and young children. Ann Emerg Med 1986;15:667–73.
27. Phillips GW, Zideman DA. Relation of infant heart to sternum: its significance in cardiopulmonary resuscitation. Lancet 1986;1:1024–5.
28. Finholt DA, Kettrick RG, Wagner HR, et al. The heart is under the lower third of the sternum. Implications for external cardiac massage. Am J Dis Child 1986;140: 646–9.
29. Clements F, McGowan J. Finger position for chest compressions in cardiac arrest in infants. Resuscitation 2000;44:43–6.
30. Houri PK, Frank LR, Menegazzi JJ, et al. A randomized, controlled trial of two-thumb vs two-finger chest compression in a swine infant model of cardiac arrest [see comment]. Prehosp Emerg Care 1997;1:65–7.
31. Dorfsman ML, Menegazzi JJ, Wadas RJ, et al. Two-thumb vs. two-finger chest compression in an infant model of prolonged cardiopulmonary resuscitation. Acad Emerg Med 2000;7:1077–82.
32. Christman C, Hemway RJ, Wyckoff MH, et al. The two-thumb is superior to the two-finger method for administering chest compressions in a manikin model of neonatal resuscitation. Arch Dis Child Fetal Neonatal Ed 2011;96:F99–101.
33. David R. Closed chest cardiac massage in the newborn infant. Pediatrics 1988; 81:552–4.
34. Todres ID, Rogers MC. Methods of external cardiac massage in the newborn infant. J Pediatr 1975;86:781–2.
35. Berg RA, Hilwig RW, Kern KB, et al. Simulated mouth-to-mouth ventilation and chest compressions (bystander cardiopulmonary resuscitation) improves outcome in a swine model of prehospital pediatric asphyxial cardiac arrest. Crit Care Med 1999;27:1893–9.
36. Berg RA, Hilwig RW, Kern KB, et al. "Bystander" chest compressions and assisted ventilation independently improve outcome from piglet asphyxial pulseless "cardiac arrest". Circulation 2000;101:1743–8.
37. Babbs CF, Nadkarni V. Optimizing chest compression to rescue ventilation ratios during one-rescuer CPR by professionals and lay persons: children are not just little adults. Resuscitation 2004;61:173–81.
38. Solevag AL, Dannevig I, Wyckoff M, et al. Extended series of cardiac compressions during CPR in a swine model of perinatal asphyxia. Resuscitation 2010; 81:1571–6.
39. Solevag AL, Dannevig I, Wyckoff M, et al. Return of spontaneous circulation with a compression:ventilation ratio of 15:2 versus 3:1 in newborn pigs with cardiac arrest due to asphyxia. Arch Dis Child Fetal Neonatal Ed 2011;96(6): F417–21.

40. Hemway RJ, Christman C, Perlman J. The 3:1 is superior to a 15:2 ratio in a newborn manikin model in terms of quality of chest compressions and number of ventilations. Arch Dis Child Fetal Neonatal Ed 2012. [Epub ahead of print].

41. Kern KB, Hilwig RW, Berg RA, et al. Importance of continuous chest compressions during cardiopulmonary resuscitation: improved outcome during a simulated single lay-rescuer scenario. Circulation 2002;105:645–9.

42. Sanders AB, Kern KB, Berg RA, et al. Survival and neurologic outcome after cardiopulmonary resuscitation with four different chest compression-ventilation ratios. Ann Emerg Med 2002;40:553–62.

43. Ewy GA, Zuercher M, Hilwig RW, et al. Improved neurological outcome with continuous chest compressions compared with 30:2 compressions-to-ventilations cardiopulmonary resuscitation in a realistic swine model of out-of-hospital cardiac arrest. Circulation 2007;116:2525–30.

44. Voogdt KG, Morrison AC, Wood FE, et al. A randomised, simulated study assessing auscultation of heart rate at birth. Resuscitation 2010;81:1000–3.

45. Wyckoff MH. Neonatal cardiopulmonary resuscitation: critical hemodynamics. NeoReviews 2010;11:e123–9.

46. Chalak LF, Barber CA, Hynan L, et al. End-tidal CO_2 detection of an audible heart rate during neonatal cardiopulmonary resuscitation after asystole in asphyxiated piglets. Pediatr Res 2011;69:401–5.

47. Turner I, Turner S. Optimum cardiopulmonary resuscitation for basic and advanced life support: a simulation study. Resuscitation 2004;62:209–17.

48. Berkowitz ID, Chantarojanasiri T, Koehler RC, et al. Blood flow during cardiopulmonary resuscitation with simultaneous compression and ventilation in infant pigs. Pediatr Res 1989;26:558–64.

49. Hou SH, Lue HC, Chu SH. Comparison of conventional and simultaneous compression-ventilation cardiopulmonary resuscitation in piglets. Jpn Circ J 1994;58:426–32.

Medications in Neonatal Resuscitation

Epinephrine and the Search for Better Alternative Strategies

Gary M. Weiner, MD[a,b,*], Susan Niermeyer, MD, MPH[c]

KEYWORDS

- Epinephrine • Adrenaline • Resuscitation • Newborn • Asphyxia neonatorum
- Vasopressin • Volume

KEY POINTS

- Epinephrine remains the primary vasopressor for use in neonatal resuscitation in response to asystole or prolonged bradycardia not resolving with adequate ventilation and chest compressions. Epinephrine increases coronary perfusion pressure primarily through peripheral vasoconstriction.

- Current neonatal resuscitation guidelines recommend prompt intravenous (IV) administration of epinephrine in a dose of 0.01 mg/kg to 0.03 mg/kg, because endotracheal administration results in unpredictable absorption and may require higher doses than the IV route. High-dose epinephrine poses additional risks to premature and asphyxiated newborn infants and does not result in better long-term survival than conventional doses.

- Intraosseous (IO) administration provides acceptable vascular access and may be a more rapid route than umbilical venous catheter (UVC) for pediatric professionals who do not have extensive neonatal experience.

- Vasopressin has been considered an alternative to epinephrine in adults, but there is insufficient evidence to recommend its use in newborn infants. Alternative vasopressors may have a role in postresuscitation stabilization.

- Future research will focus on examination of the best sequence for epinephrine administration and chest compressions and better understanding of the pathologies underlying neonatal cardiac arrest and profound bradycardia at birth. Meanwhile, close attention to preparation for delivery, emphasizing the basics of adequate ventilation and euvolemia, helps prevent the need for extensive cardiopulmonary resuscitation (CPR).

---

[a] Department of Pediatrics, St. Joseph Mercy Hospital, 5301 East Huron River Drive, Ann Arbor, MI 48106, USA; [b] Wayne State University School of Medicine, 3901 Beaubien Boulevard, Detroit, MI 48201-2196, USA; [c] Section of Neonatology, Children's Hospital Colorado, University of Colorado School of Medicine, 13121 East 19th Avenue, Mail Stop 8402, Aurora, CO 80045, USA
* Corresponding author. Department of Pediatrics, St. Joseph Mercy Hospital, 5301 East Huron River Drive, Ann Arbor, MI 48106.
E-mail address: weinerg@trinity-health.org

Clin Perinatol 39 (2012) 843–855
http://dx.doi.org/10.1016/j.clp.2012.09.005
0095-5108/12/$ – see front matter © 2012 Elsevier Inc. All rights reserved.

CASE

A primiparous woman arrives at the hospital at 37 weeks' gestation with decreased fetal movement. In triage, the monitor shows repeated late decelerations and prolonged fetal bradycardia prompts an emergent cesarean delivery. At the time of birth, the baby appears limp and apneic with a heart rate of 40 beats/minute. The health provider positions and clears the airway and stimulates and dries the baby, but she does not breathe and her heart rate remains 40 beats/minute. The health provider begins positive pressure ventilation, applies a saturation monitor to her right hand, and calls for additional help. Despite appropriate corrective steps to improve ventilation, endotracheal intubation, and coordinated chest compressions, she remains severely bradycardic. The International Liaison Committee on Resuscitation guidelines[1] and Neonatal Resuscitation Program[2] recommend epinephrine administration when positive pressure ventilation and coordinated chest compressions have not achieved a heart rate above 60 beats/minute.

1. Why would epinephrine be effective when assisted ventilation and chest compressions have failed to restore normal circulation?
2. What is the optimal route of epinephrine administration?
3. What is the optimal dose of epinephrine?
4. Should arginine vasopressin be considered instead of or in addition to epinephrine?

EPINEPHRINE

Epinephrine (adrenaline) is an endogenously produced catecholamine that stimulates all adrenergic receptors. In isolation, α receptor and β receptor stimulation may appear to cause opposing effects (**Table 1**). Ultimately, the balance between the density of each receptor type at the target tissue, the receptor's binding affinity for epinephrine, and other local factors determine the physiologic effects in vivo. Epinephrine increases heart rate, conduction velocity, and contractility by stimulating β_1 and β_2 receptors on neonatal cardiac myocytes, the sinoatrial (SA) node, and the atrioventricular (AV) node.[3–5] Its effect on peripheral vascular resistance, cardiac output, and coronary blood flow depends on the balance between β_2 receptor–stimulated coronary artery dilation and α_1 receptor–mediated and α_2 receptor–mediated vasoconstriction.

Table 1
Hemodynamic effects of neonatal adrenergic receptors

Receptor	Location	Effect
α_1	Vascular smooth muscle Coronary arteries	• Vasoconstriction
α_2	Central nervous system Presynaptic neurons Coronary arteries	• Decreased norepinephrine release • Decreased blood pressure • Vasoconstriction
β_1	SA and AV nodes Heart muscle	• Increased heart rate (chronotropy) • Increase conduction velocity (dromotropy) • Increase contractility (inotropy) • Increase myocyte relaxation (lusitropy)
β_2	Vascular smooth muscle Heart muscle	• Vasodilation • Biphasic effect on heart rate (initial increase, then decrease) • Increase contractility

WHAT DOES EPINEPHRINE DO DURING CARDIOVASCULAR COLLAPSE?
Which is More Important, Alpha or Beta Stimulation?

Epinephrine was first recommended as an agent to restore spontaneous circulation during cardiac arrest more than 100 years ago and has been widely recommended as a component of CPR guidelines in adults, children, and neonates.[6,7] Initially, epinephrine was believed effective because it increased cardiac chronotropy and inotropy through β-adrenergic stimulation. In a series of classic experiments, investigators studied the relative contribution of α-mediated and β-mediated effects by infusing selective agonists or pretreating with selective adrenergic blockade before infusing epinephrine.[8,9] Animals receiving a pure β-agonist (isoproteronol), or pretreated with an α-adrenergic blockade (phenoxybenzamine), failed to re-establish spontaneous circulation. In contrast, those who received a pure α-agonist (methoxamine), or pretreatment with β-adrenergic blockade (propranolol), were successfully resuscitated. These studies demonstrated that α-adrenergic stimulation was necessary for successful resuscitation. α-Mediated peripheral vasoconstriction increases the aortic to right atrial pressure gradient and coronary perfusion pressure.[10] When myocardial oxygen demand increases, β_2-mediated coronary vasodilation may contribute to the increased coronary perfusion.[4,11]

Epinephrine administration during asphyxia-mediated arrest

- Increases systemic vascular resistance
- Increases coronary artery perfusion pressure
- Improves blood flow to the myocardium and restores depleted ATP

Critical Coronary Perfusion Pressure

Epinephrine's crucial role in improving coronary perfusion pressure has been demonstrated in a neonatal swine model of asphyxia-induced asystole. Barber and colleagues[12] showed that successful resuscitation only occurred among animals that were able to achieve a right atrial diastolic blood pressure (DBP) of approximately 20 mm Hg. Once the cardiac rhythm had deteriorated to asystole, no subject reached the threshold DBP or was resuscitated with only positive-pressure ventilation. The combination of ventilation with coordinated compressions (3:1 ratio) rarely achieved the critical DBP or return of spontaneous circulation (ROSC). When IV epinephrine was administered in addition to ventilation and compressions, most animals reached the threshold DBP and rapidly achieved ROSC. This study is important because, if confirmed, it would lead to a significant change in the resuscitation algorithm with epinephrine administration before chest compressions.

- Among neonates with asystole, ventilation and compressions alone may not achieve the coronary perfusion pressure required for return of spontaneous circulation.

NEONATAL EPINEPHRINE ADMINISTRATION
Should Epinephrine Be Given Through an Endotracheal Tube During Neonatal Resuscitation?

All previous editions of the *Neonatal Resuscitation Textbook* recommended the endotracheal route because it was assumed that endotracheal intubation could be performed more quickly than umbilical vein catheterization. The most recent edition recommends IV administration because of concerns that endotracheal epinephrine may not be well absorbed and circulated during resuscitation.[13] There are currently no randomized controlled trials in human neonates comparing IV with endotracheal epinephrine.

Multiple case reports and case series have described successful neonatal resuscitation with endotracheal epinephrine since the 1980s[14–22]; however, questions have been raised about the quality of resuscitative efforts in these reports prior to epinephrine administration.[23–26] A recent case series among newborns in the delivery room using contemporary resuscitation standards is the best available evidence evaluating the IV and endotracheal routes.[14] In this series (n = 44), ROSC occurred in 32% (14/44) of those receiving standard dose endotracheal epinephrine (0.01 mg/kg). Among the 30 neonates who did not respond to endotracheal epinephrine, 23 (77%) subsequently had ROSC after receiving the same dose IV. Although this study indicates that endotracheal epinephrine may be effective, it suggests that it may be less effective than the same dose given IV.

- The IV route should be used for epinephrine administration as soon as access is established.
- It is reasonable to administer endotracheal epinephrine if IV access is not available.

What Is the Opimal Dose if Epinephrine Is Given by the Endotracheal Route?

The optimal dose of endotracheal epinephrine has not been established. Individual human case reports have used a wide range of epinephrine doses (0.003 mg/kg to 0.25 mg/kg). In animal models, an endotracheal dose 5 to 10 times the standard IV dose is required (0.05–0.1 mg/kg) to increase the blood epinephrine concentration[27–29] and achieve return of circulation from hypoxic arrest.[27] In a neonatal pig model of hypoxic cardiac arrest, Barber and Wyckoff[30] randomized animals to low-dose endotracheal epinephrine (0.03 mg/kg), high-dose endotracheal epinephrine (0.07 mg/kg), and standard IV epinephrine (0.01 mg/kg). The likelihood of achieving ROSC was similar between groups (ROSC 76% low-dose endotracheal tube, 89% high-dose endotracheal tube, and 91% IV) with a trend favoring IV and high-dose endotracheal administration over the low-dose endotracheal. Moreover, the low-dose endotracheal group had decreased survival 30 minutes after resuscitation (59%). If endotracheal epinephrine is given, a higher dose (0.05–0.1 mg/kg) may be needed.

Should Neonates Receive Epinephrine Through an Intraosseous Needle?

IO needles have been used for adults and children to rapidly secure access to the intravascular space since the 1940s and several reports describe infusion of emergency medications during neonatal resuscitations.[31] Two trials during simulated neonatal resuscitations have compared the placement of an IO needle with an UVC.[32,33] The studies showed that inexperienced medical students[32] and pediatric health care providers[33] could place an IO needle quickly and reliably with limited training. In each study, IO needle placement was significantly faster than UVC placement. Inexperienced providers and pediatric residents perceived the IO procedure as less difficult than UVC placement whereas neonatal specialists preferred UVC placement. This difference most likely reflects the comfort level achieved by neonatal specialists after placing many UVCs in nonemergent settings. Given the limited opportunities that many providers have to practice UVC placement, IO needle placement may be the preferred method for non-neonatal specialists and in emergency room settings.

- IO infusion is a quick and reliable method for obtaining access to the intravascular space.
- Experience with clinical outcomes of neonatal IO access is limited.
- Among non-neonatal specialists, IO access may be preferred to UVC.

Should High-Dose Intravenous Epinephrine Be Used if a Baby Does Not Improve with the Standard Dose?

The beneficial effect of epinephrine during CPR is related to increased coronary perfusion, and studies in the 1980s and 1990s indicated that higher doses of epinephrine (0.05–0.2 mg/kg) increased coronary perfusion more than standard doses.[34,35] Two case series at that time suggested that hospitalized premature newborns[36] and children[37] who had not responded to standard IV epinephrine (0.01 mg/kg) rapidly improved after high-dose (0.2 mg/kg) epinephrine. Subsequently, 2 randomized controlled trials,[38,39] including children less than 1 year of age and 3 pediatric case series,[40–42] found no statistically significant benefit from epinephrine doses above 0.03 mg/kg. In one of the randomized trials,[38] there was increased mortality among children who received high-dose epinephrine if their cardiac arrest was precipitated by asphyxia.

Animal models suggest that high-dose epinephrine may be harmful in newborns. Using a hypoxia-induced bradycardia model in neonatal lambs, Burchfield and colleagues[43] found that high-dose IV epinephrine (0.1 mg/kg) interfered with stroke volume and cardiac output. A similar animal study, using a hypoxic arrest model, found a nonstatistically significant trend favoring high-dose epinephrine (0.2 mg/kg) for ROSC; however, these animals had a higher risk for death during the immediate postresuscitation period.[44] Additional animal studies have shown that high doses may cause prolonged hypertension, tachycardia, and decreased cerebral cortical blood flow.[45,46] These adverse effects are particularly concerning among premature newborns who are already at increased risk for intracranial hemorrhage.[47]

- IV epinephrine greater than 0.03 mg/kg/dose is not recommended.
- High-dose IV epinephrine (greater than 0.05 mg/kg/dose) may cause hypertension, tachycardia, decreased cardiac output, decreased cerebral blood flow, and increased mortality.

KNOWLEDGE GAPS REGARDING EPINEPHRINE USE

Neonatal case reports, observational studies, and extrapolations from adult and animal studies comprise the evidence base for most of the current epinephrine recommendations (**Table 2**). Drawing conclusions from these studies is complicated because adrenergic receptors respond differently across mammalian species, develop at different times during gestation, and respond to epinephrine stimulation differently than adult receptors. In addition, models using intact circulation or ventricular fibrillation may not adequately replicate the hypoxic-hypercarbic cardiovascular compromise experienced by newborns. Unfortunately, the practical difficulties of organizing a randomized controlled trial for a treatment used unpredictably, emergently, and infrequently among newborns have made it difficult to effectively study epinephrine during neonatal resuscitation.

ALTERNATIVES TO EPINEPHRINE IN CARDIOPULMONARY RESUSCITATION

Despite its status as the medication most consistently included in guidelines for advanced neonatal resuscitation through the past several decades, epinephrine has limitations in its effectiveness and disadvantages that have prompted continued investigation of alternative drugs. Epinephrine increases the oxygen demands of the myocardium through its β-adrenergic effect, potentially leading to damage when hypoxia persists or myocardial perfusion and oxygen delivery are insufficient.[48] Epinephrine use, especially with repeated doses, can lead to marked hypertension,

Table 2
Epinephrine for neonatal resuscitation

Indication	Heart rate remains less than 60/min despite 30 s of effective ventilation and another 45–60 s of effective ventilation with coordinated chest compressions
Concentration	1: 10,000 = 0.1 mg/mL
Route	IV (UVC) preferred IO (alternative) Endotracheal (option while obtaining vascular access)
Preparation and labeling	1 mL syringe labeled, *IV use* OR 3–5 mL syringe labeled, *endotracheal tube use ONLY*
Dose IV or IO	0.01–0.03 mg/kg = 0.1–0.3 mL/kg Administer rapidly Flush with 0.5–1 mL normal saline
Dose endotracheal	0.05–0.1 mg/kg = 0.5–1 mL/kg Followed by positive pressure breaths

Data from Wyllie J, Perlman JM, Kattwinkel J, et al. Part 11: neonatal resuscitation: 2010 international consensus on cardiopulmonary resuscitation and emergency cardiovascular care science with treatment recommendations. Resuscitation 2010;81(Suppl 1):e260–87; and Kattwinkel J, Perlman JM, Aziz K, et al. Neonatal resuscitation: 2010 American heart association guidelines for cardiopulmonary resuscitation and emergency cardiovascular care. Pediatrics 2010;126(5):e1400–13.

which has been associated with the complication of intracranial hemorrhage in premature infants.[47]

Theoretic Advantages of Vasopressin

The ideal vasopressor for CPR should increase aortic diastolic and coronary perfusion pressure and enhance coronary and cerebral blood flow and oxygen delivery without increasing cellular oxygen demand. Vasopressin offers theoretic advantages over epinephrine because it does not significantly increase myocardial oxygen demand and its receptors are relatively unaffected by acidosis.[48] Vasopressin, also known as arginine vasopression (to distinguish it from synthetic analogs) or antidiuretic hormone, is synthesized in the hypothalamus and released into the systemic circulation from the posterior lobe of the pituitary; receptors are located on a variety of cells, including vascular smooth muscle (V1), where stimulation produces vasoconstriction (**Table 3**). Vasopressin, unlike epinephrine, is not a direct myocardial stimulant. Vasopressin causes marked vasoconstriction in skin, skeletal muscle, and mesenteric blood vessels, but at low concentrations some studies suggest vasodilatory effects

Table 3
Vasopressin receptor subtypes and mediated effects

Receptor Subtype	Location of Receptor	Effect of Receptor Stimulation
V1	Liver, vascular smooth muscle cells, platelets, central nervous system, most peripheral tissue	Vasoconstriction
V2	Kidney collecting duct cells	Osmoregulation, water retention
V3	Central nervous system (adenohypophysis)	Corticotropin (ACTH) secretion

in coronary, pulmonary, and cerebral arteries.[49] Additional effects of vasopressin include osmoregulation and water retention through action on V2 receptors in the kidney and corticotropin secretion modulated by V3 receptors within the adenohypophysis.[49] Corticotropin secretion stimulated by vasopressin may represent an important collateral effect, because increased plasma cortisol concentrations during CPR correlate with improved outcome in adults.[50]

Recent studies using a chemiluminescence assay for the stable precursor fragment C-terminal provasopressin in umbilical venous cord blood of infants with gestational ages 23 to 42 weeks showed concentrations 10-fold higher than normal adult levels in term infants and 70-fold higher in extremely preterm infants.[51] Elevations in cord plasma arginine vasopressin (mean 180 pg/mL; 95% CI, 92–350) were reported in a series of acutely asphyxiated infants with 5-minute Apgar score less than or equal to 6 and/or umbilical arterial pH less than or equal to 7.05. In one clinical series, absence of a prompt vasopressin response in critically ill neonates predicted an unfavorable clinical course.[52]

Vasopressin Use in Adult Cardiac Arrest

Vasopressin has been extensively studied in adult CPR. Previous Advanced Cardiovascular Life Support (ACLS) guidelines recommended using epinephrine or vasopressin every 5 minutes in adult cardiac arrest.[53] Three randomized controlled trials,[54–56] however, and 1 meta-analysis[57] showed no difference in overall outcomes (ROSC, survival to discharge, or neurologic outcome) for vasopressin compared with epinephrine as a first-line vasopressor during cardiac arrest. Two additional randomized controlled trials compared epinephrine in combination with vasopressin to epinephrine alone in cardiac arrest and showed no difference in ROSC, survival to discharge, or neurologic outcome.[58,59] The most recent ACLS (2010) guidelines state, "Although there is evidence that vasopressors may improve ROSC and short-term survival, there is insufficient evidence to suggest that vasopressors improve survival to discharge and neurologic outcome….Given the observed benefit in short-term outcomes, the use of epinephrine or vasopressin may be considered in adult cardiac arrest."[60]

Vasopressin in Pediatric Cardiac Arrest

Data on vasopressin in pediatric cardiac arrest are limited. Small case series reported ROSC with vasopressin or terlipressin (a synthetic vasopressin analogue) administration when standard therapy had failed[61–63]; however, a database analysis of vasopressin use for in-hospital pediatric cardiac arrest showed lower ROSC and a trend toward decreased survival at 24 hours and at discharge.[64] Pediatric Advanced Life Support guidelines state, "There is insufficient evidence for or against the administration of vasopressin or its long-acting analogue, terlipressin, in pediatric cardiac arrest."[65]

Vasopressors in Postresuscitation Stabilization

Additional studies have investigated the role of vasopressor agents for postresuscitation stabilization. Vasopressin improved hemodynamic measures (mean arterial blood pressure, requirement for other pressors, and pulmonary capillary wedge pressure) in greater than 90% of adult patients with cardiovascular failure unresponsive to standard measures after cardiac arrest.[66] In an ischemic arrest model, the combination of milrinone and vasopressin improved cardiac index at 30 minutes when compared with epinephrine or vasopressin alone or in combination.[67] Milrinone, epinephrine, and dobutamine improved cardiac output and systemic oxygen delivery in a model

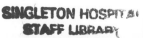

of asphyxiated newborn piglets,[68] and milrinone increased intestinal blood flow by decreasing superior mesenteric artery vascular resistance.[69]

- Vasopressin offers theoretic advantages as a vasopressor therapy for cardiac arrest.
- Vasopressin is an alternative to epinephrine for adult cardiac arrest, but there is no evidence to support its use in pediatric or neonatal CPR.
- Alternative vasopressors may have usefulness in postresuscitation stabilization of neonates.

EXPLORING NONPHARMACOLOGIC ALTERNATIVES

Going forward, the most productive alternative approach to the problem of prolonged bradycardia and/or asystole in the newly born infant may be that of prevention and therapy targeted to underlying etiology of arrest (**Table 4**). Timely delivery in the setting of fetal compromise—obstructed labor, placental insufficiency, intrauterine infection, uterine rupture, and hemorrhagic complications of pregnancy/labor—may reduce the need for CPR at delivery, acknowledging the demonstrated risk factors of antepartum hemorrhage, lack of antenatal steroids, breech position, lower gestational age and birth weight, and early-onset sepsis in extremely low-birth-weight (ELBW) infants.[70] Delayed cord clamping, especially in preterm infants, may help insure adequate

Table 4
Alternatives for prevention and therapy for persistent bradycardia or asystole during neonatal resuscitation

Alternative Approach	Mechanism of Action
Antenatal steroids	Accelerated structural/functional pulmonary maturation of fetus (more effective ventilation of ELBW infants)
Close communication between obstetric and neonatal care providers	Anticipation of need for intensive resuscitation at birth
Availability of timely cesarean section	Avoidance of prolonged fetal distress from obstructed labor, compromised placental blood supply, intrauterine infection
Team training in airway skills, vascular access, and crisis resource management	Effective ventilation of ELBW infants (by face mask and endotracheal tube), vascular access for volume expansion (as needed), and rapid differential diagnosis of etiology of prolonged bradycardia/asystole
Improved interfaces for positive-pressure ventilation of ELBW infants	Effective ventilation of ELBW infants (avoidance of bradycardia due to poor pulmonary recruitment/ventilation)
Immediate availability of emergency-release blood	Volume replacement after obstetric hemorrhage
Investigation of resuscitation with intact umbilical cord	Avoidance of bradycardia due to immediate cord compression; facilitation of placental transfusion after expansion of pulmonary circuit with ventilation and maintenance of normal circulating volume
Investigation of alternative vasopressors	Improved specificity of action and efficacy
Investigation of improved strategies for postresuscitation support	Lessening of end-organ injury

circulating volume and avoid the stimulus for bradycardia resulting from immediate clamping.[24] Emphasis on establishment of effective ventilation requires consideration of antenatal steroid therapy in preterm gestations and immediate ability to intubate in the case of a depressed infant with meconium in the amniotic fluid or extremely preterm infant with severe respiratory distress. Striking variation in the rates of delivery room CPR[70] and documentation of cardiac compressions and medication administration occurring before establishment of effective ventilation suggest the need to refocus on achieving effective bag and mask ventilation and rapid intubation when necessary.[26] If bradycardia persists or asystole is present despite effective ventilation, the presence of a full team that has practiced management of advanced resuscitations facilitates timely interventions (chest compressions and vascular access) and analysis of the underlying cause of the arrest.[71] Better understanding of underlying pathologies of bradycardia/arrest at delivery may permit future pharmacologic investigation to be directed toward more specific, targeted therapy, and postresuscitation support.[72]

- Measures to prevent bradycardia and circumstances leading to cardiac arrest should be included in delivery planning.
- Better recognition of underlying pathologies of bradycardia/cardiac arrest will permit targeted therapy.

SUMMARY

Epinephrine remains the primary vasopressor for use in neonatal resuscitation in response to asystole or prolonged bradycardia not resolving with adequate ventilation and chest compressions. Epinephrine increases coronary perfusion pressure primarily through peripheral vasoconstriction. Current neonatal resuscitation guidelines recommend prompt IV administration of epinephrine in a dose of 0.01 mg/kg to 0.03 mg/kg, because endotracheal administration results in unpredictable absorption and may require higher doses than the IV route. IO administration provides acceptable vascular access and may be a more rapid route than UVC for pediatric professionals who do not have extensive neonatal experience. High-dose epinephrine poses additional risks to premature and asphyxiated newborn infants and does not result in better long-term survival than conventional doses. Vasopressin has been considered an alternative to epinephrine in adults, but there is insufficient evidence to recommend its use in newborn infants. Alternative vasopressors may have a role in postresuscitation stabilization. Future research will focus on examination of the best sequence for epinephrine administration and chest compressions and better understanding of the pathologies underlying neonatal cardiac arrest and profound bradycardia at birth. Meanwhile, close attention to preparation for delivery, emphasizing the basics of adequate ventilation and euvolemia, helps prevent the need for extensive CPR.

REFERENCES

1. Wyllie J, Perlman JM, Kattwinkel J, et al. Part 11: neonatal resuscitation: 2010 international consensus on cardiopulmonary resuscitation and emergency cardiovascular care science with treatment recommendations. Resuscitation 2010;81(Suppl 1):e260–87.
2. Kattwinkel J, Perlman JM, Aziz K, et al. Neonatal resuscitation: 2010 American heart association guidelines for cardiopulmonary resuscitation and emergency cardiovascular care. Pediatrics 2010;126(5):e1400–13.
3. Polin RA, Fox WW, Abman SH. Fetal and neonatal physiology. 4th edition. Philadelphia: Elsevier/Saunders; 2011.

4. Kuznetsov V, Pak E, Robinson RB, et al. Beta 2-adrenergic receptor actions in neonatal and adult rat ventricular myocytes. Circ Res 1995;76(1):40–52.

5. Devic E, Xiang Y, Gould D, et al. Beta-adrenergic receptor subtype-specific signaling in cardiac myocytes from beta(1) and beta(2) adrenoceptor knockout mice. Mol Pharmacol 2001;60(3):577–83.

6. Crile G, Dolley DH. An experimental research into the resuscitation of dogs killed by anesthetics and asphyxia. J Exp Med 1906;8(6):713–25.

7. Field JM, Hazinski MF, Sayre MR, et al. Part 1: executive summary: 2010 American Heart Association Guidelines for Cardiopulmonary Resuscitation and Emergency Cardiovascular Care. Circulation 2010;122(18 Suppl 3):S640–56.

8. Redding JS, Pearson JW. Evaluation of drugs for cardiac resuscitation. Anesthesiology 1963;24:203–7.

9. Otto CW, Yakaitis RW, Blitt CD. Mechanism of action of epinephrine in resuscitation from asphyxial arrest. Crit Care Med 1981;9(5):364–5.

10. Wyckoff MH. Neonatal cardiopulmonary resuscitation: critical hemodynamics. NeoReviews 2010;11(3):e123–9.

11. Gao F, de Beer VJ, Hoekstra M, et al. Both beta1- and beta2-adrenoceptors contribute to feedforward coronary resistance vessel dilation during exercise. Am J Physiol Heart Circ Physiol 2010;298(3):H921–9.

12. Barber CA, Garcia D, Wyckoff MH. Neonatal cardiac compressions following asystole from asphyxia: beneficial or futile? Toronto: Pediatric Academic Societies; 2007. vol. 617932.7. E-PAS2007.

13. Kattwinkel J. Neonatal resuscitation textbook. 6th edition. Elk Grove Village (IL): American Academy of Pediatrics and American Heart Association; 2011.

14. Barber CA, Wyckoff MH. Use and efficacy of endotracheal versus intravenous epinephrine during neonatal cardiopulmonary resuscitation in the delivery room. Pediatrics 2006;118(3):1028–34.

15. Brimacombe J, Gandini D. Airway rescue and drug delivery in an 800 g neonate with the laryngeal mask airway. Paediatr Anaesth 1999;9(2):178.

16. Greenberg MI, Roberts JR, Baskin SI. Use of endotracheally administered epinephrine in a pediatric patient. Am J Dis Child 1981;135(8):767–8.

17. Guay J, Lortie L. An evaluation of pediatric in-hospital advanced life support interventions using the pediatric Utstein guidelines: a review of 203 cardiorespiratory arrests. Can J Anaesth 2004;51(4):373–8.

18. Jankov RP, Asztalos EV, Skidmore MB. Favourable neurological outcomes following delivery room cardiopulmonary resuscitation of infants < or = 750 g at birth. J Paediatr Child Health 2000;36(1):19–22.

19. Lindemann R. Resuscitation of the newborn. Endotracheal administration of epinephrine. Acta Paediatr Scand 1984;73(2):210–2.

20. O'Donnell AI, Gray PH, Rogers YM. Mortality and neurodevelopmental outcome for infants receiving adrenaline in neonatal resuscitation. J Paediatr Child Health 1998;34(6):551–6.

21. Polin K, Brown DH, Leikin JB. Endotracheal administration of epinephrine and atropine. Pediatr Emerg Care 1986;2(3):168–9.

22. Schwab KO, von Stockhausen HB. Plasma catecholamines after endotracheal administration of adrenaline during postnatal resuscitation. Arch Dis Child Fetal Neonatal Ed 1994;70(3):F213–7.

23. Ziino AJ, Davies MW, Davis PG. Epinephrine for the resuscitation of apparently stillborn or extremely bradycardic newborn infants. Cochrane Database Syst Rev 2011;(2):CD003849.

24. Wyllie J, Niermeyer S. The role of resuscitation drugs and placental transfusion in the delivery room management of newborn infants. Semin Fetal Neonatal Med 2008;13(6):416–23.

25. Wyckoff MH, Perlman J, Niermeyer S. Medications during resuscitation—what is the evidence? Semin Neonatol 2001;6(3):251–9.

26. Perlman JM, Risser R. Cardiopulmonary resuscitation in the delivery room. Associated clinical events. Arch Pediatr Adolesc Med 1995;149(1):20–5.

27. Jasani MS, Nadkarni VM, Finkelstein MS, et al. Effects of different techniques of endotracheal epinephrine administration in pediatric porcine hypoxic-hypercarbic cardiopulmonary arrest. Crit Care Med 1994;22(7):1174–80.

28. Kleinman ME, Oh W, Stonestreet BS. Comparison of intravenous and endotracheal epinephrine during cardiopulmonary resuscitation in newborn piglets. Crit Care Med 1999;27(12):2748–54.

29. Crespo SG, Schoffstall JM, Fuhs LR, et al. Comparison of two doses of endotracheal epinephrine in a cardiac arrest model. Ann Emerg Med 1991;20(3):230–4.

30. Barber CA, Wyckoff MH. Randomized controlled trial of endotracheal versus intravenous administration of epinephrine during neonatal cardiopulmonary resuscitation in asphyxiated piglets. Honolulu (HI): Pediatric Academic Societies; 2008. vol. E-PAS2008: 4453.12.

31. Engle WA. Intraosseous access for administration of medications in neonates. Clin Perinatol 2006;33(1):161–8, ix.

32. Abe KK, Blum GT, Yamamoto LG. Intraosseous is faster and easier than umbilical venous catheterization in newborn emergency vascular access models. Am J Emerg Med 2000;18(2):126–9.

33. Rajani AK, Chitkara R, Oehlert J, et al. Comparison of umbilical venous and intraosseous access during simulated neonatal resuscitation. Pediatrics 2011;128(4):e954–8.

34. Brown CG, Werman HA, Davis EA, et al. The effects of graded doses of epinephrine on regional myocardial blood flow during cardiopulmonary resuscitation in swine. Circulation 1987;75(2):491–7.

35. Chase PB, Kern KB, Sanders AB, et al. Effects of graded doses of epinephrine on both noninvasive and invasive measures of myocardial perfusion and blood flow during cardiopulmonary resuscitation. Crit Care Med 1993;21(3):413–9.

36. Goetting MG, Paradis NA. High dose epinephrine in refractory pediatric cardiac arrest. Crit Care Med 1989;17(12):1258–62.

37. Goetting MG, Paradis NA. High-dose epinephrine improves outcome from pediatric cardiac arrest. Ann Emerg Med 1991;20(1):22–6.

38. Perondi MB, Reis AG, Paiva EF, et al. A comparison of high-dose and standard-dose epinephrine in children with cardiac arrest [see comment]. N Engl J Med 2004;350(17):1722–30.

39. Patterson MD, Boenning DA, Klein BL, et al. The use of high-dose epinephrine for patients with out-of-hospital cardiopulmonary arrest refractory to prehospital interventions. Pediatr Emerg Care 2005;21(4):227–37.

40. Dieckmann RA, Vardis R. High-dose epinephrine in pediatric out-of-hospital cardiopulmonary arrest. Pediatrics 1995;95(6):901–13.

41. Carpenter TC, Stenmark KR. High-dose epinephrine is not superior to standard-dose epinephrine in pediatric in-hospital cardiopulmonary arrest. Pediatrics 1997;99(3):403–8.

42. Rodriguez Nunez A, Garcia C, Lopez-Herce Cid J, et al. Is high-dose epinephrine justified in cardiorespiratory arrest in children?. An Pediatr (Barc) 2005;62(2): 113–6 [in Spanish].

43. Burchfield DJ, Preziosi MP, Lucas VW, et al. Effects of graded doses of epinephrine during asphxia-induced bradycardia in newborn lambs. Resuscitation 1993; 25(3):235–44.

44. Berg RA, Otto CW, Kern KB, et al. A randomized, blinded trial of high-dose epinephrine versus standard-dose epinephrine in a swine model of pediatric asphyxial cardiac arrest. Crit Care Med 1996;24(10):1695–700.

45. Gedeborg R, Silander HC, Ronne-Engstrom E, et al. Adverse effects of high-dose epinephrine on cerebral blood flow during experimental cardiopulmonary resuscitation. Crit Care Med 2000;28(5):1423–30.

46. McCaul CL, McNamara PJ, Engelberts D, et al. Epinephrine increases mortality after brief asphyxial cardiac arrest in an in vivo rat model. Anesth Analg 2006; 102(2):542–8.

47. Bada HS. Prevention of intracranial hemorrhage. NeoReviews 2000;1:e48–53.

48. Ornato JP. Optimal vasopressor drug therapy during resuscitation. Crit Care 2008;12(2):123.

49. Treschan TA, Peters J. The vasopressin system: physiology and clinical strategies. Anesthesiology 2006;105(3):599–612 [quiz: 639–40].

50. Kornberger E, Prengel AW, Krismer A, et al. Vasopressin-mediated adrenocorticotropin release increases plasma cortisol concentrations during cardiopulmonary resuscitation. Crit Care Med 2000;28(10):3517–21.

51. Koch L, Dabek MT, Frommhold D, et al. Stable precursor fragments of vasoactive peptides in umbilical cord blood of term and preterm infants. Horm Res Paediatr 2011;76(4):234–9.

52. Antonov AG, Baibarina EN, Volobuev AI, et al. Clinical value of determining the levels of renin, aldosterone and vasopressin in newborn infants in critical conditions. Pediatriia 1990;(10):8–12 [in Russian].

53. International Liaison Committee on Resuscitation. 2005 International consensus on cardiopulmonary resuscitation and emergency cardiovascular care science with treatment recommendations. Part 4: advanced life support. Resuscitation 2005;67(2–3):213–47.

54. Lindner KH, Dirks B, Strohmenger HU, et al. Randomised comparison of epinephrine and vasopressin in patients with out-of-hospital ventricular fibrillation. Lancet 1997;349(9051):535–7.

55. Wenzel V, Krismer AC, Arntz HR, et al. A comparison of vasopressin and epinephrine for out-of-hospital cardiopulmonary resuscitation. N Engl J Med 2004;350(2): 105–13.

56. Stiell IG, Hebert PC, Wells GA, et al. Vasopressin versus epinephrine for inhospital cardiac arrest: a randomised controlled trial. Lancet 2001;358(9276):105–9.

57. Aung K, Htay T. Vasopressin for cardiac arrest: a systematic review and metaanalysis. Arch Intern Med 2005;165(1):17–24.

58. Callaway CW, Hostler D, Doshi AA, et al. Usefulness of vasopressin administered with epinephrine during out-of-hospital cardiac arrest. Am J Cardiol 2006;98(10): 1316–21.

59. Gueugniaud PY, David JS, Chanzy E, et al. Vasopressin and epinephrine vs. epinephrine alone in cardiopulmonary resuscitation. N Engl J Med 2008;359(1):21–30.

60. Morrison LJ, Deakin CD, Morley PT, et al. Part 8: advanced life support: 2010 international consensus on cardiopulmonary resuscitation and emergency cardiovascular care science with treatment recommendations. Circulation 2010; 122(16 Suppl 2):S345–421.

61. Mann K, Berg RA, Nadkarni V. Beneficial effects of vasopressin in prolonged pediatric cardiac arrest: a case series. Resuscitation 2002;52(2):149–56.

62. Matok I, Vardi A, Augarten A, et al. Beneficial effects of terlipressin in prolonged pediatric cardiopulmonary resuscitation: a case series. Crit Care Med 2007; 35(4):1161–4.
63. Gil-Anton J, Lopez-Herce J, Morteruel E, et al. Pediatric cardiac arrest refractory to advanced life support: is there a role for terlipressin? Pediatr Crit Care Med 2010;11(1):139–41.
64. Duncan JM, Meaney P, Simpson P, et al. Vasopressin for in-hospital pediatric cardiac arrest: results from the American Heart Association National Registry of Cardiopulmonary Resuscitation. Pediatr Crit Care Med 2009;10(2):191–5.
65. Kleinman ME, de Caen AR, Chameides L, et al. Part 10: pediatric basic and advanced life support: 2010 international consensus on cardiopulmonary resuscitation and emergency cardiovascular care science with treatment recommendations. Circulation 2010;122(16 Suppl 2):S466–515.
66. Mayr V, Luckner G, Jochberger S, et al. Arginine vasopressin in advanced cardiovascular failure during the post-resuscitation phase after cardiac arrest. Resuscitation 2007;72(1):35–44.
67. Palmaers T, Albrecht S, Heuser F, et al. Milrinone combined with vasopressin improves cardiac index after cardiopulmonary resuscitation in a pig model of myocardial infarction. Anesthesiology 2007;106(1):100–6.
68. Joynt C, Bigam DL, Charrois G, et al. Milrinone, dobutamine or epinephrine use in asphyxiated newborn pigs resuscitated with 100% oxygen. Intensive Care Med 2010;36(6):1058–66.
69. Joynt C, Bigam DL, Charrois G, et al. Intestinal hemodynamic effects of milrinone in asphyxiated newborn pigs after reoxygenation with 100% oxygen: a dose-response study. Shock 2009;31(3):292–9.
70. Wyckoff MH, Salhab WA, Heyne RJ, et al. Outcome of extremely low birth weight infants who received delivery room cardiopulmonary resuscitation. J Pediatr 2012;160(2):239–244.e2.
71. Sawyer T, Sierocka-Castaneda A, Chan D, et al. Deliberate practice using simulation improves neonatal resuscitation performance. Simul Healthc 2011;6(6): 327–36.
72. Sood S, Giacoia GP. Cardiopulmonary resuscitation in very low birthweight infants. Am J Perinatol 1992;9(2):130–3.

Resuscitation of Preterm Infants
Delivery Room Interventions and Their Effect on Outcomes

Colm P.F. O'Donnell, MB, FRCPI, MRCPCH, FRACP, PhD[a,b,c,d],
Georg M. Schmölzer, MD, PhD[e,f,g],*

KEYWORDS

- Infant • Newborn, • Delivery room • Resuscitation

KEY POINTS

- Mask leak and airway obstruction are common during mask ventilation.
- Airway pressure is a poor proxy for delivered tidal volume; therefore, tidal volume delivery should be monitored.
- CPAP/PEEP should be started in extremely preterm infants in the delivery room before intubation and surfactant is considered.
- Establishment of lung inflation in apneic newborns can be achieved with either shorter or longer inflation times.

INTRODUCTION

At birth, infants have airless, fluid-filled lungs. Establishing breathing and oxygenation after birth is vital for survival and long-term health. Very preterm infants often have particular difficulty in establishing effective breathing after birth because their lungs are structurally immature, surfactant-deficient, and not supported by a stiff chest

Conflict of interest: None.
GMS is supported in part by a Banting Postdoctoral Fellowship, Canadian Institute of Health Research, and an Alberta Innovates-Health Solution Clinical Fellowship.
[a] Department of Neonatology, The National Maternity Hospital, Holles Street, Dublin 2, Ireland; [b] Department of Neonatology, Our Lady's Children's Hospital, Crumlin, Dublin 12, Ireland; [c] National Children's Research Centre, Gate 5, Our Lady's Children's Hospital, Crumlin, Dublin 12, Ireland; [d] Children's Research Centre, School of Medicine and Medical Science, University College Dublin, Belfield, Dublin 4, Ireland; [e] Department of Pediatrics, University of Alberta, 10240 Kingsway Avenue Northwest, T5H 3V9, Edmonton, Canada; [f] Division of Neonatology, Department of Pediatrics, Medical University Graz, Auenbrugger platz 30, 8036 Graz, Austria; [g] Neonatal Research Group, Murdoch Childrens Research Institute, 50 Flemington Road, Parkville VIC 3052, Melbourne, Australia
* Corresponding author. Department of Newborn Medicine, Royal Alexandra Hospital, 10240 Kingsway Avenue Northwest, T5H 3V9, Edmonton, Alberta, Canada.
E-mail address: georg.schmoelzer@me.com

Clin Perinatol 39 (2012) 857–869
http://dx.doi.org/10.1016/j.clp.2012.09.010
0095-5108/12/$ – see front matter © 2012 Elsevier Inc. All rights reserved.
perinatology.theclinics.com

wall.[1] These factors also render the lungs of very preterm infants uniquely susceptible to injury. Most very preterm infants receive respiratory support in the delivery room (DR). The DR is often a stressful environment where decisions are made quickly and resuscitators need to be skilled in clinical assessment and mask ventilation.[2] However, assessment and mask ventilation are often more difficult than is widely appreciated; and it is possible that the lungs of the infants who most need support may be damaged by the support they are given.

Bronchopulmonary dysplasia (BPD) rarely develops in infants greater than 33 weeks gestation and the risk is inversely proportional to gestational age and birth weight.[3–5] Advances in neonatal care, including antenatal glucocorticoid treatment and intratracheal surfactant administration, which have dramatically reduced the severity of and mortality from respiratory distress syndrome in premature infants have not reduced the rates of oxygen dependence at 36 weeks' postmenstrual age or BPD. Neonatologists are familiar with the concept of reducing lung injury and are increasingly careful to apply ventilation strategies that are gentle to the lung in the neonatal intensive care unit (NICU). However, there has not been the same emphasis on using the same gentle approach during the first few minutes after birth.[1] During positive pressure ventilation (PPV) in the DR the lungs of preterm infants are often ventilated with little or no positive end-expiratory pressure (PEEP) and potentially injurious tidal volumes (V_T),[2,6–8] which have been shown to alter surfactant response in animal models.[9–12]

A lung-protective strategy should start immediately after birth. To facilitate the early development of an effective functional residual capacity (FRC), reduce atelectotrauma (injury from repeated opening and collapse of lung units), and improve oxygenation during the transition of preterm infants, a continuous distending pressure (PEEP or continuous positive airway pressure [CPAP]) should be applied at the initiation of respiratory support. Sustained inflations (SI), an inflating pressure higher than PEEP (typically 20–25 cm H_2O) applied for a sustained period (typically 10–20 seconds), may also aid the formation of FRC. Although PEEP helps maintain end-expiratory lung volume[13–22] and SIs are advocated as lung recruitment maneuvers, neither has been mandated in neonatal resuscitation guidelines.[23]

RESPIRATORY SUPPORT IN THE DR

The International Liaison Committee on Resuscitation and various national resuscitation guidelines recommend equipment and techniques for neonatal resuscitation.[23–25] They all agree that PPV is the cornerstone of respiratory support immediately after birth.[23–25] The purpose of PPV is to create an FRC, deliver an adequate V_T to facilitate gas exchange and stimulate breathing, while minimizing lung injury.[1] To establish FRC immediately after birth and to prevent lung collapse PEEP or CPAP should be provided.[1] Rather than focus on PEEP, however, more attention is usually paid to the peak inflating pressure. A peak inflating pressure is somewhat arbitrarily chosen with the assumption an adequate V_T will be delivered.[1,23] However, the delivered V_T is rarely measured and therefore airway pressure is not adjusted to optimize V_T delivery.[2,6]

Interfaces During Respiratory Support in the DR

Face masks and nasal prongs are used to give respiratory support to preterm infants in the DR.[26–29] Although it has been reported,[30] the laryngeal mask airway is not commonly used in preterm infants. Round silicone face masks that cover the infant's mouth and nose are used more frequently than one or two prongs inserted into a short distance into the nostrils.[1,2,15,16,28,31] Masks and prongs have potential advantages and disadvantages. Face masks seem easy to use and PEEP, CPAP, or PPV are delivered to nose and mouth. However, obstruction is common,[2,32,33] it is difficult to achieve a good face mask seal,[2–8,31,33–36] and the pressure is lost if the facemask is lifted to assess the infant. Also, considerable pressure may be applied to the infant's head by the resuscitator to achieve a good seal.[1,37]

A single nasal prong (nasopharyngeal airway, short nasal tube) can be made by shortening an endotracheal tube of an internal diameter appropriate for a preterm infant (2.5 for infants <1000 g, 3 if >1000 g), typically to 5 cm, and reinserting the connector. A single nasal prong may reduce obstruction of the airway by the tongue, the rationale for its use in children with Pierre Robin syndrome. If respiratory support is given through a single nasal prong, it is delivered to the nasopharynx. There are, however, large leaks through the mouth and contralateral nostril, which should be actively closed if PPV is given.[2–8,31,38] Although the single nasal prong does not need to be constantly held in place like a face mask, it can become dislodged or kinked resulting in loss of pressure. Care also needs to be taken that the prong is inserted into the nasopharynx perpendicular to the face, not inserted vertically up the nose because the cribriform plate could be pierced.

Studies have suggested that a single nasal prong may offer advantages over face masks in preterm infants[9–12,16,17]; randomized studies comparing them have not yet been reported. One randomized study found binasal prongs to be superior to the rarely used triangular plastic Rendell-Baker mask that was developed for inhalational anesthesia.[13–22,39] Although double prongs have been demonstrated to be superior to a single prong for delivering nasal CPAP in the NICU, their use has not been compared in the DR.[1,23,40] Although double prongs are more difficult to secure and keep in the nose than a single nasal prong, the experience of Columbia Hospital in New York demonstrates that bilateral nasal Hudson prongs can be used effectively to apply CPAP and PEEP immediately after birth.[1,23–25,41]

Ventilation Devices for Respiratory Support in the DR

Self-inflating bags, flow-inflating bags, and T-pieces are recommended for use in the DR.[13–25] Although each has potential advantages and disadvantages, there is currently little evidence to guide clinicians' choice of ventilation device.[1,23,27] A self-inflating bag does not provide PEEP or CPAP.[1,42] Although an attached PEEP-valve provides inconsistent PEEP during PPV, CPAP cannot be delivered.[1,23,29,43–45] Variable and operator-dependent PEEP may be provided with a flow-inflating bag.[1,2,6,23,46] T-piece devices allow operators to consistently deliver predetermined level of PEEP and CPAP.[26–29,43] SIs can be delivered more accurately with a T-piece device than with a flow-inflating bag.[30,43,47,48]

Davies and colleagues[49] compared two self-inflating bags, the (no longer available) Samson resuscitator and Laerdal resuscitator, during PPV of 20 term or near-term asphyxiated newborns. Although infants resuscitated with the Laerdal resuscitator had significantly improved arterial blood gases, no significant difference in any short- or long-term outcomes were observed.[49] In a randomized study of 104 extremely low birth weight infants, Finer[22] compared CPAP-PEEP with no CPAP-PEEP during PPV using a T-piece device. Overall the rates of intubation, death, and BPD were similar in both groups.[22] Dawson and colleagues[29] randomized 80 preterm infants less than 29 weeks' gestation to receive PPV with either a T-piece device with PEEP or a self-inflating bag without a PEEP valve. There was no significant difference in oxygen saturation or heart rate at 5 minutes after birth or in mortality, rate of intubation, or BPD between the groups.[29] A larger study comparing the T-piece and self-inflating bag is ongoing.

Mask Ventilation in the DR

Correct positioning of the infant's head and neck during mask ventilation is crucial.[50] Several factors can reduce the effectiveness of mask ventilation, including poor face mask technique resulting in leak or airway obstruction, spontaneous movements of the baby, movements by or distraction of the resuscitator, and such procedures as changing the wraps or fitting a hat.[32,33,51] Mannequin and DR studies have shown that mask PPV is difficult and mask leak and airway obstruction are common problems during PPV.[2,32,33,35,36,50,52] Leak and obstruction are usually not recognized unless CO_2 detectors or respiratory function monitors (RFM) (**Fig. 1**) are used.[1,32,33]

Mask Leak

Mannequin and human observational studies reported wide variation in measured mask leak (see **Fig. 1B**).[2,33,35,36,52] O'Donnell and colleagues[3–5,36] reported large mask leaks during PPV in a mannequin model. Wood and colleagues[1,35] compared two commonly used face masks and reported similar mask leaks in a mannequin. A mannequin study demonstrated that operators were able to reduce mask leak during PPV when flow waves were observed on a RFM.[2,6–8,53] In a recent randomized control trial Schmölzer and colleagues[8–12] compared the effect of having an RFM visible or not during mask PPV in infants less than 32 weeks in the DR. When resuscitators were able to observe displayed flow waves, mask leak was significantly reduced from 54% to 37%.[8,13–22] In addition, significantly more infants left the DR on CPAP and significantly fewer infants were intubated and required oxygen at 5 minutes after birth.[8,23] Although some short-term outcomes were significantly improved, no differences in any long-term outcomes were observed.[8,23–25] However, a significant reduction in endotracheal intubation and oxygen use is promising and might indicate that flow wave guidance to reduce mask leak can decrease rate of endotracheal intubation.

Airway Obstruction

Two observational studies reported that the airway of preterm infants is frequently obstructed during PPV in the DR.[23–25,32,33] Using a colorimetric CO_2-detector, Finer and colleagues[1,32] found airway obstruction in 75% of infants receiving PPV in the DR. Although CO_2-detectors are very useful devices to assess effective ventilation, they cannot differentiate between an inadequate V_T, airway obstruction or circulatory failure. In contrast, an RFM that displays flow and V_T signals allows one to distinguish between mask leak and airway obstruction (see **Fig. 1C**).[1,33,34] A recent observational study in the DR showed that severe airway obstruction, defined as a reduction in V_T of more than 75%, occurs in 25% of infants receiving mask ventilation.[1,23,33] Current resuscitation manuals suggest that airway obstruction may be caused by manual compression of the soft tissues of the neck, tongue, and thus the trachea, or hyperextension or flexion of the head.[2,6,23,50] In addition, obstruction may be caused by the face mask being held on the face so tightly that it obstructs the mouth and nose.[23,26–29,50] Resuscitation guidelines recommend various airway maneuvers to maintain upper airway patency during PPV.[23,30] However, none of these maneuvers has been systematically evaluated during PPV in newly born infants[2,15,16,23,28,31,50] and it remains unanswered whether airway obstruction is caused by the facemask being held too tightly over the face or by soft tissue compression.

V_T Delivery

A low V_T may be insufficient to achieve adequate gas exchange resulting in hypercapnia, whereas excessive V_T may cause hypocapnia and lung injury from

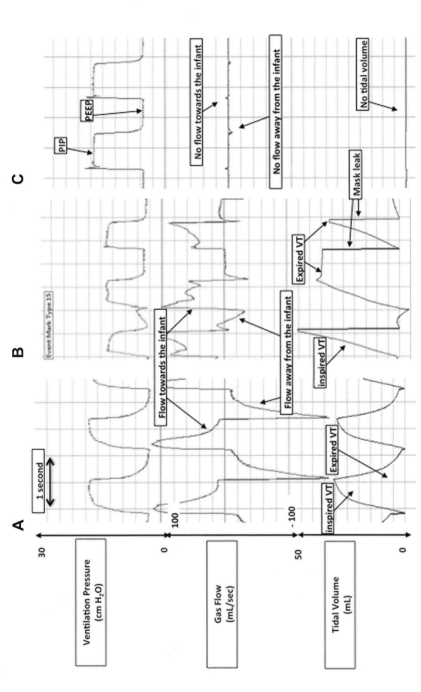

Fig. 1. Positive pressure ventilation in a 28-week-old preterm infant. (A) Mask ventilation with no leak. However, the delivered V_T is around 25 mL/kg. (B) PPV with mask leak of around 90% to 100% is delivered compared with total airway obstruction (C). PIP, peak inflating pressure.

overstretching (volutrauma). Low and excessive V_T promote release of inflammatory mediators, which contribute to BPD.[10,32,33,54] Abnormal CO_2 content (hypocapnia or hypercapnia) can cause cardiovascular dysfunction. Clinicians struggle to achieve a balance between aerating the distal gas exchange units (alveoli) without overdistending the lung and causing injury.[1,2,6–8,31,33–36]

Animals studies have shown that lung injury can occur during resuscitation with just a few large manual inflations with V_T up to 40 mL/kg.[9,11,37,55,56] Similar V_T have been recently reported during resuscitation of preterm infants.[2–7,31,38] Dreyfuss and coworkers[16,17,57] and Hernandez and coworkers[39,58] showed in animal models that lung injury was predominantly caused by high V_T ventilation and not by high pressure per se. Many lesions occurred within 2 minutes of starting ventilation. However, if V_T was controlled so the lungs did not overdistend, little or no injury occurred.[1,40,58] During PPV a peak inflation pressure is chosen with the assumption that this will deliver an adequate V_T. However, the delivered V_T is rarely measured and therefore airway pressure is not adjusted to optimize V_T delivery (see **Fig. 1**A).[1,2,6,34,41,59] Studies using a lung simulator demonstrated that operators are able to adjust to compliance changes faster when V_T was displayed on an RFM rather than airway pressure.[13–23,60,61] In a randomized control trial Schmölzer and colleagues[8,23,27] compared V_T guidance with clinical assessment during mask PPV in the DR in preterm infants less than 32 weeks gestation. The delivered median V_T was similar in both groups (5.7 mL/kg in the RFM visible group vs 5.6 mL/kg in the RFM masked group).[1,8,42] However, both the proportion of infants with a V_T greater than 8 mL/kg (0.81; 95% confidence interval, 0.67–0.98) and the mean/median mask leak was a significantly lower when the RFM was visible (37% vs 54%; $P = .01$).[1,8,29,43–45] This is promising because animal studies have shown that V_T greater than 8 mL/kg contributes to lung injury.[1,10,12,23,46] In addition, Tracy and coworkers[29,43,62] reported that most preterm infants receiving PPV in the DR are overventilated and had hypocapnia with $Paco_2$ less than 25 mm Hg. Abnormal CO_2 content (hypocapnia or hypercapnia) has been shown to cause cardiovascular dysfunction and is a known risk factor for brain injury.

Sustained Inflation

Establishment of lung inflation in apneic newborns can be achieved with either shorter or longer inflation times.[23,43,47,48] In a small series of asphyxiated term infants, a prolonged initial inflation of 5 seconds showed a twofold increase in FRC compared with PPV alone.[18,49,63] However, no randomized clinical trials have evaluated the use of SI or different duration of inflations in term babies. Nevertheless, initial SI is commonly taught and used.

In preterm infants a lung protective strategy should start at birth to support lung fluid clearance and to establish FRC. In anesthetized preterm rabbits that were not breathing spontaneously and were ventilated through an endotracheal tube immediately after birth, a prolonged SI of 20 seconds coupled with PEEP caused a rapid increase in FRC. Ventilation with PEEP alone (ie, no SI) also resulted in a rapid increase in FRC; but neither ventilation with an SI without PEEP, nor ventilation without an SI or PEEP, resulted in FRC formation.[49,64,65] Evidence for the use of SI in human preterm infants comes from cohort and randomized studies.[14–16,22] Lindner and coworkers[15,22] reported a dramatic reduction in the rate of DR intubation (from 84% to 40%) and increase in the proportion of extremely low birth weight infants never intubated during their admission at their institution (from 7% to 25%) after the introduction of a series of interventions in the DR that included giving a 15-second SI. Similarly, Lista and colleagues[14,29] demonstrated reductions in the rates of mechanical ventilation (51% vs 75%), surfactant (45% vs 61%), and postnatal steroid (10% vs 25%) use, and BPD in survivors (7% vs 25%); and in the mean duration of mechanical ventilation (5 vs 11 days) and oxygen therapy (21 vs 31 days) among infants less than 32 weeks when an initial 15-second SI was given in addition to PPV in the DR. Harling and colleagues[29,66] randomized 52 preterm infants to an initial 5-second SI at the start of PPV or not, and did not find a difference in cytokines measured in bronchoalveolar lavage fluid. Lindner and coworkers[15,50] randomized 61 infants less than 29 weeks given respiratory support through a single nasal prong in the DR to receive either a 15-second SI or PPV. Overall no difference in mortality, severe intraventricular hemorrhage, or BPD was observed. However, between 30% and 40% of preterm infants did not require intubation or mechanical ventilation within the first 48 hours after birth.[15,32,33,51] Te Pas and colleagues[2,16,32,33,35,36,50,52] randomized 207 infants less than 33 weeks to receive either a 10-second SI followed by nasal CPAP with a T-piece through a single nasal prong or mask PPV with self-inflating bag without an attached PEEP-valve. Infants randomized to SI/CPAP were less frequently intubated in the first 72 hours, were ventilated for a shorter duration, and had a reduced rate of BPD.[16]

Although these studies suggest that an initial SI has the potential to reduce the need for mechanical ventilation and BPD, the results should be interpreted with caution. The cohort studies are subject to confounders and can at best suggest an association between the use of an SI and improved outcomes. For example, the study of Lindner reported that many aspects of DR care changed over time, the use of SI being just one element. Harling's and Lindner's randomized studies were small and not adequately powered to detect differences in important clinical outcomes. In addition, Harling used an SI shorter than that demonstrated to have benefits in animal models. The intervention studied by te Pas had several elements, of which the use of an SI was just one. Consequently, it is not possible to determine how much, if any, of the differences observed between the groups is caused by the use of an SI. The infants studied by te Pas and colleagues[15,16] were on average 500 g heavier than those studied by Lindner. Larger studies of SI in preterm infants are ongoing.

CPAP versus Routine Intubation

Many observational studies have documented an association between lower rates of BPD and increased use of early CPAP.[22,41,67–69] Avery and coworkers[41] reported BPD rates in eight NICUs in the United States in an era before the widespread use of antenatal steroids and the introduction of surfactant. The rate of BPD was much lower in one center where CPAP was used in preference to mechanical ventilation compared with centers where infants were routinely ventilated.[41] Van Marter and coworkers[67] similarly showed a large difference in the prevalence of BPD between the centers (4% at Columbia vs 22% in Boston) in the postsurfactant era, despite similar mortality rates. These studies prompted large randomized control trials enrolled of CPAP or endotracheal intubation at birth.[19,20] The COIN trial randomized 610 spontaneously breathing infants of 25 to 28 weeks gestation who had signs of respiratory distress at 5 minutes of life to receive either CPAP or endotracheal intubation. Although the risk of dying or being treated with oxygen at 28 days of life was lower among infants randomized to CPAP (odds ratio, 0.63; 95% confidence interval, 0.46–0.88; $P = .006$), the difference in the proportion of infants who had died or were treated with oxygen at 36 weeks' corrected gestational age was not significant between the groups (CPAP 33.9% vs intubation 38.9%). Infants in the CPAP group required fewer days of ventilation and the use of surfactant was halved[20]; however, more infants treated with nasal CPAP developed pneumothorax (9% vs 3%).[20] The SUPPORT trial randomized 1316 infants between 24 and 28 weeks to receive CPAP or endotracheal intubation and surfactant. Overall, mortality (47.8% and 51%, respectively) and BPD rates were similar between the CPAP and the surfactant group. Infants randomized to CPAP were intubated less frequently, ventilated for a shorter duration, and received post-natal corticosteroids for BPD less frequently.[19] There was no difference in the rate of air leak between the groups (CPAP 6.8% vs intubation 7.4%). In the Delivery Room Management trial, infants 26 to 29 week's gestation were randomized to nasal CPAP, to intubation-surfactant-extubation within 30 minutes to nasal CPAP, or to intubation for prophylactic surfactant and mechanical ventilation for at least 6 hours. Recruitment was stopped when 648 of a planned sample of 876 had been enrolled. The differences in death or moderate-severe BPD (nasal CPAP 4.1% vs intubation-surfactant-extubation 7% vs prophylactic surfactant 7.2%) and in pneumothorax (5.4% vs 3.2 vs 4.8%) observed among the groups were not significantly. Among infants randomized to nasal CPAP, 48% were managed without intubation and ventilation and 54% without surfactant. The results from these studies suggest that preterm infants should start on CPAP in the DR before intubation and surfactant is considered.

MONITORING OF BODY TEMPERATURE DURING NEONATAL STABILIZATION

It was traditionally recommended that, to prevent them from becoming cold, all infants should be placed under radiant heat, dried with towels, and covered with warmed towels and a hat after birth.[70] Despite these measures, hypothermia on admission to the NICU remained common and was associated with increased mortality among extremely preterm infants.[71] Although it is not clear whether this association is coincidental (sick babies who are more likely to die spend longer being resuscitated in the DR where they get cold) or causal (hypothermia increases the risk of dying), it is generally agreed that hypothermia should be avoided in preterm infants.

Polyethylene wrapping is used to prevent hypothermia in preterm infants. This exploits a simple principle, that polyethylene allows radiant heat to be transmitted but reduces evaporative heat loss. Randomized trials demonstrated that preterm infants placed in food-grade polyethylene bags without first drying them had higher mean temperature on admission to NICU compared with infants who were dried and wrapped with towels.[72,73] These studies led to the International Liaison Committee on Resuscitation recommending their use for extremely preterm infants.[74] However, about one-third of infants randomized to polyethylene bags had a temperature less than 36.5°C on admission to the NICU in these studies, whereas less than 10% had temperature greater than 37.5°C.[72,73]

Exothermic mattresses are also used as an additional heat source to prevent hypothermia in preterm infants. These mattresses are filled with sodium acetate gel and heat is produced when a disk within the mattress is snapped causing the gel to crystallize. Cohort studies have demonstrated that hypothermia is reduced when exothermic mattresses are used in conjunction with polyethylene bags, but that babies are more often hyperthermic on admission.[75,76] Although there are less data about the effects of hyperthermia on preterm infants, it is also thought to be something to be avoided.[74] In a recent study, extremely preterm infants randomized to be placed on an exothermic mattress (not in a polyethylene bag) had a higher mean admission temperature on admission than infants randomized to polyethylene bag.[77] Most infants in both groups, however, had admission temp less than 36.5°C. A recent quasi-randomized study showed that preterm infants, some of whom were placed in polyethylene bags, had a higher mean admission temperature if they were placed on an exothermic mattress.[78] Again, hypothermia was common in both groups and hyperthermia occurred rarely.

Other DR interventions have also been studied. A randomized study showed that infants treated with a polyethylene cap had similar mean admission temperature to infants in polyethylene bags, and that both were higher to infants who were dried and wrapped in towels.[78] In addition, a cohort study showed that using warmed and humidified gases for respiratory support in the DR is associated with increased temperatures on admission to the NICU.[79] Although the long-term effects of hypothermia and hyperthermia among preterm infants are not clear and merit further study, randomized studies to define the best strategy for achieving admission temperature in the normal range (eg, polyethylene bag with or without exothermic mattress) are warranted.

SUMMARY

Despite advances in neonatal care, the rate of oxygen dependence at 36 weeks' postmenstrual age or BPD has not fallen. A lung-protective strategy should start immediately after birth to establish a FRC, reduce volutrauma and atelectotrauma, facilitate gas exchange, and improve oxygenation during neonatal transition.

REFERENCES

1. Schmölzer GM, Pas te AB, Davis P, et al. Reducing lung injury during neonatal resuscitation of preterm infants. J Pediatr 2008;153:741–5.
2. Schmölzer GM, Kamlin CO, O'Donnell CP, et al. Assessment of tidal volume and gas leak during mask ventilation of preterm infants in the delivery room. Arch Dis Child Fetal Neonatal Ed 2010;95:F393–7.
3. Baraldi E, Filippone M. Chronic lung disease after premature birth. N Engl J Med 2007;357:1946–55.
4. Jobe AH, Bancalari E. Bronchopulmonary dysplasia. Am J Respir Crit Care Med 2001;163:1723.
5. Jobe AH. The new BPD. Neoreviews 2006;7:e531–45.
6. Poulton DA, Schmölzer GM, Morley CJ, et al. Assessment of chest rise during mask ventilation of preterm infants in the delivery room. Resuscitation 2011;82: 175–9.
7. Schmölzer GM, Kamlin CO, Dawson JA, et al. Tidal volume delivery during surfactant administration in the delivery room. Intensive Care Med 2011;37: 1833–9.
8. Schmölzer GM, Morley CJ, Wong C, et al. Respiratory function monitor guidance of mask ventilation in the delivery room: a feasibility study. J Pediatr 2012;160. 377–381.e2.
9. Björklund LJ, Ingimarsson J, Curstedt T, et al. Manual ventilation with a few large breaths at birth compromises the therapeutic effect of subsequent surfactant replacement in immature lambs. Pediatr Res 1997;42:348–55.
10. Hillman NH, Moss TJ, Kallapur SG, et al. Brief, large tidal volume ventilation initiates lung injury and a systemic response in fetal sheep. Am J Respir Crit Care Med 2007;176:575–81.
11. Hillman NH, Kallapur SG, Pillow JJ, et al. Airway injury from initiating ventilation in preterm sheep. Pediatr Res 2010;67:60–5.
12. Polglase GR, Hillman NH, Pillow JJ, et al. Positive end-expiratory pressure and tidal volume during initial ventilation of preterm lambs. Pediatr Res 2008;64:517–22.

13. Duff JP, Rosychuk RJ, Joffe AR. The safety and efficacy of sustained inflations as a lung recruitment maneuver in pediatric intensive care unit patients. Intensive Care Med 2007;33:1778–86.

14. Lista G, Fontana P, Castoldi F, et al. Does sustained lung inflation at birth improve outcome of preterm infants at risk for respiratory distress syndrome. Neonatology 2011;99:45–50.

15. Lindner W, Vossbeck S, Hummler H, et al. Delivery room management of extremely low birth weight infants: spontaneous breathing or intubation? Pediatrics 1999;103:961–7.

16. Pas te AB, Walther FJ. A randomized, controlled trial of delivery-room respiratory management in very preterm infants. Pediatrics 2007;120:322–9.

17. Fuchs H, Lindner W, Buschko A, et al. Cerebral oxygenation in very low birth weight infants supported with sustained lung inflations after birth. Pediatr Res 2011;70:176–80.

18. Boon AW, Milner AD, Hopkin IE. Lung expansion, tidal exchange, and formation of the functional residual capacity during resuscitation of asphyxiated neonates. J Pediatr 1979;95:1031–6.

19. Finer NN, Carlo WA, Walsh MC, et al, SUPPORT Study Group of the Eunice Kennedy Shriver NICHD Neonatal Research Network. Early CPAP versus surfactant in extremely preterm infants. N Engl J Med 2010;362:1970–9.

20. Morley CJ, Davis PG, Doyle LW, et al. Nasal CPAP or intubation at birth for very preterm infants. N Engl J Med 2008;358:700–8.

21. Morley CJ. Continuous distending pressure. Arch Dis Child Fetal Neonatal Ed 1999;81:F152.

22. Finer NN. Delivery room continuous positive airway pressure/positive end-expiratory pressure in extremely low birth weight infants: a feasibility trial. Pediatrics 2004;114:651–7.

23. Kattwinkel J, Perlman JM, Aziz K, et al. Part 15: neonatal resuscitation: 2010 American Heart Association guidelines for cardiopulmonary resuscitation and emergency cardiovascular care. Circulation 2010;122:S909–19.

24. Nolan JP, Soar J, Zideman DA, et al. European Resuscitation Council guidelines for resuscitation 2010 section 1. Executive summary. Resuscitation 2010;81:1219–76.

25. Schmölzer GM, Resch B, Schwindt JC. Standards zur Versorgung von reifen Neugeborenen in Österreich. Monatsschr Kinderheilkd 2011;29(159):1235–43.

26. Singhal N, McMillan DD, Yee WH, et al. Evaluation of the effectiveness of the standardized neonatal resuscitation program. J Perinatol 2001;21:388–92.

27. Hawkes CP, Ryan CA, Dempsey EM. Comparison of the T-piece resuscitator with other neonatal manual ventilation devices: a qualitative review. Resuscitation 2012;83(7):797–802.

28. Lindner W, Högel J, Pohlandt F. Sustained pressure—controlled inflation or intermittent mandatory ventilation in preterm infants in the delivery room? A randomized, controlled trial on initial respiratory support via nasopharyngeal tube. Acta Paediatr 2005;94:303–9.

29. Dawson JA, Schmölzer GM, Kamlin CO, et al. Oxygenation with T-piece versus self-inflating bag for ventilation of extremely preterm infants at birth: a randomized controlled trial. J Pediatr 2011;158:912–8.

30. Brimacombe J, Gandini D. Airway rescue and drug delivery in an 800 g neonate with the laryngeal mask airway. Paediatr Anaesth 1999;9:178.

31. Schmölzer GM, Morley CJ. Equipment and technology for continuous positive airway pressure during neonatal. Noninvasive mechanical ventilation: theory, equipment, and clinical applications. Heidelberg: Springer Verlag; 2010. p. 335–41.

32. Finer NN, Rich W, Wang C, et al. Airway obstruction during mask ventilation of very low birth weight infants during neonatal resuscitation. Pediatrics 2009;123:865–9.
33. Schmölzer GM, Dawson JA, Kamlin CO, et al. Airway obstruction and gas leak during mask ventilation of preterm infants in the delivery room. Arch Dis Child Fetal Neonatal Ed 2011;96:F254–7.
34. Schmölzer GM, Kamlin CO, Dawson JA, et al. Respiratory monitoring of neonatal resuscitation. Arch Dis Child Fetal Neonatal Ed 2010;95:F295–303.
35. Wood FE, Morley CJ, Dawson JA, et al. Assessing the effectiveness of two round neonatal resuscitation masks: study 1. Arch Dis Child Fetal Neonatal Ed 2008;93: F235–7.
36. O'Donnell CP. Neonatal resuscitation 2: an evaluation of manual ventilation devices and face masks. Arch Dis Child Fetal Neonatal Ed 2005;90:F392–6.
37. van Vonderen JJ, Kleijn TA, Schilleman K, et al. Compressive force applied to a manikin's head during mask ventilation. Arch Dis Child Fetal Neonatal Ed 2012;97(4):F254–8.
38. Morley CJ, Davis P. Continuous positive airway pressure: current controversies. Curr Opin Pediatr 2004;16:141–5.
39. Capasso L, Capasso A, Raimondi F, et al. A randomized trial comparing oxygen delivery on intermittent positive pressure with nasal cannulae versus facial mask in neonatal primary resuscitation. Acta Paediatr 2005;94:197–200.
40. Davis P, Davies M, Faber B. A randomised controlled trial of two methods of delivering nasal continuous positive airway pressure after extubation to infants weighing less than 1000 g: binasal (Hudson) versus single nasal prongs. Arch Dis Child Fetal Neonatal Ed 2001;85:F82–5.
41. Avery ME, Tooley WH, Keller JB, et al. Is chronic lung disease in low birth weight infants preventable? A survey of eight centers. Pediatrics 1987;79:26–30.
42. Morley CJ, Dawson JA, Stewart MJ, et al. The effect of a PEEP valve on a Laerdal neonatal self-inflating resuscitation bag. J Paediatr Child Health 2010;46:51–6.
43. Bennett S, Finer NN, Rich W, et al. A comparison of three neonatal resuscitation devices. Resuscitation 2005;67:113–8.
44. Finer NN, Barrington KJ, Al-Fadley F, et al. Limitations of self-inflating resuscitators. Pediatrics 1986;77:417.
45. Oddie S, Wyllie J, Scally A. Use of self-inflating bags for neonatal resuscitation. Resuscitation 2005;67:109–12.
46. Dawson JA, Gerber A, Kamlin OO, et al. Providing PEEP during neonatal resuscitation: which device is best? J Paediatr Child Health 2011;47:698–703.
47. Klingenberg C, Dawson JA, Gerber A, et al. Sustained inflations: comparing three neonatal resuscitation devices. Neonatology 2011;100:78–84.
48. Field D, Milner AD, Hopkin IE. Efficiency of manual resuscitators at birth. Arch Dis Child 1986;61:300–2.
49. Davies VA, Rothberg AD, Argent AC, et al. A comparison of two resuscitators in the management of birth asphyxia. S Afr Med J 1985;68:19–22.
50. Chua C, Schmölzer GM, Davis PG. Airway manoeuvres to achieve upper airway patency during mask ventilation in newborn infants: an historical perspective. Resuscitation 2012;83:411–6.
51. Schilleman K, Siew ML, Lopriore E, et al. Auditing resuscitation of preterm infants at birth by recording video and physiological parameters. Resuscitation 2012;83: 1135–9.
52. Schilleman K, Witlox RS, Lopriore E, et al. Leak and obstruction with mask ventilation during simulated neonatal resuscitation. Arch Dis Child Fetal Neonatal Ed 2010;95:F398–402.

53. Wood FE, Morley CJ, Dawson JA, et al. A respiratory function monitor improves mask ventilation. Arch Dis Child Fetal Neonatal Ed 2008;93:F380–1.
54. Lista G, Colnaghi M, Castoldi F, et al. Impact of targeted-volume ventilation on lung inflammatory response in preterm infants with respiratory distress syndrome (RDS). Pediatr Pulmonol 2004;37:510–4.
55. Björklund L, Ingimarsson J, Curstedt T, et al. Lung recruitment at birth does not improve lung function in immature lambs receiving surfactant. Acta Anaesthesiol Scand 2001;45:986–93.
56. Wada K, Jobe AH, Ikegami M. Tidal volume effects on surfactant treatment responses with the initiation of ventilation in preterm lambs. J Appl Physiol 1997;83:1054–61.
57. Dreyfuss D, Basset G, Soler P, et al. Intermittent positive-pressure hyperventilation with high inflation pressures produces pulmonary microvascular injury in rats. Am Rev Respir Dis 1985;132:880–4.
58. Hernandez LA, Peevy KJ, Moise AA, et al. Chest wall restriction limits high airway pressure-induced lung injury in young rabbits. J Appl Physiol 1989;66:2364–8.
59. Schmölzer GM, Morley CJ, Davis PG. Respiratory function monitoring to reduce mortality and morbidity in newborn infants receiving resuscitation. Cochrane Database Syst Rev 2010;(9):CD008437.
60. Kattwinkel J, Stewart C, Walsh B, et al. Responding to compliance changes in a lung model during manual ventilation: perhaps volume, rather than pressure, should be displayed. Pediatrics 2009;123:e465–70.
61. Bowman TA, Paget-Brown A, Carroll J, et al. Sensing and responding to compliance changes during manual ventilation using a lung model: can we teach healthcare providers to improve? J Pediatr 2012;160:372–6.
62. Tracy MB. How safe is intermittent positive pressure ventilation in preterm babies ventilated from delivery to newborn intensive care unit? Arch Dis Child Fetal Neonatal Ed 2004;89:84F–7F.
63. Vyas H, Milner AD, Hopkin IE, et al. Physiologic responses to prolonged and slow-rise inflation in the resuscitation of the asphyxiated newborn infant. J Pediatr 1981;99:635–9.
64. Pas te AB, Siew M, Wallace MJ, et al. Effect of sustained inflation length on establishing functional residual capacity at birth in ventilated premature rabbits. Pediatr Res 2009;66:295–300.
65. Siew ML, Pas te AB, Wallace MJ, et al. Positive end-expiratory pressure enhances development of a functional residual capacity in preterm rabbits ventilated from birth. J Appl Physiol 2009;106:1487–93.
66. Harling AE. Does sustained lung inflation at resuscitation reduce lung injury in the preterm infant? Arch Dis Child Fetal Neonatal Ed 2005;90:F406–10.
67. Van Marter LJ, Allred EN, Pagano M, et al. Do clinical markers of barotrauma and oxygen toxicity explain interhospital variation in rates of chronic lung disease? Pediatrics 2000;105:1194–201.
68. Ammari A, Suri M, Milisavljevic V, et al. Variables associated with the early failure of nasal CPAP in very low birth weight infants. J Pediatr 2005;147:341–7.
69. Booth C, Premkumar MH, Yannoulis A, et al. Sustainable use of continuous positive airway pressure in extremely preterm infants during the first week after delivery. Arch Dis Child Fetal Neonatal Ed 2006;91:F398–402.
70. Niermeyer S, Kattwinkel J, Van Reempts P, et al. Contributors and reviewers for the neonatal resuscitation guidelines. International guidelines for neonatal resuscitation. An excerpt from the guidelines 2000 for cardiopulmonary resuscitation

and emergency cardiovascular care: international consensus on science. Pediatrics 2000;106:e29.

71. Costeloe K, Hennessy E, Gibson AT, et al. The EPICure study: outcomes to discharge from hospital for infants born at the threshold of viability. Pediatrics 2000;106:659–71.

72. Vohra S, Frent G, Campbell V, et al. Effect of polyethylene occlusive skin wrapping on heat loss in very low birth weight infants at delivery: a randomized trial. J Pediatr 1999;134:547–51.

73. Vohra S, Roberts RS, Zhang B, et al. Heat loss prevention (HeLP) in the delivery room: a randomized controlled trial of polyethylene occlusive skin wrapping in very preterm infants. J Pediatr 2004;145:750–3.

74. Perlman JM, Wyllie J, Kattwinkel J, et al. Part 11: neonatal resuscitation: 2010 international consensus on cardiopulmonary resuscitation and emergency cardiovascular care science with treatment recommendations. Circulation 2010; 122:S516–38.

75. Singh A, Duckett J, Newton T, et al. Improving neonatal unit admission temperatures in preterm babies: exothermic mattresses, polythene bags or a traditional approach&quest. J Perinatol 2009;30:45–9.

76. Ibrahim CP, Yoxall CW. Use of self-heating gel mattresses eliminates admission hypothermia in infants born below 28 weeks gestation. Eur J Pediatr 2009;169: 795–9.

77. Simon P, Dannaway D, Bright B, et al. Thermal defense of extremely low gestational age newborns during resuscitation: exothermic mattresses vs polyethylene wrap. J Perinatol 2010;31:33–7.

78. Chawla S, Amaram A, Gopal SP, et al. Safety and efficacy of Trans-warmer mattress for preterm neonates: results of a randomized controlled trial. J Perinatol 2011;31:780–4.

79. Pas te AB, Lopriore E, Dito I, et al. Humidified and heated air during stabilization at birth improves temperature in preterm infants. Pediatrics 2010;125:e1427–32.

Infants with Prenatally Diagnosed Anomalies

Special Approaches to Preparation and Resuscitation

Christopher E. Colby, MD[a],*, William A. Carey, MD[a],
Yair J. Blumenfeld, MD[b], Susan R. Hintz, MD, MS Epi[c]

KEYWORDS

- Congenital anomalies • Fetal • Prenatal diagnosis • Delivery room • Cardiac
- Abdominal wall defect • Neural tube defect • Congenital diaphragmatic hernia

KEY POINTS

- A multidisciplinary coordinated approach to care of the fetus is essential to optimize outcomes.
- Information gained during the prenatal period may have significant implications for the care the newborn receives once delivered.
- Data is available on the "best practices" for initial resuscitation and newborn care for many common anomalies.
- A comprehensive plan of the care a newborn with anomalies may be shared with families during prenatal consultation.

THE IMPORTANCE OF A MULTIDISCIPLINARY APPROACH TO THE CONTINUUM OF COMPLEX FETAL CARE

As care providers for pregnant women and their children, the ultimate goal is always a "healthy mommy" and a "healthy baby." However, when a fetal anomaly is diagnosed prenatally the goal becomes achieving the best possible outcome for the neonate without compromising the mother's health. The actual management of

[a] Department of Pediatrics, Neonatal Medicine, Mayo Clinic, 200 First Street SW, Rochester, MN 55905, USA; [b] Department of Obstetrics and Gynecology, Division of Maternal-Fetal Medicine, Stanford University School of Medicine, Lucile Packard Children's Hospital, 300 Pasteur Drive, Stanford, CA 94305, USA; [c] Department of Pediatrics, Division of Neonatal and Developmental Medicine, Stanford University School of Medicine, The Center for Fetal and Maternal Health, Lucile Packard Children's Hospital, 750 Welch Road, Palo Alto, CA 94304, USA
* Corresponding author.
E-mail address: colby.christopher@mayo.edu

Clin Perinatol 39 (2012) 871–887
http://dx.doi.org/10.1016/j.clp.2012.09.012   perinatology.theclinics.com

pregnancies complicated by fetal anomalies requires a robust multidisciplinary approach that begins at the very onset of diagnosis and continues well into postnatal life. Multidisciplinary complex fetal management teams include maternal-fetal medicine, neonatology, genetics, fetal and pediatric imaging, virtually every pediatric medical and surgical subspecialty, and medical social work. Despite great advances in prenatal diagnosis, from ultrasound (US), magnetic resonance imaging (MRI), microarray prenatal genetic testing, and noninvasive prenatal diagnosis,[1] the presumptive diagnosis of a fetal anomaly is often only confirmed after delivery, and the functional and neurodevelopmental outcomes for the child cannot be perfectly predicted during the neonatal period. This uncertainty by itself adds a complex dimension to an already complex clinical, social, ethical, and economic scenario. Over the years, the authors have developed an individualized approach to each new diagnosis, fetal clinical management challenge, and family. They counsel patients objectively without superimposing their own views and predispositions, and with an evidence-based approach whenever possible. They have learned that pregnancy "success" is defined differently for each family, and that expectant mothers' decisions differ even when the fetal and neonatal outcome is likely to be poor. This article reviews general considerations for prenatal diagnosis of fetal anomalies, pregnancy management, and special approaches for resuscitation and immediate care of the newborn with known congenital anomalies. The article is far too brief to provide comprehensive guidelines for all specific anomalies, but rather gives an overview and basic framework to approach these complex cases.

DELINEATING FETAL ANOMALIES IN UTERO, MANAGEMENT OF THE PREGNANCY, FETAL SURVEILLANCE

Fetal Diagnosis

Congenital anomalies include malformations, which are abnormalities of tissue development, and deformities, which are abnormalities caused by mechanical stressors, such as oligohydramnios or amniotic bands. Anomalies can be isolated, or a part of a more global syndrome, often with an underlying genetic cause. The mainstay of prenatal diagnosis is still a routine prenatal US.[2] Anatomic surveys are often performed at 18 to 22 weeks gestation and most anomalies can be detected with two-dimensional US. The benefit of three-dimensional and four-dimensional US in the initial detection of fetal anomalies is unclear but there is little doubt that these advanced modalities are beneficial in determining the extent of some lesions as is the case for craniofacial defects, and skeletal defects.[3–5] Three-dimensional and four-dimensional US are also useful in overcoming technical barriers, such as fetal position, and surface-rendering imaging of various lesions may assist in the presentation and counseling of expectant patients.[5] Advanced US techniques including pulse-wave and color Doppler assessment assist in determining the effects of the lesion on the fetal cardiovascular system, and surveillance of fetal well-being.[6] Furthermore, it is important to recognize that despite advances in US, fetal anomalies may be missed or misdiagnosed in utero.[7]

With the introduction of routine first trimester nuchal translucency assessment for fetal aneuploidy the focus of prenatal US has shifted toward earlier diagnosis of fetal anomalies, even as early as the first trimester.[8] Although many malformations can be detected early in gestation, including those of the central nervous system (CNS), cardiovascular system, skeletal system, abdominal wall defects, and others, it is important to remember that a "normal" first trimester US should not be equated with a "normal" anatomic survey.[9]

Recent advances in prenatal MRI have made this modality an important adjunct tool in the diagnosis, characterization, and management of fetal anomalies. Benefits of MRI over US include more detailed and improved visualization of the fetal CNS (especially in the third trimester when US views are limited by calcifications of the calvarium); volume assessment of fetal lung tissue and masses; and assessment of visceral involvement. Unlike US, MRI is limited by fetal movement, is much more costly, and requires specialized expertise in ascertaining and interpreting imaging, thus largely limiting application of fetal MRI to tertiary care centers.

One of the first questions that arise at the time of diagnosis of a fetal anomaly is whether the suspected defect is isolated, or a part of a more global genetic mutation or syndrome, which is important for antepartum counseling, intrapartum management, and postnatal care. A multidisciplinary discussion with a prenatal geneticist is vital so that expectant patients are presented with all prenatal diagnostic options including genetic testing. The mainstay of prenatal genetic testing is a fetal karyotype, performed after chorionic villus sampling or amniocentesis; yet, it is important to counsel patients about the limitations of karyotype. Consideration for additional genetic tests, such as molecular sequencing of specific genes, fluorescent in-situ hybridization for microdeletions, or a more detailed assessment by microarray technology, should be performed with the input of a perinatal geneticist so that patients understand the risks, benefits, and limitation of each technique. Use of noninvasive prenatal diagnosis methods, such as cell-free fetal DNA, have been largely limited to trisomy 18 and 21.[1] Future advances in noninvasive prenatal genetic technology may allow for the identification of specific gene mutations or microdeletions.

Fetal Surveillance

Fetal anomalies may be associated with changes in fetal and maternal health over the course of pregnancy, which may subsequently impact management decisions. Examples include increasing size of bronchopulmonary malformations (BPMs) and associated changes in other fetal findings, fetal hydrops that can evolve across several fetal fluid cavities, and fetal cardiac arrhythmias that may have variable response to treatment resulting in altered fetal condition. Each of these may carry prognostic implications, and may alter the antepartum management and timing and mode of delivery. Close surveillance by US and other modalities is therefore crucial. Assessment of fetal well-being can be achieved with nonstress testing or biophysical profile. Results from these tests may determine consideration for early delivery, as is the case with worsening intrauterine growth restriction or fetal hydrops.

In general, close surveillance by a maternal-fetal medicine specialist (perinatologist), who often assumes the primary obstetric care responsibility, is warranted. In addition to routine obstetric care, perinatologists can offer an enhanced understanding of diagnosis and management of possible associated adverse obstetric complications. Ongoing communication with neonatology is critical in counseling expectant mothers and families about the postnatal course, for direction in developing a delivery and immediate care plan, and coordinating and interpreting input from other pediatric subspecialists. The neonatologist is the primary caretaker for the infant in the delivery room and in the neonatal intensive care unit (NICU), and thus often has the role to manage and synchronize all aspects of the multidisciplinary team, particularly in the most complex cases.

Maternal Issues Complicating Antenatal Management and Delivery

The risk of certain adverse pregnancy outcomes is increased in the setting of certain fetal anomalies. Fetal hydrops and polyhydramnios from a range of fetal causes can be associated with the so-called "mirror syndrome," whereby the mother develops edema and severe preeclampsia, a condition that may be life threatening.[10] Polyhydramnios caused by a variety of fetal anomalies can lead to preterm labor and preterm premature rupture of membranes. A substantial additive risk for certain fetal anomalies is premature delivery, either spontaneously because of the complications described previously or because of intervention for worsening fetal status near term.

Timing and Mode of Delivery

Planning for delivery is one of the most important aspects of the antepartum management of pregnancies complicated by fetal anomalies. The importance of input from all members of the multidisciplinary team cannot be understated. Decisions regarding timing and mode are often altered by the expected need for complex postnatal resuscitation. In general, spontaneous labor and vaginal delivery is the goal because this carries the lowest risk of maternal morbidity. However, medical and other requirements may supersede. For example, if immediate neonatal surgical intervention is anticipated, such as complete heart block potentially requiring pacemaker or obstructive cardiac lesions expected to require immediate catheterization, a planned cesarean delivery may be required. A planned induction may be of benefit in cases where the patient lives distant from the tertiary center where delivery is required to ensure appropriate maternal and neonatal care.

Recent reports have highlighted the risks of late preterm (34–37 weeks) and even early term (37–39 weeks) gestation compared with those delivered at 39 weeks gestation.[11] These data apply primarily to "elective" deliveries but the authors have made attempts to mitigate this risk whenever possible even in cases of pregnancies complicated by fetal anomalies. However, it is important to recognize that the goal of optimal fetal outcome is not only affected by the gestational age of delivery, but also by the location of institution and the team that is immediately available for resuscitation.[12]

DELIVERY, RESUSCITATION, AND APPROACH TO IMMEDIATE NEONATAL MANAGEMENT BY ANOMALY CATEGORIES
Congenital Heart Disease

Planning for delivery
Given advances in prenatal screening, genetic diagnosis, and fetal echocardiography, it is possible to anticipate the needs of a neonate with congenital heart disease (CHD). However, prenatal US misses some fetuses with even significant cyanotic CHD because of such factors as lesion type, fetal position, and sonographer expertise.[7] When a prenatal diagnosis is made, consultation by a multidisciplinary team including perinatology, pediatric cardiology, neonatology, and genetics should occur to develop an evidence-based plan for fetal surveillance, delivery planning, and management of the neonate on delivery.

Timing and mode of delivery
An important determinant of the outcomes of complex CHD is the clinical condition of the neonate before corrective surgery.[13,14] It is critical that delivery occur at a medical center capable of optimal intrapartum monitoring and neonatal resuscitation, evaluation, and management. Expectant mothers who live at a distance should be considered for induction of labor at 39 weeks gestation (or at least after 37 weeks gestation) if vaginal delivery is appropriate, or for planned cesarean delivery or more complex multidisciplinary delivery as required. It should be noted that earlier gestational age is an independent risk factor for adverse short-term and neurodevelopmental outcomes in

neonates with CHD,[15,16] and it is rare that early delivery must be performed for fetal indications but this can occur (eg, hydrops fetalis).

In a tertiary or quaternary care hospital with immediate availability of experienced neonatologists, pediatric cardiologists, and cardiovascular surgeons, spontaneous labor and vaginal delivery can frequently be recommended for a range of fetal CHD, including those with ductal-dependent circulation. The likelihood of fetal intolerance of labor in such cases may not be dramatically increased and many women can achieve a successful vaginal delivery.[17] However, for a subgroup prenatally suspected to be at high risk for need of immediate intervention (eg, d-transposition of the great vessels with restrictive atrial septal defect [ASD] or ductus arteriosus, hypoplastic left heart syndrome [HLHS] with restrictive ASD, or severe fetal bradycardia) a planned cesarean delivery with a multidisciplinary team in attendance, and in some cases, an operating room team assembled and awaiting delivery, may be required. Some have suggested ex utero intrapartum therapy (EXIT) to extracorporeal membrane oxygenation (ECMO) as a strategy for cases of HLHS with highly restrictive ASD.[18]

Delivery room resuscitation and anticipated immediate NICU needs
Each hospital has a specific approach to physical location and team duty assignments for the "resuscitation room" within or adjacent to the delivery room, and for the NICU. Therefore, the plans for each space noted here and in subsequent sections may vary. Particularly when the heart malformation is predicted to be cyanotic, delivery room preparations should include laryngoscope and appropriate endotracheal tubes; preparation of umbilical venous and arterial catheters; and prostaglandin E_1 infusion, as indicated by the patient's diagnosis. As with any high-risk delivery, the appropriate team must be assembled, with responsibilities for each member clearly assigned in advance.

In most cases of even complex, ductal-dependent fetal CHD, the infant does not require respiratory resuscitation or advanced airway management. The neonatology team can obtain vascular access, and prostaglandin E_1 infused at a low dose (0.01–0.025 μg/kg/min) to maintain patency of the ductus arteriosus. Because prostaglandin E_1 infusions may induce apnea in the neonate, endotracheal intubation may be required, but the authors have found this to occur rarely. Development of increasing respiratory distress, cyanosis, and impaired systemic perfusion despite appropriate management are ominous signs, which may indicate prenatally unanticipated complications including restrictive ASD in the setting of HLHS or transposition of the great vessels with intact ventricular septum, or total anomalous pulmonary venous return.

Characterizing the anomaly and additional neonatal evaluation
Comprehensive cardiac assessment should be performed on arrival of the neonate to the NICU, including conventional chest radiography, electrocardiography, and echocardiography. In addition to confirming or refining the prenatal diagnosis of CHD, echocardiography can provide evidence of unexpected serious complications before they manifest clinically. In tertiary care institutions with integrated multidisciplinary fetal management teams, the cardiology team is alerted to the impending delivery, and can perform a first echocardiogram simultaneous with the initial admission preparations by the neonatology team; both teams then provide a coordinated, early postnatal update for mother and family.

As with other major congenital anomalies, it is important to determine whether CHD exists in isolation or as part of a constellation of anomalies suggestive of a genetic syndrome. Thorough physical examination and review of initial radiographs for evidence of other malformations are important first steps in this process. If dysmorphic features are suspected, consultation with a geneticist is indicated. In addition, further subspecialty consultation, evaluations, and genetic testing (eg, fluorescent in-situ hybridization for 22q11 deletion) may be recommended based on the specific cardiac lesion or family history.

Intrathoracic Masses

Planning for delivery

Although congenital diaphragmatic hernia (CDH) and BPMs (including congenital cystic adenomatoid malformation [CCAM] and bronchopulmonary sequestrations) are embryologically and anatomically distinct, they may similarly affect fetal development, threaten fetal well-being, and cause severe respiratory failure in the infant. In the case of CDH, determination of liver position, measurement of the lung/head ratio by US or MRI, and presence of other anomalies provide prognostic information for a multidisciplinary team including perinatology, neonatology, and pediatric surgery, and in discussions with parents.[19–22] To date, no randomized trials of fetal surgical intervention for CDH has shown benefit over standard postnatal therapy,[23] but several trials of fetoscopic tracheal occlusion targeting the most severe cases are ongoing in Europe, South America, and the United States (ClinicalTrials.gov). The CCAM volume ratio has been used to identify fetal patients with CCAM at highest risk for development of hydrops, need for extremely close surveillance, and consideration for fetal intervention. Some cases of CCAM, especially those that are microcystic, may be amenable to treatment with antenatal corticosteroids.[24] However, even large fetal BPMs can reduce significantly in size prenatally to virtually undetectable by US,[25] an evolution that may alter the need to recommend delivery at a tertiary center.

Timing and mode of delivery

Because infants with CDH or very large BPM can present with severe respiratory failure on delivery, it is essential that delivery occur at a tertiary care center with the capacity for advanced neonatal resuscitation and neonatal respiratory and cardiac management, immediate availability pediatric surgery, and ECMO. It is most common for induction of labor to be scheduled with a plan for vaginal delivery, unless there are obstetric contraindications. Precise timing of delivery has been debated[26,27]; in general, the authors target 39 weeks, and have a low threshold for earlier delivery or planned cesarean in severe cases. If hydrops develops, consideration for early delivery may be required. It should be noted that some institutions have suggested an EXIT to ECMO strategy for the most severe CDH cases, EXIT to resection for extremely large BPM persisting through late gestation, or those with developing hydrops.[18,23,25,28]

Delivery room resuscitation and anticipated immediate NICU needs

Preparing for the delivery of a neonate with CDH or persistently very large BPM requires a comprehensive management plan from delivery room to NICU. The delivery room team should include physicians, nurses, and respiratory therapists experienced in advanced neonatal resuscitation. The presence of a pharmacist to assist with sedative and emergency medication administration should be considered. All members of the team should be aware of the most recent fetal imaging findings, including evolving hydrops, and prepared for implications to resuscitation. For CDH in particular, the use of bag-mask positive airway pressure should be avoided, and immediate intubation and low-pressure ventilation should be initiated. A nasogastric tube should be placed quickly to continuous suction. Thoracostomy tubes and drainage equipment should be readily available in the delivery room.

For infants with CDH, who are at high risk for pulmonary hypertension and hypercarbia, an umbilical artery catheter should be placed for continuous blood pressure monitoring and frequent blood gas analysis. Central venous access should also be obtained for inotropic infusions and total parenteral nutrition. Routine respiratory management of CDH has evolved over years to a "gentle ventilation" approach, including permissive hypercapnia and emphasis on limiting airway pressure and volutrauma,[29] and use of high-frequency oscillatory ventilation if conventional ventilation maneuvers produce inadequate response to meet goals. Many tertiary centers offer a trial of inhaled nitric oxide before a decision to institute ECMO. Surfactant is not given unless the infant is preterm with evidence of respiratory distress syndrome.[30] The approach to timing of surgical repair has also changed significantly over the decades, from immediate surgery in the past, to the current approach of delayed repair to allow for evaluation, stabilization, and resolution of significant pulmonary vascular reactivity.

For infants with large BPM, many but not all require ventilatory support after delivery. Infants with extremely large BPM, even without hydrops, may also rarely require ECMO. When clinically indicated by respiratory distress because of the mass, surgical resection is undertaken during the initial neonatal admission. In the absence of respiratory distress, surgery can be delayed for several months, and the infant is discharged with follow-up.

Characterizing the anomaly and additional neonatal evaluation

Routine chest radiograph should be performed for any infant with prenatally diagnosed intrathoracic mass. For infants with CDH, serial chest radiograph is required. Echocardiography is an important tool in the management of the infant with CDH to evaluate for potentially associated CHD, and for assessment and surveillance of pulmonary hypertension and right heart failure. Advanced imaging with MRI is usually not feasible for infants with CDH during the immediate neonatal period because of clinical instability, but bedside abdominal and thoracic US can further characterize findings noted on prenatal imaging. Congenital diaphragmatic hernia may be associated with other significant congenital anomalies, occasionally as part of a genetic syndrome. Consultation with a geneticist should be sought if other anomalies are discovered or dysmorphic features are suspected. Infants with BPM often are sufficiently stable to undergo preoperative imaging in the radiology suite if needed during the NICU course. Computed tomography (CT) and MRI both have been used to delineate the location, airway connectivity, and vasculature of these masses before surgery. In the absence of respiratory distress associated with BPM, CT or MRI is delayed to closer to the time of planned resection.

Fetal Airway Obstruction and High Risk for Neonatal Airway Obstruction

Planning for delivery

Fetal airway obstruction may occur at any level of the airway, and may be caused by several etiologies including external compression (eg, cervical teratoma, cervical lymphatic malformation) or intrinsic structural abnormalities (eg, tracheal or laryngeal stenosis or atresia). Fetuses with severe micrognathia may be at significant risk for airway obstruction at delivery, and the anatomy of the jaw may make securing an oropharyngeal airway extremely difficult.

Cervical lymphatic malformations (often referred to as cystic hygromas) presenting early in gestation are associated with a high rate of associated anomalies, hydrops, and fetal demise. Those presenting in the third trimester are less likely to be associated with these adverse findings; nevertheless a detailed search for anomalies and other causes for nonimmune hydrops should be performed in all cases.[31] Cervical teratomas are rare, but generally large and bulky, and significantly threaten fetal airway.[32] Congenital high airway obstruction syndrome (CHAOS) caused by congenital laryngeal atresia and tracheal atresia may be suspected when large echogenic fetal lungs and inverted or flat hemidiaphragms are seen on prenatal US in the presence of polyhydramnios.[33] Each of these distal obstructions may present with life-threatening respiratory distress that may not be remedied without creation of a surgical airway. Fetal MRI has been used as an adjunct diagnostic tool with US to allow more detailed visualization of the airways in these cases, and to allow the care teams for the expectant mother, fetus, and newborn to better assess the need for complex delivery room scenarios.[34] Although originally refined for deliveries after fetal surgical procedures, EXIT has been used as a delivery strategy to allow for the airway to be secured while remaining on placental support.[18,35] Micrognathia occurs most commonly and may be readily identified on antenatal US, particularly with three-dimensional and four-dimensional US. The degree to which prenatally observed micrognathia causes difficulties in obtaining an airway postnatally is challenging to predict. Given the high association with other anomalies, it is also extremely important that a thorough fetal evaluation has occurred before multidisciplinary counseling and consideration of the most appropriate delivery plan.

Timing and mode of delivery

All cases of suspected fetal airway obstruction should be referred for prenatal multidisciplinary evaluation and delivered at a tertiary care center with highly specialized neonatology, pediatric surgery, and pediatric otorhinolaryngology staff available at delivery. In the most severe cases, an EXIT delivery should be considered. The decision to recommend EXIT is a complex one, influenced by multiple maternal and fetal factors. It is critical to understand the complete findings of the fetal patient. If the airway anomaly is an isolated finding, EXIT may offer a life-saving tool. It is not simply an "enhanced cesarean delivery"; the mother is under deep anesthesia, and the uterus must remain relaxed so as to maintain uteroplacental circulation. EXIT requires a specialized perinatology and obstetric anesthesia team, in combination with expanded physician and nursing teams from neonatology, pediatric surgery, otorhinolaryngology, and pediatric anesthesiology. Detailed multidisciplinary consultation among subspecialists and with the expectant mother and family are necessary, relating all relevant risks and benefits for the EXIT procedure. Timing of delivery depends fetal health, development of hydrops, and progression of polyhydramnios leading to preterm labor. In CHAOS, approximately one-third of cases are thought to spontaneously perforate during the fetal course and decompress with resolution or stabilization of hydrops. Induction of labor at term gestation may be indicated in mild to moderate micrognathia, especially when the expectant mother lives at a distance from the tertiary center. In more concerning micrognathia cases, there is usually a low threshold for a planned cesarean delivery so that pediatric anesthesia and otorhinolaryngologist are available in the delivery room to perform an endoscopic airway examination or emergency tracheostomy. In all cases of suspected severe airway compromise, is advisable to prepare an ECMO circuit and alert the appropriate ECMO support services in advance of delivery.

Delivery room resuscitation and anticipated immediate NICU needs

If an EXIT procedure is planned, team preparation should begin well in advance of the delivery date, and contingency strategies in place in case delivery must be moved forward emergently. Roles for each member of the team must be determined, order of events reviewed, and algorithm and equipment list created. These complex deliveries usually take place in operating rooms that are not familiar to team members, therefore the details are important; how many people will be allowed in the room, who will stand where, how long will be allowed for each airway attempt before moving to the next phase and what team will be responsible for each, and even how long it will take to return to the NICU. Direct laryngoscopy and oropharyngeal intubation while on placental support is the optimal neonatal outcome for the EXIT procedure, but may require moving to rigid bronchoscopy, then retrograde intubation by tracheostomy with limited neck dissection, and finally even formal tracheostomy.[18,35]

Infants considered to have only mild or moderate micrognathia may also require advanced airway management on delivery. The resuscitation team should be familiar with the principles of positioning and trained in the use of a range of airway devices (eg, oral airway, laryngeal mask airway). All of these devices, sized according to the estimated fetal weight, should be immediately available at the time of delivery, as should a flow-inflating bag, facial mask, and endotracheal tube. The NICU staff responsible for the care of a neonate with severe micrognathia should be briefed on how to use ancillary airway devices, such as an oral airway and laryngeal mask airway. Once the pharyngeal obstruction has been relieved or bypassed, standard respiratory support measures should be sufficient to maintain adequate oxygenation and ventilation in affected neonates. Neonates affected by laryngeal or tracheal atresia who have survived resuscitation require mechanical ventilation for a variable period of time, depending on the gestational age at birth, the state of lung development, capillary leak, and presence or absence of hydrops fetalis. For those with CHAOS, because of stretch injury in utero caused by lung overdistention, diaphragmatic function may be impaired for many months.

Characterizing the anomaly and additional neonatal evaluation

Whether or not micrognathia is associated with other oropharyngeal anomalies, evaluation by a pediatric otorhinolaryngologist is essential. Physical and endoscopic examinations may help determine how best to position and feed an affected neonate and whether surgical interventions are required (eg, tracheostomy and gastrostomy). Micrognathia is often accompanied by retroglossia and cleft palate, a complex of findings referred to as Pierre Robin syndrome. The finding of micrognathia is highly associated with other anomalies and genetic or other syndromes; therefore, consultation with a geneticist or dysmorphologist is important to a complete neonatal evaluation. Although laryngeal atresia and tracheal atresia are best characterized by endoscopic examination, CT and MRI may be useful to assess the tracheobronchial anatomy and lung parenchyma.[33] Most cases of CHAOS are isolated, except for those associated with Fraser syndrome.[36] Infants with cervical teratoma are at risk for hypothyroidism and hypoparathyroidism and should be serially monitored. In the longer-term, they should be followed with serial alpha fetoprotein levels because of the potential for teratoma reoccurrence and the rare possibility of malignant transformation. In all cases of severe airway obstruction and ongoing respiratory compromise, infants ideally should be cared for in a center with specialized nutritional, occupational, developmental, and respiratory therapy services to optimize functional, growth, and developmental outcomes.

Encephalocele and Myelomeningocele

Planning for delivery

Encephalocele and myelomeningocele require prenatal multidisciplinary coordination with a team including pediatric neurosurgery. Although these can be identified by prenatal US as early as the first trimester, adjunct imaging with fetal MRI can reveal additional important CNS or other anomalies[37] that may affect prognosis.

Encephalocele is often associated with other anomalies, in the CNS and elsewhere, and a clear understanding of the severity and extent of other fetal findings is necessary to guide counseling and management.[38] Most myelomeningoceles are isolated, but have a range of associated intracranial findings including Chiari II malformations. Recent evidence suggests that prenatal repair of myelomeningocele may improve motor outcomes and reduces the need for ventricular shunting through very early childhood, and therefore referral of the mother for fetal surgery may be considered in selected cases.[39] However, open fetal surgery is associated with severe maternal morbidity and risk for premature delivery.

Timing and mode of delivery

Myelomeningocele and encephalocele pose very different challenges to the delivering obstetrician and the neonatal resuscitation team.[40] For both, the expectant mother should be referred for counseling and delivery planning at a site with an experienced, multidisciplinary team. Even in the case of encephalocele with a very poor predicated outcome, genetics, neurologic, developmental, and neurosurgical care may be required. For encephalocele, the recommended route of delivery is determined largely by prognostic factors, which include the extent of brain tissue in the herniated sac, hydrocephalus, and presence of other anomalies. In cases of extremely poor prognosis and parental decision to offer comfort care, delivery decisions should focus on minimizing maternal risk, and vaginal delivery should be offered. However, cesarean delivery should be considered when prognosis is guarded but unclear, parents wish to proceed with full intervention, or the encephalocele size is likely to cause challenges to vaginal delivery. Although delivery route for myelomeningocele is typically by cesarean delivery, the optimal route is controversial. Some centers have advocated for vaginal delivery in cases of very small lesions.

Delivery room and anticipated immediate NICU needs

Neonates with encephaolceles may require no more than routine resuscitative measures. However, spontaneous ventilation may be impaired because of airway obstruction or central apnea. Therefore, it is important that clear discussions between the expectant mother and a multidisciplinary group including medical social work, and an understanding of the family wishes occur well before delivery. Infants with myelomeningocele generally do not have respiratory distress, but the resuscitation team should nonetheless be prepared for advanced respiratory support efforts. On delivery, the neonate should be placed in prone or side-lying position to protect the exposed neural elements and prevent rupture of the membrane covering the defect. Sterile saline-soaked gauze should cover the defect, after which a plastic wrap covering should be applied. Empiric antibiotics should be initiated once a blood culture has been obtained. During all of these maneuvers, latex-free material must be used because of the high rate of latex allergy in these patients.

After admission to the NICU, a thorough physical examination assessing the level and extent of the defect, observation of lower extremity movement, anal wink, and other anomalies should be performed. A neurosurgical consult should be obtained. Latex precautions are essential in the management of myelomeningocele even after repair of the defect.

Characterizing the anomaly and additional neonatal evaluation

Particularly in cases of encephalocele, medical genetics consultation should be considered to determine whether the lesion is isolated or part of a syndrome, to obtain karyotype if not done prenatally, and for future pregnancy counseling. For myelomeningocele, closure of open defects occurs within 1 to 2 days. Serial cranial US should be obtained on admission to the NICU and in the days after repair to evaluate the evolution of hydrocephalus and whether shunt is required. Brain and spine MRI should be obtained at some point during initial hospitalization for patients with myelomeningocele. Neurosurgical evaluation and consultation is also critical in encephalocele cases, even for those in which prognosis is predicted to be very poor because elective surgery may be undertaken to facilitate care. Nearly all patients with myelomeningocele have bladder dysfunction. Renal bladder US should be performed soon after delivery and with serial follow-up. Urology, orthopedic surgery, and physical and occupational therapy should be consulted. Referral for follow-up should be made to a multidisciplinary spina bifida clinic with expertise in the range of complications associated with myelomeningocele (www.spinabifidaassociation.org).

Abdominal Wall Defects

Planning for delivery

Omphalocele and gastroschisis require coordination of care by a multidisciplinary team including perinatology, perinatal genetics, neonatology, and pediatric surgery. Imaging by fetal US may also identify associated congenital anomalies and involvement of additional protrusion of viscera, such as the liver in cases of giant omphalocele. Given the strong association of omphalocele with other malformations (50%–70%) and chromosomal abnormalities (30%–60%) a comprehensive fetal evaluation including echocardiogram and karyotype is indicated. Not surprisingly, a normal fetal karyotype portends a better outcome for neonates with omphalocele.[41] Delivery should be at a tertiary care center with availability of neonatologist and pediatric surgeons experienced in the care of abdominal wall defects.

Timing and mode of delivery

Although omphalocele and gastroschisis develop between the third and sixth weeks of gestation, their anatomic origins are distinct. Nevertheless, omphalocele and gastroschisis are managed similarly in advance of delivery. The timing of delivery is determined by fetal well-being and may be influenced by the apparent integrity of the intestines. In cases of gastroschisis, bowel dilation is a known risk factor for poor intestinal outcomes, although it is not clear whether this should prompt preterm delivery.[42] Recent data suggest that delivery by 37 weeks gestation should be considered in cases of gastroschisis because of the increased risk of meconium staining, intrauterine growth restriction, and stillbirth near term,[43,44] although a small randomized trial suggested no benefit to elective delivery at 36 weeks.[45] Likewise, the optimal mode of delivery remains controversial, although evidence suggests vaginal delivery is safe in gastroschisis.[46] For omphalocele with liver in the sac, cesarean delivery has been advocated because of concern for liver injury during delivery.[47]

Delivery room and anticipated immediate NICU needs

As is the case with all complex deliveries, the resuscitation team should have a briefing before a gastroschisis or omphalocele delivery to clarify the role of each member. Although attention may be focused on the extra-abdominal viscera, it is important to emphasize the fundamentals of neonatal resuscitation to optimize outcomes. Thermoregulation and fluid losses deserve special attention, because the neonate may lose considerable heat through the exposed viscera, and insensible fluid loss is significant. Likewise, approach to respiratory distress may be a challenge. Intubation may be indicated during early resuscitation, because bag-mask ventilation may distend the intestines with air making reduction of the bowel more difficult. Of note, giant omphalocele, defined broadly as defect size larger than 5 cm and liver in the sac, has been associated with increased risk for respiratory distress and pulmonary hypoplasia.[48] For all infants with abdominal wall defects, a large-caliber suction catheter should be passed into the stomach and placed to suction to assist in intestinal decompression.

Beyond these fundamental aspects of resuscitation, team members must work to protect the abdominal contents, particularly for gastroschisis. One option is to place a sterile plastic bag over the lower extremities and trunk of the newborn to the level of the nipple line. Another option to maintain bowel integrity is to apply warm, sterile saline-soaked gauze loosely around the lower abdomen and defect, which is then wrapped in plastic wrap to limit insensible losses. Excessive wet dressings should be avoided because of thermoregulation issues. Peripheral vascular access should be quickly obtained, and is preferred to umbilical catheterization to preserve the surgical field for placement of the abdominal contents into a silo, if indicated.[49] A peripherally inserted central catheter should also be placed in the NICU to provide for adequate total parenteral nutrition while awaiting return of bowel function. Heart rate, blood pressure, and peripheral perfusion should be closely monitored. The significant fluid requirements and risk for hypovolemia and hypoperfusion, particularly for the infant with gastroschisis, should not be underestimated. Crystalloid and colloid boluses may be required in the initial resuscitation over the first hours. In the first 24 hours, infants with gastroschisis may require two to three times the maintenance fluids expected for a normal newborn. Intravenous antibiotics are given in the NICU.

Neonates with omphalocele or gastroschisis require evaluation by a pediatric surgeon immediately after birth. Very small defects of either type may be reduced and surgically closed primarily. Larger gastroschisis defects may require containment of the viscera within a plastic silo secured with a spring-loaded base. Some sites have moved to using this staged, initial nonsurgical silo approach for most cases.[47] This approach, which results in reduction over days to weeks depending on the size of the defect, is thought to limit significant increased intra-abdominal pressure, allowing for avoidance of intubation or reduced time on mechanical ventilation, and theoretically reducing risk for ischemic bowel injury. If silo approach is undertaken, the NICU team must frequently assess the health of the bowel by visual inspection. Any sign of intestinal hypoperfusion (eg, dusky appearance) should be brought urgently to the surgeon's attention. Fluid loss around the base of the silo must be carefully noted and accounted for in the fluid management plan. When the defect is closed primarily or after staged silo reduction, it is critically important to monitor the patient's intra-abdominal pressure. Evidence of poor perfusion to the lower extremities, decreasing urine output, and oliguria are ominous signs that may indicate advanced hypovolemia or compartment syndrome.

Similar to the evolving approach to gastroschisis, neonates with moderate or large omphalocele may be treated with an initial nonoperative approach in which sulfadiazine dressings are applied to the membrane and changed periodically. This approach, previously used only in cases of multiple anomalies or if the infant was judged so unstable as not to tolerate surgery, uses a topical therapy followed by use of a compression bandage to reduce the abdominal contents gradually into the peritoneum. This option results in gradual epithelialization of the omphalocele sac, a process that may take months to complete and be continued after discharge. In the case of giant omphalocele, this approach may need to be augmented by specially created silos and abdominal splints, but may result in reduced morbidities.[50]

Characterizing the anomaly and additional neonatal evaluation

Neonates with omphalocele and gastroschisis require careful, comprehensive investigations in the NICU. All neonates with omphalocele should be assessed by a geneticist because of its frequent association with other anomalies, and as part of a broader syndrome including Beckwith-Wiedemann. Up to 30% of patients with omphalocele have chromosomal anomalies. Given the implications for family counseling and for future pregnancies, consultation by a medical genetics team is indicated.[51] Screening echocardiography, renal US, and imaging for other midline defects (eg, cranial US) is warranted. As the postrepair course unfolds, the neonatologist must remain vigilant and have a high index of suspicion for anatomic obstruction (eg, malrotation, intestinal atresia) and necrotizing enterocolitis in patients with abdominal wall defects.[52,53]

Skeletal Dysplasia

Planning for delivery
Abnormal skeletal development may be fairly well characterized by prenatal US, although the precise diagnosis may not be achieved until genetic studies postnatally. Skeletal dysplasia is most often suspected by the detection of curved, fractured, or shortened femurs, because this long bone is commonly measured on routine prenatal US. The skeletal dysplasias are a diverse and heterogeneous group of more than 350 disorders; therefore, once suspected, additional two-dimensional and three-dimensional US evaluation (including all long bones, cranium, facial profile, mandible, clavicle, scapula, chest circumference, and hands and feet), consideration for additional imaging including fetal MRI (eg, for vertebral visualization), and consultation with a perinatologist and perinatal geneticist are critical.[54] The two most commonly identified prenatally diagnosed skeletal dysplasias are atophoric dysplasia (TD) and osteogenesis imperfect (OI).[55] The challenge for the multidisciplinary team is to determine whether the skeletal dysplasia is likely to be lethal in the perinatal period, which is associated with significant pulmonary hypoplasia because of thoracic dysplasia. Thus, it is crucial to consult with perinatologists and perinatal geneticists with expertise in diagnosing skeletal dysplasias; this may require requesting remote evaluation of prenatal imaging. In experienced hands, when numerous specific US measurements are performed, prediction of perinatal lethality for prenatally detected skeletal dysplasia is highly accurate.[54,55] In the current era, prenatal molecular testing may be recommended in light of specific US findings, which may further improve diagnostic accuracy (eg, FGFR3 analysis for TD; COL1A1 and COL1A2 analysis for OI). Coordination of care and counseling between the perinatologist, neonatologist, geneticist, and pediatric orthopedic surgeon facilitates a consistent message for the expectant mother and family of the affected fetus.

Timing and mode of delivery
Coordination of care also promotes high-quality, patient-centered care at the time of delivery. As fetal information is clarified, all neonatal providers involved in the mother's care must understand whether intensive care or palliative care measures will be provided on delivery. This decision must be predicated on the best available diagnostic information, outcomes data, and on-going, open discussions with the expectant mother and family of the affected fetus in a multidisciplinary setting. There are challenges to delivery planning for the most commonly prenatally diagnosed skeletal dysplasias. For TD, polyhydramnios and premature labor frequently complicates the pregnancy, and cephalopelvic disproportion complicates delivery. A short and rigid fetal neck, coupled with an abnormal skull and hydrocephalus, may make cesarean delivery necessary for the safety of the mother, despite a grave prognosis for the fetus. In a review of 167 fetuses with suspected OI, cesarean section delivery was not found to decrease fracture rates for infants with nonperinatal lethal type OI or prolong survival for those with perinatal lethal OI.[56] The most common reason for cesarean delivery in that series was malpresentation at labor. Thus, many sites have instituted

a general approach to reserve cesarean delivery in cases of suspected OI for maternal and obstetric indications.

Delivery room and anticipated immediate NICU needs

The resuscitation of a newborn with skeletal dysplasia may require special consideration of pulmonary hypoplasia or bone fragility. A predelivery briefing between all obstetric, genetics, and neonatal providers enables the resuscitation team to understand the current status of the fetus and most likely diagnosis. In cases where full resuscitative measures will be undertaken, preparing for airway management must include assembling the appropriately sized laryngoscope and endotracheal tube, and discussing the potential use of higher peak inspiratory pressures in the event the infant shows signs of pulmonary hypoplasia and restrictive lung disease.[57] It is especially important to anticipate pneumothorax in such cases. This possibility for intervention, and other potential advanced resuscitative measures, must be discussed during consultations with the expectant mother and family in advance of delivery to determine their wishes for escalation of care.

Although no specific guidelines are established for the initial special considerations for the newborn with suspected non-lethal OI, careful handling of the newborn is appropriate. Despite the concern for the immediate development of additional fractures, resuscitation may include chest compressions without the development of rib fractures.[58]

If the newborn with clinically significant skeletal dysplasia survives the initial assessment and resuscitation, admission to the NICU is appropriate. In some cases, advanced level of respiratory support may be required in the setting of pulmonary hypoplasia, so the NICU team should anticipate and prepare for this by designating a high-frequency oscillator for use by the patient. In more stable infants with suspected skeletal dysplasias, complex multidisciplinary diagnostic and care planning may also be required. Close communication with the family is necessary to update them on the newborn's response to intensive care. Education of the bedside providers regarding the appropriate care of a patient with prenatal fractures may prevent further fractures and model safe behaviors for the family.

Characterizing the anomaly and additional neonatal evaluation

Whether or not a diagnosis was made prenatally, consultation with a geneticist is indicated. The differential diagnosis for this broad spectrum of anomalies is extensive and requires a combination of thorough physical and radiographic examination, biochemical investigation (metabolic, peroxisomal, calcium, phosphate and albumin), and genetic molecular testing.[59]

The newborn with skeletal dysplasia who survives the initial hospitalization also needs longitudinal care in a multidisciplinary model. Pharmacologic therapy may be considered for severe OI.[60] Health maintenance guidelines for achondroplasia have been developed and are available to family and medical providers.[61]

REFERENCES

1. Verweij EJ, van den Oever JM, de Boer MA, et al. Diagnostic accuracy of noninvasive detection of fetal trisomy 21 in maternal blood: a systematic review. Fetal Diagn Ther 2012;31:81–6.
2. American Institute of Ultrasound in Medicine. American Institute of Ultrasound in Medicine practice guideline for the performance of obstetric ultrasound examinations. J Ultrasound Med 2010;29:157–66.

3. Merz E, Abramowicz JS. 3D/4D ultrasound in prenatal diagnosis. Is it time for routine use? Clin Obstet Gynecol 2012;55:336–51.

4. Cassart M, Massez A, Cos T, et al. Contribution of three-dimensional computed tomography in the assessment of fetal skeletal dysplasia. Ultrasound Obstet Gynecol 2007;29:537–43.

5. Chen CP, Shih JC, Hsu CY, et al. Prenatal three-dimensional/four-dimensional sonographic demonstration of facial dysmorphisms associated with holoprosencephaly. J Clin Ultrasound 2005;33:312–8.

6. Yagel S, Kivilevitch Z, Cohen SM, et al. The fetal venous system, part I: normal embryology, anatomy, hemodynamics, ultrasound evaluation and Doppler investigation. Ultrasound Obstet Gynecol 2010;35:741–50.

7. Friedberg MK, Silverman NH, Moon-Grady AJ, et al. Prenatal detection of congenital heart disease. J Pediatr 2009;155:26–34.

8. Malone FD, Canick JA, Ball RH, et al, First- and Second-Trimester Evaluation of Risk (FASTER) Research Consortium. First-trimester or second-trimester screening, or both, for Down's syndrome. N Engl J Med 2005;10(353):2001–11.

9. Whitworth M, Bricker L, Neilson JP, et al. Ultrasound for fetal assessment in early pregnancy. Cochrane Database Syst Rev 2010;(4):CD007058.

10. Braun T, Brauer M, Fuchs I, et al. Mirror syndrome: a systematic review of fetal associated conditions, maternal presentation and perinatal outcome. Fetal Diagn Ther 2010;27:191–203.

11. Tita AT, Lai Y, Landon MB, et al, Eunice Kennedy Shriver National Institute of Child Health, Human Development (NICHD) Maternal-Fetal Medicine Units Network (MFMU). Timing of elective repeat cesarean delivery at term and maternal perioperative outcomes. Obstet Gynecol 2011;117(2 Pt 1):280–6.

12. Calisti A, Oriolo L, Giannino G, et al. Delivery in a tertiary center with co-located surgical facilities makes the difference among neonates with prenatally diagnosed major abnormalities. J Matern Fetal Neonatal Med 2012;25(9):1735–7.

13. Fuller S, Nord AS, Gerdes M, et al. Predictors of impaired neurodevelopmental outcomes at one year of age after infant cardiac surgery. Eur J Cardiothorac Surg 2009;36(1):40–7.

14. Mahle WT, Clancy RR, Moss EM, et al. Neurodevelopmental outcome and lifestyle assessment in school-aged and adolescent children with hypoplastic left heart syndrome. Pediatrics 2000;105(5):1082–9.

15. Goff DA, Luan X, Gerdes M, et al. Younger gestational age is associated with worse neurodevelopmental outcomes after cardiac surgery in infancy. J Thorac Cardiovasc Surg 2012;143(3):535–42.

16. Costello JM, Polito A, Brown DW, et al. Birth before 39 weeks gestation is associated with worse outcomes in neonates with heart disease. Pediatrics 2010;126:e277–84.

17. Peterson AL, Quartermain MD, Ades A, et al. Impact of mode of delivery on markers of perinatal hemodynamics in infants with hypoplastic left heart syndrome. J Pediatr 2011;159(1):64–9.

18. Marwan A, Crombleholme TM. The EXIT procedure: principles, pitfalls, and progress. Semin Pediatr Surg 2006;15:107–15.

19. Jani J, Keller RL, Benachi A, et al. Antenatal-CDH-Registry Group. Prenatal prediction of survival in isolated left-sided diaphragmatic hernia. Ultrasound Obstet Gynecol 2006;27(1):18–22.

20. Jani J, Nicolaides KH, Keller RL, et al, Antenatal-CDH-Registry Group. Observed to expected lung area to head circumference ratio in the prediction of survival in fetuses with isolated diaphragmatic hernia. Ultrasound Obstet Gynecol 2007;30(1):67–71.

21. Hedrick HL, Danzer E, Merchant A, et al. Liver position and lung-to-head ratio for prediction of extracorporeal member oxygenation and survival in isolated left congenital diaphragmatic hernia. Am J Obstet Gynecol 2007;197:422.e1–4.

22. Kilian AK, Schaible T, Hofmann V, et al. Congenital diaphragmatic hernia: predictive value of MRI relative lung-to-head ratio compared with MRI fetal lung volume and sonographic lung-to-head ratio. AJR Am J Roentgenol 2009; 192(1):153–8.

23. Hedrick HL. Management of prenatally diagnosed congenital diaphragmatic hernia. Semin Fetal Neonatal Med 2010;15:21–7.

24. Curran PF, Jelin EB, Rand L, et al. Prenatal steroids for microcystic congenital cystic adenomatoid malformations. J Pediatr Surg 2010;45(1):145–50.

25. Adzick NS. Management of fetal lung lesions. Clin Perinatol 2009;36:363–76.

26. Hutcheon JA, Butler B, Lisonkova S, et al. Timing of delivery for pregnancies with congenital diaphragmatic hernia. BJOG 2010;117:1658–62.

27. Stevens TP, van Wingaarden E, Ackerman KG, et al, The CDH Study Group. Timing of delivery and survival rates for infants with prenatal diagnoses of congenital diaphragmatic hernia. Pediatrics 2009;123:494–502.

28. Cass DL, Olutoye OO, Cassady CI, et al. Prenatal diagnosis and outcome of fetal lung masses. J Pediatr Surg 2011;46:292–8.

29. Kays D, Langham M, Ledbetter D Jr, et al. Detrimental effects of standard medical therapy in congenital diaphragmatic hernia. Ann Surg 1999;230:340–8.

30. Van Meurs KP, CDH Study Group. Is surfactant therapy beneficial in the treatment of the term newborn infant with congenital diaphragmatic hernia? J Pediatr 2004; 145:312–6.

31. Gedikbasi A, Gul A, Sargin A, et al. Cystic hygroma and lymphangioma: associated findings, perinatal outcome, and prognostic factors in live-born infants. Arch Gynecol Obstet 2007;276:491–8.

32. Berge SJ, von Lindern JJ, Appel T. Diagnosis and management of cervical teratomas. Br J Oral Maxillofac Surg 2004;42:41–5.

33. Mong A, Johnson AM, Kramer SS, et al. Congenital high airway obstruction syndrome: MR/US findings, effect on management, and outcome. Pediatr Radiol 2008;38(11):1171–9.

34. Courtier J, Poder L, Wang ZJ, et al. Fetal tracheolaryngeal airway obstruction: prenatal evaluation by sonography and MRI. Pediatr Radiol 2010;40(11):1800–5.

35. Liechty KW. Ex-utero intrapartum therapy. Semin Fetal Neonatal Med 2010;15: 34–9.

36. Schauer GM, Dunn LK, Godmilow L. Prenatal diagnosis of Fraser syndrome at 18.5 weeks' gestation, with autopsy findings at 19 weeks. Am J Med Genet 1990;37:583–91.

37. Saleem SN, Said AH, Abdel-Raouf M, et al. Fetal MRI in the evaluation of fetuses referred for sonographically suspected neuro tube defects: impact on diagnosis and management decisions. Neuroradiology 2009;41:761–8.

38. Siffel C, Wong LY, Olney RS, et al. Survival of infants diagnosed with encephalocele in Atlanta 1979-1998. Paediatr Perinat Epidemiol 2003;17:40–8.

39. Adzick NS, Thom EA, Spong CY, et al, MOMS Investigators. A randomized trial of prenatal versus postnatal repair of myelomeningocele. N Engl J Med 2011; 364(11):993–1004.

40. Lo BW, Kulkarni AV, Rutka JT, et al. Clinical predictors of developmental outcome in patients with cephaloceles. J Neurosurg Pediatr 2008;2:254–7.

41. Heider AL, Strauss RA, Kuller JA. Omphalocele: clinical outcomes in cases with normal karyotypes. Am J Obstet Gynecol 2004;190(1):135–41.

42. Piper HG, Jaksic T. The impact of prenatal bowel dilation on clinical outcomes in neonates with gastroschisis. J Pediatr Surg 2006;41(5):897–900.
43. Santiago-Munoz PC, McIntire DD, Barber RG, et al. Outcomes of pregnancies with fetal gastroschisis. Obstet Gynecol 2007;110(3):663–8.
44. Lausman AY, Langer JC, Tai M, et al. Gastroschisis: what is the average gestational age of spontaneous delivery? J Pediatr Surg 2007;42(11):1816–21.
45. Logge HL, Mason GC, Thornton JG, et al. A randomized controlled trial of elective preterm delivery of fetuses with gastroschisis. J Pediatr Surg 2005;40:1726–31.
46. Abdel-Latif ME, Bolisetty S, Abeywardana S, et al, Australian, New Zealand Neonatal Network. Mode of delivery and neonatal survival of infants with gastroschisis in Australia and New Zealand. J Pediatr Surg 2008;43(9):1685–90.
47. Christison-Lagay ER, Kelleher CM, Langer JC. Neonatal abdominal wall defects. Semin Fetal Neonatal Med 2011;16:164–72.
48. Kamata SN, Usui N, Sawai T, et al. Prenatal detection of pulmonary hypoplasia in giant omphalocele. Pediatr Surg Int 2008;24:107e11–8.
49. Anderson J, Leonard D, Braner DA, et al. Umbilical vascular catheterization. N Engl J Med 2008;359:e18.
50. Lee SL, Beyer TD, Kim SS, et al. Initial nonoperative management and delayed closure for treatment of giant omphaloceles. J Pediatr Surg 2006;41(11):1846–9.
51. Paidas MJ, Crombleholme TM, Robertson FM. Prenatal diagnosis and management of the fetus with an abdominal wall defect. Semin Perinatol 1994;18:196–214.
52. Kronfi R, Bradnock TJ, Sabharwal A. Intestinal atresia in association with gastroschisis: a 26-year review. Pediatr Surg Int 2010;26(9):891–4.
53. Oldham KT, Coran AG, Drongowski RA, et al. The development of necrotizing enterocolitits following repair of gastroschisis: a surprisingly high incidence. J Pediatr Surg 1988;23(10):945–9.
54. Krakow D, Lachman RS, Rimoin DL. Guidelines for the prenatal diagnosis of fetal skeletal dysplasias. Genet Med 2009;11:127–33.
55. Schramm T, Gloning KP, Minderer S, et al. Prenatal sonographic diagnosis of skeletal dysplasias. Ultrasound Obstet Gynecol 2009;34:160–70.
56. Cubert R, Cheng E, Mack S, et al. Osteogenesis imperfecta: mode of delivery and neonatal outcome. Obstet Gynecol 2001;97(1):66–9.
57. Mogayzel PJ, Marcus CL. Skeletal dysplasia and their effect on the respiratory system. Paediatr Respir Rev 2001;2(4):365–71.
58. Sewell RD, Steinberg MA. Chest compressions in an infant with osteogenesis imperfecta type II: no new rib fractures. Pediatrics 2000;106(5):E71.
59. Hurst JA, Firth HV, Smithson S. Skeletal dysplasia. Semin Fetal Neonatal Med 2005;10:233–41.
60. Poltkin H, Racuh F, Bishop NJ, et al. Pamidronate treatment of sever osteogenesis imperfecta in children under 3 years of age. J Clin Endocrinol Metab 2000;85:1846–50.
61. Trotter TI, Hall JG, Committee on Genetics. Health supervision for children with achondroplasia [Erratum appears in Pediatrics 2005;116(6):1615]. Pediatrics 2005;116:771–83.

Optimal Timing for Clamping the Umbilical Cord After Birth

Tonse N.K. Raju, MD, DCh[a],*, Nalini Singhal, MD, DCh[b]

KEYWORDS

- Early cord clamping • Delayed cord clamping • Umbilical cord milking

KEY POINTS

- Evolving data indicate that cord clamping about 30 to 60 seconds after all births may be of benefit for all infants. For term infants, this offers higher iron stores, and decreases iron deficiency anemia, a major issue in low-income and middle-income countries. Because of this, the World Health Organization (WHO) has recommended delayed cord clamping for all infants after birth in low-income and middle-income countries.[1,2] In preterm infants, a delay in cord clamping increases hemoglobin concentration and systemic blood pressure, reduces the need for blood transfusions, and reduces the frequency of all grades of intraventricular hemorrhage.
- The benefits of delayed cord clamping in all term infants in industrialized countries, however, need to be weighed against the possibility of more infants developing jaundice and needing phototherapy, especially in settings where early discharge is commonly practiced.
- Milking of the umbilical cord seems to provide similar benefits as delaying umbilical cord clamping. Moreover, either of these procedures do not adversely affect any of the immediate birth outcomes, such as Apgar scores, umbilical cord pH, or respiratory distress.
- Although maternal outcomes have not been rigorously studied, the incidence of postpartum hemorrhage or retained placenta does not increase with delayed cord clamping.

Another thing very injurious to the child, is the tying and cutting of the navel string too soon; which should always be left till the child has not only repeatedly breathed but till all pulsation in the cord ceases. As otherwise the child is much weaker than it ought to be, a portion of the blood being left in the placenta, which ought to have been in the child…

—*Erasmus Darwin*[3]

Most mammals in the animal kingdom wait until the expulsion of the placenta to sever the umbilical cord from a newborn after delivery. In humans, the attendant aiding the

[a] Eunice Kennedy Shriver National Institute of Child Health and Human Development, National Institutes of Health, 6100 Executive Boulevard, 4B03, Bethesda, MD 20892, USA; [b] University of Calgary, 2888 Shaganappi Trail Northwest, Calgary, Alberta T3B 6C8, Canada
* Corresponding author.
E-mail address: rajut@mail.nih.gov

Clin Perinatol 39 (2012) 889–900
http://dx.doi.org/10.1016/j.clp.2012.09.006
0095-5108/12/$ – see front matter Published by Elsevier Inc.

perinatology.theclinics.com

delivery clamps and severs the umbilical cord, much before the placenta is delivered—often within a few seconds of an infant's birth. However, the optimal timing for clamping of the umbilical cord in human infants after birth has remained controversial.

The practice of early cord clamping started in the twentieth century, with an increasing number of women opting for hospital births and an increasing number of obstetricians conducting such deliveries. Before the mid-1950s, the term, *early clamping*, was loosely defined as cord clamping approximately 1 minute after birth, and *late clamping* was usually reserved for clamping done more than 5 minutes after birth. In a series of studies on blood volume changes after birth performed by investigators in Sweden, the United States, and Canada, it was reported that in healthy term infants, more than 90% of blood volume is achieved within the first few breaths infants take after birth.[4] Because of these findings and the lack of specific recommendations on the optimal timing, the interval between birth and cord clamping began to be shortened.

THE PROS AND CONS OF EARLY VERSUS DELAYED CLAMPING

At present, in most deliveries, cord clamping is performed soon after birth, often before 10 to 15 seconds after birth, with the baby maintained at or below the level of the placenta. This practice probably evolved with intent to carryout resuscitation of preterm and depressed term infants as soon after birth as possible. The benefit of immediate cord clamping after birth, however, has not been demonstrated. In addition to the timing of cord clamping, the location of the baby at or below the level of the introitus affects placental transfusion.

Because of many demonstrated benefits from delaying cord clamping, in recent years, several international organizations and entities have recommended this practice (**Table 1**), albeit with a caveat, "if (or whenever) possible."[1,2,5–7] According to a European consensus, delayed cord clamping is the first step of resuscitation for infants at risk for respiratory distress syndrome.[6]

There are valid concerns, however, about universally adopting delayed cord clamping. Some of the concerns are that there can be a delay in performing timely resuscitation when needed, that the practice may interfere with attempts to collect cord blood for banking purposes, and that it may increase the potential for excessive placental transfusion, leading to neonatal polycythemia, especially in pregnancies with risk factors, such as maternal diabetes, severe intrauterine growth restriction, and living in high altitudes.

Yet, equally valid counterpoints have been proposed to support delayed cord clamping. Because the placenta continues to perform gas exchange after delivery, sick and preterm infants are likely to benefit most from additional blood volume derived from a delay in cord clamping—echoing the recommendation of the European expert consensus.[6] The American Congress of Obstetricians and Gynecologists opined that the routine practice of umbilical cord clamping should not be altered for the collection of cord blood for banking.[8] Neonatal polycythemia has not been observed at higher frequencies among infants in delayed cord clamping groups in several systematic reviews and in large randomized controlled studies.[9–13]

PHYSIOLOGIC RATIONALE

A series of physiologic studies between 1960 and 1980 showed that factors facilitating placental-to-neonatal blood transfusion include initiation of extrauterine breathing, gravity, and the position of the infants relative to the placenta; the time of clamping of the umbilical cord; the patency of the umbilical blood vessels; and uterine contractions.[3,14] Recent experimental works in pregnant sheep have provided additional

Table 1
International organizations statements on optimal timing for clamping umbilical cord

Organizations and/or Professional Societies and Scientific Groups	Statement	References
WHO	In preterm infants, delaying cord clamping by 30–120 s seems associated with less need for blood transfusion and less intraventricular hemorrhage. The beneficial effects of delayed cord clamping may yield the greatest benefits in settings where access to health care is limited. For term infants: to reduce the risk of postpartum hemorrhage in the mother, WHO recommends clamping the cord after the approximately 3 min after birth. For infants, there is growing evidence that delayed cord clamping is beneficial and can improve the iron status for up to 6 months after birth. This may be particularly relevant for infants living in low-resource settings with less access to iron-rich foods.	[1,2]
Society of Obstetricians and Gynaecologists of Canada	Whenever possible, delaying cord clamping by at least 60 s is preferred to clamping because there is less intraventricular hemorrhage and less need for transfusion in those with late clamping.	[5]
European Association of Perinatal Medicine	If possible, delay clamping of the umbilical cord for at least 30–45 s with the baby held below the mother to promote placento-fetal transfusion: evidence grade A.	[6]
International Liaison Committee on Resuscitation	Delay in umbilical cord clamping for at least 1 min is recommended for newborn infants not requiring resuscitation. There is insufficient evidence to support or refute a recommendation to delay cord clamping in babies requiring resuscitation.	[7]

insights into the dynamics of transitional circulation after birth, breathing, and cord clamping. After umbilical cord clamping, the right ventricle filling volume drops abruptly (due to cessation of umbilical venous blood flow into the right ventricle), leading to a drop in right ventricle output by approximately 50%. Cord clamping that leads to umbilical arterial occlusion causes a marked increase in left ventricular afterload from a lack of low-resistance placental circulation[15–18] and increased left ventricular diameter at the end of diastole,[19] potentially leading to a drop in cardiac output (discussed later).

Many physiologic benefits have been documented in clinical studies, too, from delayed cord clamping. Preterm infants in a delayed cord clamping group had significantly higher superior vena cava blood flow and greater right ventricular output and stroke volumes that persisted up to 48 hours after birth.[19] Baenziger and colleagues[20] showed higher values for mean regional cerebral tissue oxygenation in a delayed cord clamping group at 4 hours of age (69.9% vs 65.5%), which persisted at 24 hours of age (71.3% vs 68.1%).

Another concern often expressed is the potential delay in resuscitating an infant born after emergency instrument delivery due to fetal distress and/or perinatal asphyxia. It is precisely in such situations that delayed cord clamping has potential to be beneficial. Fetal distress, secondary to intrauterine cord compression, leads to selective clamping of the thin-walled umbilical vein carrying oxygenated blood from the placenta to the fetus, without occluding the thicker-walled umbilical arteries carrying deoxygenated blood from the fetus to the placenta.[21] Because the latter blood has no chance of returning to the fetus, fetal oxygenated blood volume gets depleted. According to Hutchon,[21] a delayed cord clamping (40 seconds has been a standard in his unit) and additional placental transfusion can be immensely beneficial for infants born with a history of fetal distress from umbilical cord compression; this should be deemed the first step of neonatal resuscitation.

An additional issue to be considered is the immediate establishment of pulmonary ventilation. Based on fetal/neonatal lamb experiments, Hooper proposes the following 3 scenarios that might be encountered in clinical settings (S.B. Hooper, PhD, personal communications, 2012).

1. The best scenario is that infants start breathing soon after birth and the umbilical cord is clamped at least 30 to 60 seconds after establishing pulmonary ventilation. The importance of pulmonary ventilation is that it stimulates a decrease in pulmonary vascular resistance and an increase in pulmonary blood flow after birth. This is necessary to replace the venous return to the left ventricle that is lost after cord occlusion. During fetal life, umbilical venous blood flow via the foramen ovale had been an important factor contributing to the filling of left atrium and left ventricle, thus maintaining optimal cardiac output. Thus, the sequence of events (described previously) postnatally facilitates an increase in pulmonary venous return carrying oxygenated blood, establishing adequate left atrial and left ventricular filling and cardiac output, leading to a smooth cardiovascular transition.

2. Although not ideal, an acceptable scenario is that infants breathe and cry soon after birth, and the cord is also clamped right at that time. Here, too, the cardiovascular transition may proceed seemingly smoothly (which happens in most term infants), despite a diminished blood volume and a fall in right ventricular filling due to immediate cord clamping. Because of lung aeration, however, and possibly the existence of adequate capacitance in a healthy term infant, the left ventricular output may not be affected.

3. The worst scenario is that infants do not breathe immediately after birth, and the umbilical cord is occluded soon after birth. The extent of adverse events would then depend on, among other things (eg, pre-existing cardiac failure, pulmonary compliance, degree of pulmonary hypertension and so forth), the effectiveness of the bag-and-mask ventilation. Because the umbilical venous flow into the right heart (containing oxygenated blood from the placenta) drops by approximately 50% on cord occlusion, flow through the foramen ovale into the left heart must also drop proportionately. If assisted ventilation does not establish proper aeration of the lungs for whatever reason, pulmonary vascular resistance remains high, preventing the normal increase of pulmonary blood flow and return of oxygenated blood via the pulmonary veins into the left atrium. These events lead to a significant drop in left ventricular output. Then, if the caregivers opt to administer fluid boluses in rapid sequence, a stage may be set to increase the likelihood of intraventricular hemorrhage, especially in very preterm infants, with an already maximally vasodilated cerebral vascular bed superimposed on an immature cerebral autoregulatory systems.

TERM NEWBORNS

It is estimated that 3.6 billion people in the world are iron deficient and 2 billion of them have overt iron deficiency anemia.[22] Iron deficiency anemia is also highly prevalent in women of reproductive age and children under 5 years of age in low-income and middle-income countries. In areas of the world where maternal iron deficiency anemia is common, up to 30% of infants have iron deficiency anemia. In industrialized countries, iron deficiency is prevented by iron supplementation, a practice that is difficult to implement in low-resources settings. Many studies dating back several decades have confirmed that delayed umbilical cord clamping at birth enhances red cell mass and improves iron status during infancy.[9,23–29] In term infants, 1-minute delay in cord clamping after birth leads to an additional 80 mL of blood from the placenta to an infant's circulation, which increases to approximately 100 mL by 3 minutes after birth. This additional blood (plasma and the red cell mass) adds to extra iron, amounting to 40 mg/kg to 50 mg/kg of body weight. Such supplemental iron from placental transfusion, combined with the approximately 75 mg/kg of body iron present at birth in a full-term newborn, may help prevent iron deficiency during the first year of life.[30]

Several studies have documented that in term infants, delaying cord clamping leads to higher hemoglobin/hematocrit soon after birth, which persists up to 4 to 6 months of age.[12,13,29–39] The mean hemoglobin advantage was between 2 g/dL to 3 g/dL. In another study, the circulating ferritin levels remained higher in infants in the late clamping group until 6 months: weighted mean difference $+11.8\,\mu g/L$ (95% CI, 4.07–19.53).[30]

Although none of the studies of delayed cord clamping has reported an increased risk of clinically significant polycythemia due to delayed cord clamping, the relationship between delayed cord clamping and polycythemia, hyperbilirubinemia, and phototherapy requirements has not been consistent. The investigators of a meta-analysis of 1762 infants reported significantly higher rates of phototherapy (relative risk [RR] 1.69; 95% CI, 1.08–2.63) and clinical jaundice[9] in infants in the delayed cord clamping group. Indications for phototherapy in different reports, however, were not described. Moreover, the studies that reported polycythemia did not report increased need for phototherapy. The studies that reported increased need for phototherapy also reported similar levels of bilirubin in the early and delayed cord clamping group. **Box 1** provides a list of reported benefits from delayed cord clamping in term infants.

PRETERM NEWBORNS

In a systematic review of 10 trials of early versus delayed cord clamping in 454 preterm infants under 37 weeks' gestation, no statistically significant differences were found between the groups in cord blood pH (weighted mean difference, 0.01; 95% CI, −0.03–0.05), Apgar scores (RR for 5-min Apgar <8, 1.17; 95% CI, 0.62–2.20), and temperature on admission (weighted mean difference, 0.14°C; 95% CI, −0.31−0.03).[8]

The only study to the authors' knowledge that evaluated the feasibility of neonatal resuscitation with the cord still attached to the placenta also measured infant blood volume and concluded that delayed cord clamping resulted in higher blood volumes.[40]

Box 1
Reported benefits of delayed cord clamping: term infants

- Higher hemoglobin at 4–12 months of age
- Improved serum ferritin during the first year
- Improved total body iron stores at 1 year of age
- Improved survival from malaria in endemic regions
- Lower circulating lead levels in regions with high air pollution
  - Competitive effect between iron and lead

Several studies have documented higher blood pressure and higher red blood cell volume and hemoglobin.[10,18,40–47] The benefits of delayed cord clamping included a reduced need for blood transfusions for treating low blood pressure (RR 0.39; 95% CI, 0.18–0.85) and anemia (RR 0.49; 95% CI, 0.31–0.81).[46]

In their systematic review, Rabe and colleagues[9] reported that in 7 of 10 trials, the incidence of any grade of intraventricular hemorrhage was significantly lower in the delayed cord clamping groups (P<.002). The incidence of intraventricular hemorrhage was 47 of 164 (28.7%) in the early cord clamping groups compared with 27 of 165 (16.4%) in the delayed cord clamping groups, for an increased RR of 1.90 (95% CI, 1.27–2.84) with early cord clamping. Considering that the infant death rate was similar between 2 groups (RR 1.40, 95% CI, 0.59–3.32 between early versus late cord clamping groups), an approximately 2-fold reduced risk for intraventricular hemorrhage with delayed cord clamping should be deemed an important benefit. In none of the reports was there an increased need for exchange transfusion for polycythemia, and/or hyperbilirubinemia.

Rabe and colleagues[48] recently updated their systematic review on cord clamping in 738 preterm infants born between 24 and 36 weeks of gestation among the 15 eligible studies for review. The maximum delay in cord clamping was 180 seconds. The investigators concluded that delaying cord clamping was associated with fewer infants requiring transfusions for anemia (7 trials, 392 infants; RR 0.61; 95% CI, 0.46–0.81) and for low blood pressure (4 trials with estimable data for 90 infants; RR 0.52; 95% CI, 0.28–0.94) and reduced frequency of any (all grades) of intraventricular hemorrhage diagnosed by cranial ultrasound (10 trials, 539 infants; RR 0.59; 95% CI, 0.41–0.85) compared with immediate clamping groups. There were no clear differences among the groups for infant death, severe (grade 3 to 4) intraventricular hemorrhage, and periventricular leukomalacia. For several of these outcomes, however, reporting was incomplete, and the estimates provided wide CIs. Outcomes after discharge from the hospital was reported in only 1 small study; no significant differences between the groups (n = 58) in mean Bayley Scales of Infant Development II scores at 7 months of age corrected for prematurity.[48] **Box 2** provides a list of reported benefits from delayed cord clamping in preterm infants.

UMBILICAL CORD MILKING

There are only a few reports of milking of the umbilical cord, which include one clinical trial and a secondary analysis from the same trial,[49,50] a randomized controlled trial,[50]

Box 2
Reported benefits from delayed cord clamping: preterm infants

- Higher circulating blood volume for 24–48 hours
- Fewer blood transfusions
- Better systemic blood pressure
- Reduced need for inotropic support
- Increased blood flow in the superior vena cava
- Increased left ventricular output
- Higher cerebral oxygenation index
- Lower frequency of any intracranial hemorrhage
  - No difference in rates of severe intraventricular hemorrhage

and a study assessing cerebral oxygenation.[51] Hosono and colleagues[49,50] compared milking of a 20-cm segment of the umbilical cord 2 to 3 times, with immediate cord clamping in preterm singleton infants born between 24 and 28 weeks. They found significantly higher initial hemoglobin concentrations, higher mean systemic blood pressure, reduced need for blood transfusions, and higher urine output during the first 72 hours in the cord milked group compared with the immediate cord clamping group. The milked group also required a shorter duration of supplemental oxygen and mechanical ventilation.

Rabe and colleagues[52] conducted the only randomized controlled trial comparing repeated milking of the umbilical cord (4 times) and 30 seconds' delayed cord clamping in 58 preterm infants born between 24 and $32^{6/7}$ weeks of gestation. Infants in both groups had similar concentrations of hemoglobin levels after birth.

In a study involving 50 stable preterm infants at less than 29 weeks of gestation, Takami and colleagues[51] assessed cardiac functions, including left ventricular output and measured cerebral perfusion and cerebral oxygen extraction at specified intervals between 3 and 72 hours of age, using near-infrared spectroscopy. In 26 infants, milking of the cord had been performed according to a pre-existing protocol, and in 24, this was not done (the timing of the cord clamping was not provided). The study found that at 24 hours of age, compared with the controls, infants in the umbilical cord milked group had higher left ventricular end-diastolic dimension, left ventricular cardiac output, superior vena cava flow, and cerebral tissue oxygenation index. The investigators interpreted these positive benefits as secondary to improved cardiac functions and left ventricular preload. More studies are needed to evaluate the potential benefits and risks of umbilical cord milking, however, especially in comparison with delayed cord clamping.

MATERNAL OUTCOMES

A 2008 Cochrane review assessed the effect of cord clamping in term births on maternal and fetal outcomes in 11 clinical trials involving 2989 mothers and their babies.[10] Reviewers found no significant differences in postpartum hemorrhage between the early cord clamping (clamping within 1 minute after birth) and late cord clamping groups (clamping at least 1 minute after birth or after cessation of cord pulsation) in any of the 5 trials (2236 women) that measured this outcome (RR for postpartum hemorrhage 500 mL or more, 1.22; 95% CI, 0.96–1.55).

SUMMARY

According to WHO recommendation, delayed cord clamping in low-income and middle-income countries may be beneficial,[1,2] because many studies have documented improved iron stores during the first half of infancy, especially in resources-limited settings, where iron deficiency anemia is highly prevalent. The benefits of delayed cord clamping in all term infants in industrialized countries, however, need to be weighed against the possible need for more infants developing jaundice and needing phototherapy, especially in settings where early discharge is commonly practiced.

In addition, there does not seem to be any difference between infants receiving early versus delayed cord clamping with respect to immediate birth outcomes, such as Apgar scores, umbilical cord pH, or respiratory distress. Although maternal outcomes have not been rigorously studied, the incidence of postpartum hemorrhage is reported as similar between immediate and late cord clamping groups.

There is evidence, however, to support delayed cord clamping in preterm infants. As with term infants, delaying cord clamping 30 to 60 seconds after birth with the baby at a level below the placenta is associated with neonatal benefits, including improved transitional circulation, better establishment of red cell volume, and decreased need for blood transfusion. The single most important clinical benefit for preterm infants is the possibility of an approximately 50% reduction in intraventricular hemorrhage. The timing of umbilical cord clamping should not be altered for the purpose of collecting cord blood for banking.[5]

Box 3
Unresolved issues

Maternal care
- What is the best time to clamp the cord in relation to administration of uterotonic drugs in active management of the second stage of labor?
- How can cord clamping time in cases of maternal hemorrhage best be optimized?
- Should the cord clamping time be different in women positive for HIV?

Resuscitation
- How can the infant's position in relation to placenta be consistently maintained, especially in cesarean deliveries?
- Can resuscitation with the umbilical cord still attached to the undelivered placenta be carried out?
- How can the timing of birth and the timing of various steps of neonatal resuscitation, including the recording of the Apgar scores, be recorded?

Cord clamping
- How long a delay is ideal—30 seconds, 60 seconds, or other durations, depending on infant condition?
- What should be the location of baby while clamping the cord in relation to the placenta in cesarean sections?
- Should the exact time of cord clamping be documented in all births?
- Up to what lower gestational age can benefits from delayed cord clamping be demonstrated?

Clamping versus milking of the cord?
- Are there differential benefits between milking and delayed clamping?
- What is the appropriate length of the cord to be milked?
- How fast and how many times is milking appropriate?

At-risk infants
- What should be the standard for cord clamping in births at high altitudes?
- What should be done in infants with a risk for fetal polycythemia (eg, infants with severe intrauterine growth restriction, infants of diabetic mothers, and infants large or small for gestational age)?

Guidelines and education
- There is a need to develop standardized protocols
- Clinicians should maintain data on outcomes and report them periodically for collective learning
- All guidelines need to revised as new evidences evolve

FUTURE RESEARCH

Several unresolved issues related to optimal time for cord clamping are listed in **Box 3**. Although many randomized controlled trials have evaluated the benefits of delayed versus immediate cord clamping in term and preterm infants, the ideal timing for cord clamping has yet to be established. Further studies are also needed to evaluate the optimal timing of cord clamping, especially in relation to the management of the third stage of labor in relation to cord clamping and the timing of cord clamping in relation to the initiation of voluntary or assisted ventilation in the neonate. The ideal time for clamping the umbilical cord after cesarean delivery versus vaginal births is also an important area for future research because premature infants, who may benefit most from delayed cord clamping, are more likely to be born via cesarean delivery from a mother who may have other medical and obstetric complications.

Larger clinical trials are needed to investigate the effect of delayed cord clamping on infants delivered at less than 28 weeks' gestation. Further investigation is required to evaluate management of cord clamping in high-risk pregnancies whose infants are prone to develop polycythemia. The risks of umbilical cord milking remain unknown, and more studies are needed to compare milking of the umbilical cord with delayed cord clamping. The value of enhanced stem cell and plasma transfusion due to delayed cord clamping with respect to immediate and long-term immunity, host defense, and repair is another important area for future research.

ACKNOWLEDGMENTS

We thank Stuart B. Hooper, PhD, Department of Physiology, Faculty of Medicine, Nursing & Health Sciences, Monash University, Australia, for his valuable input concerning the physiologic consequences of cord clamping in relation to ventilation, and Professor Heike Rabe, Senior Clinical Lecturer, Brighton and Sussex Medical School, UK, for providing the text of her latest systematic review on cord clamping in preterm infants.

REFERENCES

1. Ceriani Cernadas JM. Early versus delayed umbilical cord clamping in preterm infants: RHL commentary (last revised: 7 March 2006). The WHO Reproductive Health Library. Geneva (Switzerland): World Health Organization; 2006. Available at: http://apps.who.int/rhl/pregnancy_childbirth/childbirth/3rd_stage/jccom/en/last. Accessed June 13, 2012.
2. The WHO Reproductive Health Library: Optimal timing of cord clamping for the prevention of iron deficiency anaemia in infants The World Health Organization (last update 2 March 2012). Available at: http://www.who.int/elena/titles/cord_clamping/en/last. Accessed June 13, 2012.
3. Dunn PM. Dr Erasmus Darwin (1731–1802) of Lichfield and placental respiration. Arch Dis Child Fetal Neonatal Ed 2003;88:F346–8.
4. Philip AG, Saigal S. When should we clamp the umbilical cord? Neoreviews 2004; 5:e142–54.
5. No 235 SOGC Clinical Practice Guideline. Active management of the third stage of labour: prevention and treatment of postpartum hemorrhage. Ottawa, Canada: Society of Obstetricians and Gynaecologists of Canada; 2009.
6. Sweet DG, Carnielli V, Greisen G, et al. European consensus guidelines on the management of neonatal respiratory distress syndrome in preterm infants—2010 update. Neonatology 2010;97:402–17.

7. Perlman JM, Wyllie J, Kattwinkel J, et al. Part 11: neonatal resuscitation: 2010 International consensus on cardiopulmonary resuscitation and emergency cardiovascular care science with treatment recommendations. Circulation 2010;122:S516–38.

8. No. 399 ACOG Committee Opinion. Umbilical cord blood banking. ACOG Committee Opinion No. 399. American College of Obstetricians and Gynecologists. Obstet Gynecol 2008;111:475–7.

9. Rabe H, Reynolds GJ, Diaz-Rossello JL. A systematic review and meta-analysis of a brief delay in clamping the umbilical cord of preterm infants. Neonatology 2008;93:138–44.

10. McDonald SJ, Middleton P. Effect of timing of umbilical cord clamping of term infants on maternal and neonatal outcomes. Cochrane Database Syst Rev 2008;(2):CD004074.

11. Mathew JL. Timing of umbilical cord clamping in term and preterm deliveries and infant and maternal outcomes: a systematic review of randomized controlled trials. Indian Pediatr 2011;48:123–9.

12. Van Rheenen P, Brabin BJ. Late umbilical cord-clamping as an intervention for reducing iron deficiency anaemia in term infants in developing and industrialised countries: a systematic review. Ann Trop Paediatr 2004;24(1):3–16.

13. Van Rheenen P, de Moor L, Eschbach S, et al. Delayed cord clamping and haemoglobin levels in infancy: a randomised controlled trial in term babies. Trop Med Int Health 2007;12:603–16.

14. Yao AC, Lind J. Effect of early and late cord clamping on systolic-time Intervals of newborn-infant. Acta Paediatr Scand 1977;66:489–93.

15. Polglase GR, Morley CJ, Crossley KJ, et al. Positive end-expiratory pressure differentially alters pulmonary hemodynamics and oxygenation in ventilated, very premature lambs. J Appl Phys 2005;99:1453–61.

16. Polglase GR, Wallace MJ, Morgan DL, et al. Increases in lung expansion alter pulmonary hemodynamics in fetal sheep. J Appl Phys 2006;101:273–82.

17. Crossley KJ, Allison BJ, Polglase GR, et al. Dynamic changes in blood flow through the ductus arteriosus at birth. J Physiol 2009;587:4695–703.

18. Zaramella P, Freato F, Quaresima V, et al. Early versus late cord clamping: effects on peripheral blood flow and cardiac function in term infants. Early Hum Dev 2008;84:195–200.

19. Sommers R, Stonestreet BS, Oh W, et al. Hemodynamic effects of delayed cord clamping in premature infants. Pediatrics 2012;129:e667–72.

20. Baenziger O, Stolkin F, Keel M, et al. The influence of the timing of cord clamping on postnatal cerebral oxygenation in preterm neonates: a randomized, controlled trial. Pediatrics 2007;119:455–9.

21. Hutchon DJ. Delayed cord clamping may be beneficial in rich settings. BMJ 2006;333:1073.

22. DeMaeyer E, Adiels-Tegman M. The prevalence of anemia in the world. World Health Stat Q 1985;38:302–16.

23. Geethanath RM, Ramji S, Thirupuram S, et al. Effect of timing of cord clamping on the iron status of infants at 3 months. Indian Pediatr 1997;34:103–6.

24. Grajeda R, PerezEscamilla R, Dewey KG. Delayed clamping of the umbilical cord improves hematologic status of Guatemalan infants at 2 months of age. Am J Clin Nutr 1997;65:425–31.

25. Mercer J, Erickson-Owens D. Delayed cord clamping increases infants' iron stores. Lancet 2006;367:1956–8.

26. Jahazi A, Kordi M, Mirbehbahani NB, et al. The effect of early and late umbilical cord clamping on neonatal hematocrit. J Perinatol 2008;28:523–5.

27. Jaleel R, Deeba F, Khan A. Timing of umbilical cord clamping and neonatal hae-matological status. J Pak Med Assoc 2009;59:468–70.
28. Linderkamp O, Nelle M, Kraus M, et al. The effect of early and late cord-clamping on blood-viscosity and other hemorheological parameters in full-term neonates. Acta Paediatr 1992;81:745–50.
29. Pisacane A. Neonatal prevention of iron deficiency—placental transfusion is a cheap and physiological solution. British Medical Journal 1996;312(7024):136–7.
30. Eichenbaum-Pikser G, Zasloff JS. Delayed clamping of the umbilical cord: a review with implications for practice. J Midwifery Womens Health 2009;54: 321–6.
31. Hutton EK, Hassan ES. Late vs early clamping of the umbilical cord in full-term neonates: systematic review and meta-analysis of controlled trials. JAMA 2007; 297:1241–52.
32. Linderkamp O. Blood rheology in the newborn infant. Baillieres Clin Haematol 1987;1987(1):801–25.
33. Ceriani Cernadas JM, Carroli G, Pellegrini L, et al. The effect of timing of cord clamping on neonatal venous hematocrit values and clinical outcome at term: a randomized, controlled trial. Pediatrics 2006;117:e778–86.
34. Chaparro CM, Fornes R, Neufeld LM, et al. Early umbilical cord clamping contrib-utes to elevated blood lead levels among infants with higher lead exposure. J Pediatr 2007;151:506–12.
35. Chaparro CM, Neufeld LM, Alavez GT, et al. Effect of timing of umbilical cord clamping on iron status in Mexican infants: a randomised controlled trial. Lancet 2006;367:1997–2004.
36. Chaparro CM. Timing of umbilical cord clamping: effect on iron endowment of the newborn and later iron status. Nutr Rev 2011;69(Suppl 1):S30–6.
37. van Rheenen P. Delayed cord clamping and improved infant outcomes. BMJ 2011;343:d7127.
38. van Rheenen PF, Brabin BJ. A practical approach to timing cord clamping in resource poor settings. BMJ 2006;333:954–8.
39. van Rheenen PF, Brabin BJ. Effect of timing of cord clamping on neonatal venous hematocrit values and clinical outcome at term: a randomized, controlled trial. Pediatrics 2006;118:1317–8.
40. Aladangady N, McHugh S, Aitchison TC, et al. Infants' blood volume in a controlled trial of placental transfusion at preterm delivery. Pediatrics 2006; 117:93–8.
41. Kugelman A, Borenstein-Levin L, Riskin A, et al. Immediate versus delayed umbil-ical cord clamping in premature neonates born <35 weeks: a prospective, randomized, controlled study. Am J Perinatol 2007;24:307–15.
42. van Rheenen PF, Gruschke S, Brabin BJ. Delayed umbilical cord clamping for reducing anaemia in low birth weight infants: implications for developing coun-tries. Ann Trop Paediatr 2006;26:157–67.
43. Emhamed MO, van Rheenen P, Brabin BJ. The early effects of delayed cord clamping in term infants born to Libyan mothers. Trop Doct 2004;34(4):218–22.
44. Venâncio SI, Levy RB, Saldiva SR, et al. Effects of delayed cord clamping on hemoglobin and ferritin levels in infants at three months of age. Cad Saude Pub-lica 2008;24(Suppl 2):S323–31.
45. Strauss RG, Mock DM, Johnson K, et al. Circulating RBC volume, measured with biotinylated RBCs, is superior to the Hct to document the hematologic effects of delayed versus immediate umbilical cord clamping in preterm neonates. Transfu-sion 2003;43:1168–72.

46. Ultee CA, Van Der Deure J, Swart J, et al. Delayed cord clamping in preterm infants delivered at 34-36 weeks' gestation: a randomised controlled trial. Arch Dis Child Fetal Neonatal Ed 2008;93:F20–3.

47. Ibrahim HM, Krouskop RW, Lewis DF, et al. Placental transfusion: umbilical cord clamping and preterm infants. J Perinatol 2000;20:351–4.

48. Rabe H, Diaz-Rossello JL, Duley L, et al. Effect of timing of umbilical cord clamping and other strategies to influence placental transfusion at preterm birth on maternal and infant outcomes. Cochrane Database Syst Rev 2012;(8):CD003248. http://dx.doi.org/10.1002/14651858.CD003248.pub3.

49. Hosono S, Mugishima H, Fujita H, et al. Umbilical cord milking reduces the need for red cell transfusions and improves neonatal adaptation in infants born at less than 29 weeks' gestation: a randomised controlled trial. Arch Dis Child Fetal Neonatal Ed 2008;93:F14–9.

50. Hosono S, Mugishima H, Fujita H, et al. Blood pressure and urine output during the first 120 h of life in infants born at less than 29 weeks' gestation related to umbilical cord milking. Arch Dis Child Fetal Neonatal Ed 2009;94:F328–31.

51. Takami T, Suganami Y, Sunohara D, et al. Umbilical cord milking stabilizes cerebral oxygenation and perfusion in infants born before 29 weeks of gestation. J Pediatr 2012;161:742–7.

52. Rabe H, Jewison A, Alvarez RF, et al. Milking compared with delayed cord clamping to increase placental transfusion in preterm neonates. Obstet Gynecol 2010; 117(2):205–11.

Neonatal Stabilization and Postresuscitation Care

Steven A. Ringer, MD, PhD[a], Khalid Aziz, MA, MEd(IT), FRCPC[b],*

KEYWORDS

- Neonatal resuscitation • Neonatal stabilization • Education • Post-resuscitation care
- Neonatal mortality

KEY POINTS

- Neonatal resuscitation alone does not address most causes of neonatal mortality, such as prematurity, low birth weight, respiratory distress, and infections. To address these, care-givers need to be trained in both neonatal resuscitation and stabilization.
- Neonatal stabilization requires caregivers to evaluate whether babies are at-risk or unwell, to decide what interventions are required, and to act on those decisions.
- A number of programs address neonatal stabilization in a variety of levels of care in both well-resourced and limited health care environments. They address institutional, clinical, and human factors to varying degrees.
- This article suggests a shift in clinical, educational and implementation science from a focus on resuscitation to one on the resuscitation-stabilization continuum.

INTRODUCTION

Neonatal mortality continues to be a significant health concern across the world. Of note, preterm birth complications, intrapartum-related complications, and sepsis or meningitis are the leading causes of neonatal death.[1] Although effective neonatal resuscitation training for health providers is vital for improved survival, one should not underestimate the need for training in neonatal care and stabilization after birth to identify and manage these conditions.

Conflicts of interest: Dr Aziz is an author of the *Acute Care of at-Risk Newborns* textbook and volunteers as Board Member of the ACoRN Neonatal Society, a not-for-profit society that owns copyright to the ACoRN Program. He makes no financial gain from ACoRN materials. He has no other conflicts to declare. Dr Ringer is a member of the Newborn Resuscitation Program Steering Committee of the American Academy of Pediatrics and an Assistant Editor of the *Textbook of Neonatal Resuscitation,* 6th edition. He makes no financial gain from these activities, and has no other conflicts to declare.

[a] Department of Newborn Medicine, Harvard Medical School, Brigham and Women's Hospital, 75 Francis Street, Boston, MA 02492, USA; [b] Department of Pediatrics, University of Alberta, DTC5027 Royal Alexandra Hospital, 10240 Kingsway, Edmonton AB, Canada T5H 3V5
* Corresponding author.
E-mail address: khalid.aziz@ualberta.ca

Clin Perinatol 39 (2012) 901–918
http://dx.doi.org/10.1016/j.clp.2012.09.007
0095-5108/12/$ – see front matter © 2012 Elsevier Inc. All rights reserved.

Health care providers around the world, irrespective of level of care, are faced with the possibility that a baby may be at-risk or unwell at birth or soon after. It should also be appreciated that most babies in the world are born outside high-risk neonatal centers, even in countries with highly developed perinatal services. For example, in Alberta, Canada, with a highly regionalized health care system, only one-quarter of babies are born in level III centers, with the remainder born in an assortment of level II and I units (K. Aziz, personal communication, August 2012). In many countries, such as Ethiopia, 9 of 10 babies are born at home.[2] Even when born in hospital, rural facilities in China have been shown to have up to 4 times the neonatal mortality of urban perinatal centers.[3] Clearly, outside high-risk centers, health care providers have limitations in how they might respond to an at-risk or unwell baby; these limitations may be, first, in their ability to recognize risk for or signs of illness; second, in access to training and resources to provide this care; or third, in transportation to where the care may be provided.

How valuable is a neonatal resuscitation program if, a few minutes after effective resuscitation, a health care provider is unable to identify at-risk or sick babies, and unable to provide effective stabilization? In answering this question, it seems clear that 2 populations of patients are important: those requiring postresuscitation care, and those who are well at birth but may become ill. Among babies who require substantial resuscitation but seemingly recover by 5 minutes of age, Frazier and Werthammer[4] found that 62% had short-term complications requiring evaluation and treatment. Even among babies whose resuscitation needs at birth are less pronounced, the need for assessment and treatment often continues.

This article describes the key principles of effective stabilization, evaluation, and initial postbirth treatment. We focus primarily on the term and late preterm infants.

IDENTIFYING BABIES WHO ARE UNWELL OR AT RISK FOR BECOMING UNWELL

Looking at the leading causes of neonatal death worldwide, many of them may be identifiable before birth, or very shortly after. We know that approximately 1 in 10 babies in the world are born preterm[1]; we are often well aware of intrapartum complications, such as abruption and antepartum bleeding; and neonatal sepsis, pneumonia, and meningitis all present with very abnormal clinical signs.

In developing an approach to help caregivers appropriately care for babies after birth, a reasonable first step is to educate them about the risk factors for instability. Knowing, for example, that short gestation or maternal fever is more likely to lead to a preterm or sick baby may lead to earlier intervention in labor, or perhaps transfer to a birthing center with adequate resources. This approach has been successfully protocolized in North America for the prevention of early-onset sepsis.[5] After birth, for example, providers should clearly identify low birth weight as a warning sign of future instability, even if the child is well.

Triage is one of the most important aspects of health care provider training. In neonatal resuscitation we have identified "vital" signs that determine whether a baby should remain in its mother's arms or should be introduced to the initial steps of resuscitation: providers are trained that a baby is well if the baby is breathing, active, and developing normal color and tone. Similarly, providers may be taught the "vital signs for stabilization" as a means of triage.

What might these "vital signs for stabilization" be? As with resuscitation, they should reflect a transition to extrauterine vital organ function. Respiratory stability might be indicated by lack of distress and a regular, quiet breathing pattern. Cardiovascular stability might be confirmed by normal heart rate, color, and perfusion. A baby who is alert and responsive, with normal activity, waking for feeds, would be neurologically stable. The absence of significant emesis, diarrhea, or abdominal distension would support stable alimentary function. Integrity of the skin, and normal skin turgor and color would indicate stability, as might a normal body temperature; one might add absence of signs of dehydration. Such a checklist of "vital signs for stabilization" would require validation through rigorous clinical studies to confirm their relative value in confirming normality, and predicting a normal outcome. A number of validated clinical acuity scores for newborns, such as transport risk index of physiologic stability (TRIPS)[6] and clinical risk index for babies (CRIB)[7] have used such indicators of stability, and would be a good starting point for establishing the "vital signs of stabilization."

Internationally, the World Health Organization (WHO) and the United Nations Children Fund (UNICEF)[8,9] have developed educational programs to address the immediate care of the newborn, based on the principles of identifying babies who are eligible for normal newborn care, and those who will require stabilization. Evidence from the field suggests that elements of these programs, as well as the programs themselves, reduced neonatal mortality[10]; such validated programs would be another source for the "vital signs of stabilization."

EDUCATION PROGRAMS FOR SICK BABIES

Just as resuscitation program algorithms divide interventions into initial triage, then support of the airway, followed by assisted breathing and then circulatory support, stabilization programs need structure. Most programs address key organ systems in sequence, often recognizing that respiratory stability is a priority after resuscitation.

In addition to the WHO-UNICEF normal newborn care program,[8] there are a number of educational programs that facilitate stabilization. These differ slightly in their approaches and target different types of provider or institution (as shown in **Table 1**). They do, however, generally follow the same principles: identify the sick baby, sort out which organ system is unstable, and address the instability systematically. They include the following:

- Integrated Management of Neonatal and Childhood Illness (IMNCI)[8]
- Pregnancy, childbirth, postpartum, and newborn care. A guide for essential practice[9]
- Perinatal Continuing Education Program[11]
- S.T.A.B.L.E[12]
- Acute Care of at-Risk Newborns (ACoRN)[13]

Each program has been evaluated to varying degrees, largely with respect to the effect on learners and practice, rather than outcome.[10,14–16] The utility of these approaches lies in ensuring that caregivers can quickly assess the major areas of concern during stabilization, and provide care that is tailored to the individual infant's needs. The following section reviews each of the major components of stabilization after resuscitation.

SYSTEM-SPECIFIC AND ORGAN-SPECIFIC ISSUES RELATING TO STABILIZATION
Postresuscitation Observation

Following resuscitation at birth, the initial triage decision focuses on which babies need more intensive observation, and which can be observed in conjunction with their mother in the usual postpartum or nursery setting. Most infants who require some resuscitation at birth will quickly stabilize and can remain with their parents.

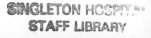

Table 1
Neonatal stabilization programs

Program	Source	Target	Content
IMNCI (Integrated Management of Neonatal and Childhood Illness)[9]	WHO-UNICEF (India)	Community-based and facility-based health care providers. Low resourced environments and referral facilities.	Identification of an unwell infant for transfer to a facility. Focus on feeding, jaundice, infection, and diarrhea.
Pregnancy, childbirth, postpartum, and newborn care. A guide for essential practice[8]	WHO, UNPF, UNICEF, The World Bank	Health care professionals caring for well babies. Low resourced environments.	Care of the well baby, with identification, early treatment, and transfer of an unwell infant. Focus on resuscitation, feeding, jaundice, temperature, infection, immunization/prevention.
Perinatal Continuing Education Program (PCEP)[11]	University of Virginia	Interprofessional perinatal health care teams in well-resourced health care systems	Comprehensive institution-based neonatal care as might be found in the United States or Canada
S T A.B.L.E.[12]	The S.T.A.B.L.E. Program, Utah, USA	Postresuscitation/pretransport stabilization by health care professionals in well-resourced health care systems	System-based approach to evaluation and immediate management: S = Sugar and Safe care T = Temperature A = Airway B = Blood pressure L = Laboratory work E = Emotional support
Acute Care of at-Risk Newborns (ACoRN)[13]	ACoRN Neonatal Society, Canada	Interprofessional teams at level 1, 2, and 3 perinatal centers in well-resourced health care systems	System-based approach to identification of the at-risk or unwell baby and immediate management by area of concern (respiratory, cardiovascular, neurologic, surgical, intake, temperature, and infection)

Abbreviations: UNICEF, United National Children's Fund; UNPF, United Nations Population Fund; WHO, World Health Organization.

Continuing observation in a high-dependency area is necessary for any infant requiring resuscitation who then continues to have abnormal signs or symptoms, especially if there is a need for ongoing support. Observation is also warranted for infants with historical risks for infection,[17] or who are at risk for side effects of maternal medication. Although less common, infants with prenatally diagnosed disorders that might result in a problem with transition (such as a possible aortic coarctation or renal anomalies) should be more closely monitored in the period after birth.

Observation may consist simply of regular visual inspection, with assessment of heart rate, respiratory rate, and temperature at intervals. It could be augmented with cardiorespiratory and arterial saturation monitoring. Glucose testing may also be considered. Institutions and caregivers who provide perinatal services, irrespective of level of care, should have contingencies for observation of sick or at-risk babies.

Observation is particularly important for babies whose initial needs are more complex. The principles of newborn resuscitation, as articulated by the Neonatal Resuscitation Program of the American Academy of Pediatrics/American Heart Association, stress that the primary focus during resuscitation should be on the support of breathing and ventilation.[18] In general, the number of babies who need a particular level of intervention decreases as the complexity of the intervention increases. For most babies, therefore, their needs during resuscitation rarely exceed a brief period of positive pressure ventilation. For those who do require ventilatory support immediately following birth, postresuscitation observation would identify significant complications, such as respiratory distress or hypoxic ischemic encephalopathy.

The length and site of the observation period depends on the clinical status and can range from several minutes to a few hours as babies transition. In most instances, problems with transition resolve fairly quickly after birth, and the period of more intensive observation can be safely concluded. Once this has occurred and any necessary laboratory evaluation has been completed, the infant can be safely monitored in the well nursery or mother's bedside for the duration of postpartum care. For some infants, the resolution of even relatively mild symptoms may occur slowly, and it is challenging to determine how long to wait before admitting the baby to a neonatal unit. The decision becomes more complex when the capabilities of the birthing environment are limited, and transport is being considered. At the same time, it is usually unwise to prolong the observation period in the hope that resolution is coming soon. This may delay further care, and unnecessarily tie up resources.

It is recommended that each perinatal service or institution have guidelines for a maximum period of initial observation, after which a decision on admission or transfer should be made. In most situations, a baby who fails to have normal "vital signs of stabilization" within 4 hours should be admitted to a unit able to provide higher level of care.

Respiratory Distress

The most common immediate concern in the unstable newborn is whether breathing is adequate. Respiratory distress has been described to occur after birth in approximately 1% of term infants, and may be 3 to 5 times as common in late preterm infants.[19] In most situations, respiratory stability (or instability) may be confirmed by clinical examination. Health care providers should be trained to recognize that a healthy baby has normal color and respiratory rate, requires no supplemental oxygen or respiratory support, and breathes quietly and effortlessly. The ACoRN Program advocates a respiratory score to identify the severity of distress. The ACoRN Respiratory Score has been validated in term and late preterm infants[20]; use of this score should not, however, preclude practitioners from establishing the signs of distress clinically. One benefit of the score is the categorization of respiratory distress into mild, moderate, and severe, facilitating clinical responses or consultation in keeping with illness severity.

If there are signs of respiratory instability, oxygen saturation should be monitored and supplemental oxygen administered to maintain normal levels.[21] Given the risk of aspiration, feeding should be deferred while the severity and cause are being ascertained. A chest radiograph may be helpful in establishing the cause of respiratory distress. Blood gases should be measured if the oxygen requirement is persistent or increasing, there are signs of diminished perfusion, or acidosis is suspected. Further care depends on an assessment of the underlying etiology as well as the clinical course: increasing respiratory distress after birth may be life threatening and requires care by trained neonatal practitioners in an appropriate level of care.

The most common causes of respiratory distress immediately after birth are listed in **Box 1**. These can usually be distinguished on the basis of clinical presentation, associated factors, radiographs and laboratory tests.

Transient tachypnea of the newborn (TTN) occurs in approximately 5 in 1000 term births, and with greater frequency in late preterm infants.[22] It usually causes "mild" respiratory distress. It is caused by incomplete resorption of pulmonary fluid at birth, resulting in transient pulmonary edema. TTN is more common following cesarean section, especially with no labor. It is more common in males and shows a genetic predisposition, for example in families with a history of asthma. It is also seen more frequently in macrosomic babies and in infants of diabetic mothers. Infants with TTN are usually term or late preterm, and present within 6 hours of birth with tachypnea, sometimes with respiratory rates as high as 120 breaths per minute. Grunting, flaring, and retractions may occur. Signs are usually mild, and the need for supplemental oxygen is usually minimal (Fio_2 <0.4), if at all. The anteroposterior diameter of the chest is typically increased, with apparent hyperinflation.

TTN is a self-limiting condition and does not normally require investigation. It should improve with time, and resolve in 24 hours or so. If done, the baby's complete blood count (CBC) is usually normal, and blood gases are unremarkable. A chest radiograph is also optional, and may show mild pulmonary edema including prominent interlobar fissures and streakiness in the perihilar regions. Air leak is rare. Caution should be used in interpreting radiographs taken within an hour or 2 of birth, as they may show infiltrates that will rapidly clear on their own.

Box 1
Common causes of respiratory distress after birth

Respiratory distress syndrome (RDS)

Transient tachypnea of the newborn (TTN)

Pneumonia

Persistent pulmonary hypertension of the newborn (PPHN)

Meconium aspiration syndrome (MAS)

Cyanotic congenital heart disease

Malformation (diaphragmatic hernia, cystic adenomatoid malformation)

Pneumothorax

Polycythemia

Metabolic acidosis

Respiratory distress syndrome (RDS) is increasingly common with increasing prematurity, occurring in 5% of late preterm babies.[23] It causes respiratory distress that may progress from mild to moderate to severe over 12 to 48 hours. RDS is caused by a deficiency of pulmonary surfactant, and many cases includes some element of persistent pulmonary hypertension, especially at late preterm gestational age. The presentation typically includes tachypnea with grunting, flaring, and retractions, often with limited chest expansion characteristic of decreased pulmonary compliance and decreased lung volumes. Respiratory distress may be mild initially, with increasing oxygen requirements and distress as atelectasis becomes more widespread in both lungs. Apnea is a serious complication.

The classical findings on the chest radiograph include decreased lung volumes and diffuse homogeneous "ground glass" appearance and air bronchograms. RDS may be complicated by lobar collapse or air leak (pneumothorax or pneumomediastinum). Blood gases typically reveal hypoxemia and hypercapnea, and (at first) minimal or no metabolic acidosis. Initial care may be supportive with oxygen or continuous positive airway pressure. Endotracheal intubation may be required. Endotracheal instillation of surfactant is effective in preventing both deterioration and death from RDS: a variety of treatment strategies have been studied, including prophylaxis, early rescue, and late rescue.[24–26] Care of babies with RDS is best provided in centers familiar with its management.

Pneumonia may present with symptoms and radiographic findings that are indistinguishable from RDS or TTN.[27] A history revealing risk factors for infection, such as maternal fever, preterm labor, or prolonged rupture of membranes, should lower the threshold for investigation and treatment with antibiotics, especially if the oxygen requirement is increasing or exceeds an Fio_2 of 0.4.

Persistent pulmonary hypertension of the newborn (PPHN) should be suspected when there is a need for oxygen supplementation without another clear explanation (irrespective of severity of respiratory distress), or when a baby with severe respiratory distress does not respond to ventilation and oxygen therapy.[28,29] On physical examination, the second heart sound may be accentuated, and there is typically evidence of right to left shunting, manifested by a differential in oxygen saturation or Po_2 between "preductal" measurements from the right upper extremity and "post ductal" measurements from the lower extremities. The chest radiograph may be entirely normal, or may confirm concurrent RDS or pneumonia. Initial therapy includes oxygen, correction of acidosis if present, and ensuring that the blood pressure remains normal.

Meconium aspiration syndrome (MAS) is suspected when there is a history of meconium staining of the amniotic fluid, especially if the baby is depressed at birth and requires resuscitation.[30,31] Of concern is babies with MAS and severe respiratory distress; those with mild to moderate distress may improve spontaneously. The initial presentation includes tachypnea and hypoxemia requiring supplemental oxygen, and the anteroposterior diameter of the chest is often increased. The chest radiograph is usually abnormal, with patchy or flocculent infiltrates and evidence of hyperinflation due to air trapping. The risk of air leak is increased, and there may be evidence of PPHN. Continued monitoring is necessary, and more extensive therapy or referral may be required.

The diagnosis of a congenital lung malformation or pneumothorax should be suspected when a baby has tachypnea and distress along with a significant requirement for supplemental oxygen.[32,33] Spontaneous pneumothorax may have minimal signs in healthy, term babies. Small lesions may cause minimal distress and may be missed at birth. With larger lesions, the baby may be in shock. The trachea and heart may be displaced from their normal positions, and examination of the lung fields may reveal absent breath sounds on one side, or even bowel sounds in the chest. The radiograph is usually diagnostic.

As for pneumothoraces, more than half resolve spontaneously with supportive management.[34] In the remainder, needle thoracostomy may be curative, although an indwelling thoracostomy tube may be required if air leak continues or recurs. It should be remembered that pneumothoraces may be secondary to other underlying lung diseases, such as RDS or MAS, with associated PPHN. For symptomatic lung malformations, immediate consultation with a pediatric surgeon is indicated.

Congenital heart disease may present with significant respiratory compromise and shock when the underlying abnormality is a left-sided duct-dependent lesion. Congenital cyanotic heart disease is suspected when there is cyanosis in the absence of significant respiratory distress, especially if the cyanosis is unresponsive to oxygen therapy.[35] Babies typically have tachypnea without significant distress, and historical factors associated with diagnoses of RDS, TTN, or pneumonia are usually absent. Although not always present, a murmur noted on physical examination should increase suspicion.[36] Prompt evaluation by a cardiologist, including a diagnostic echocardiogram, is warranted so that emergent therapy, such as prostaglandin E1, can be administered and additional care needs determined.[37]

Cardiovascular Insufficiency

The cardiovascular status of the infant can be evaluated clinically. In addition to having normal respiratory status, healthy babies are centrally pink, well perfused, warm to touch, and have palpable peripheral pulses of normal rate and rhythm. Perfusion is evaluated by assessment of capillary refill, peripheral pulses, skin color, and skin temperature, recognizing that other factors, such as stress or environmental temperature, influence findings. The definition of "normal" blood pressure levels is the subject of debate,[38,39] and there are limited data supporting any particular values. In late preterm and term infants, normal mean blood pressures are generally considered to be in the range of 35 to 45 mm Hg.

Two key mechanisms of cardiovascular instability are low perfusion states, or shock, and congenital cyanotic heart disease.

Shock in the neonatal period can result from several causes, as listed in **Box 2**. They are usually divided into 3 categories: hypovolemic, because of blood loss or severe dehydration; distributive, because of vasodilation; and cardiogenic, because of myocardial dysfunction or obstructive cardiac lesions.[40] The diagnosis is usually suspected based on associated clinical or historical factors. For example, an infant who was markedly depressed at birth and required full resuscitation is at risk for cardiogenic shock from myocardial dysfunction, whereas an infant with signs of subgaleal hemorrhage is at risk for developing hypovolemic shock from blood loss.

Initially, the presentation of shock may be insidious, as compensatory mechanisms, such as tachycardia and peripheral vasoconstriction, keep systemic blood pressure in the normal range. Over time, however, these mechanisms may fail, resulting in tissue hypoperfusion and end-organ injury. Careful evaluation will increase the likelihood of early and effective intervention, preventing serious complications. The development of metabolic acidosis is often an important signal of evolving tissue hypoperfusion, so the measurement of blood gases is usually indicated until shock is ruled out or treated.

Initial therapy includes the administration of 10 to 20 mL/kg of a crystalloid solution (such as normal saline). Colloid infusions, such as albumin, are not thought to be superior during volume resuscitation, an exception being blood transfusion for significant blood loss. In cases in which cardiogenic shock is suspected, the administration of large volumes of crystalloid may result in cardiac failure, but the initial boluses can

---

Box 2
Shock presenting after birth

Hypovolemic

    Placental hemorrhage

    Fetal to maternal hemorrhage

    Twin-twin transfusion

    Internal hemorrhage (intracranial, pulmonary, subgaleal, intra-abdominal)

Distributive

    Sepsis

    Maternal medications

Cardiogenic

    Intrapartum asphyxia

    Congenital cardiac malformation (Ebstein anomaly)

    Sepsis

---

be safely given. It is most important to monitor the response to therapy, and any ongoing fluid losses. Successful treatment should result in improvement in tachycardia and perfusion, and normalization of the blood pressure. Over time, the degree of metabolic acidosis should improve, although it may paradoxically worsen initially, as improved tissue perfusion results in distribution of lactic acid in the bloodstream. If there is limited or no response, additional fluid boluses should be administered, and, depending on the underlying etiology, the use of sympathomimetic amines such as dopamine, dobutamine, or epinephrine.

Refractory shock unresponsive to volume expanders, pressors, or inotropes requires expert consultation and evaluation to determine and exclude unusual causation. Pericardial tamponade should be considered in babies with central vascular lines whose tips are placed in the thorax. Late presentation of shock may be caused by infections, duct-dependent left-sided congenital heart lesions (such as coarctation of the aorta), adrenal crises, and metabolic disorders. Expert consultation may result in a recommendation for echocardiography, prostaglandin therapy, hydrocortisone, antibiotics, or specific metabolic cocktails.

Congenital cyanotic heart disease is described in the respiratory section.

Neurologic Instability

Healthy newborns have healthy sleep-wake states, responding appropriately to the environment and handling. They have normal tone and activity, with no abnormal movements. When they cry, they settle with comfort or feeding. A baby who is poorly responsive or "depressed" after resuscitation should be monitored. Although most infants recover uneventfully, vigilance for signs of encephalopathy is warranted. These signs include alteration in conscious level, abnormalities in cranial nerve function, hypotonia, loss of reflexes, or occurrence of seizures. The presence of encephalopathy alone does not imply a specific etiology, whether it is reversible, or when it may have occurred, but it does prompt the need for additional evaluation and consideration of effective therapies.

Hypoxic ischemic encephalopathy (HIE) occurs as the consequence of impaired delivery of metabolic substrate to the brain. It occurs in its moderate to severe form after 1 to 3 per 1000 deliveries, and is associated with cord pH lower than 7.00, low Apgar scores, and prolonged respiratory support after birth.[41] Several studies have demonstrated that therapeutic hypothermia to 33 to 34°C for 72 hours may reduce the degree of brain injury in infants with moderate or severe HIE attributable to an injury that has occurred proximate to birth.[42] It is important to rapidly exclude other causes of encephalopathy, such as meningitis and hypoglycemia, before instituting cooling; during this time, overwarming of the infant should be avoided. Although studies are ongoing to assess the impact of earlier or later initiation, the effectiveness of this therapy is currently felt to depend on initiation within 6 hours of birth, so early evaluation and consideration of this therapy is important.[43] Timely evaluation is even more important if the infant must be transported to another facility for care.

Therapeutic hypothermia should be considered when specific factors are identified. Different protocols may vary somewhat as to inclusion criteria, but all of them are based on those used in major randomized controlled trials. Typical inclusion criteria are listed in **Box 3**. If an infant appears to meet criteria, immediate consultation with a referral center familiar with therapeutic hypothermia is indicated. During the evaluation period, it may be beneficial to turn off the heat on the overhead warmer to allow passive cooling and to avoid the detrimental effects of hyperthermia in this group of patients. However, it is important to ensure that the patient's temperature does not drop below recommended levels.

HIE is often accompanied by dysfunction in other end-organs, including the kidneys, liver, and heart. Close attention to this will ensure that fluid and medication administration is adjusted accordingly.

Neonatal seizures occur in 1 to 5 in 1000 live births.[44,45] HIE is a significant risk factor, but other treatable conditions, such as hypoglycemia, electrolyte disturbance, and meningitis, should always be considered. Seizures may be difficult to recognize clinically, and classically continue despite holding or restraining the affected limb, or holding the baby. Initial therapy currently includes phenobarbital, with the addition of phenytoin or fosphenytoin as needed. When these agents fail to adequately control

---

Box 3
Inclusion criteria for therapeutic hypothermia

Gestational age ≥36 weeks and birth weight ≥2000 g.

AND

Evidence of at least 1 of the following:

History of acute perinatal event (placental abruption, cord prolapse, and/or category III fetal heart rate tracing)

History before delivery of a Biophysical Profile <6/10 (4/8) within 6 hours of birth

Cord arterial pH ≤7.0 or calculated base deficit ≥16 mEq/L

AND

Evidence of at least 1 of the following:

Apgar score ≤5 at 10 minutes

Postnatal arterial blood gas pH at <1 hour of ≤7.0 or calculated base deficit ≥16 mEq/L

Continued need for ventilation initiated at birth and continued for at least 10 minutes

AND

Evidence of neonatal encephalopathy on physical examination.

seizures, therapy with benzodiazepines is indicated. Refractory seizures require expert consultation.

Metabolic Instability

Infants who have required resuscitation are more likely to have some degree of metabolic or respiratory acidosis after birth, depending on the particular clinical situation. Assessment of blood gases is warranted when there is persistent respiratory distress, suspicion or evidence of hypoperfusion or shock, or concern that hypoxic ischemic injury may have occurred. Some mild degree of metabolic acidosis is normal after birth and does not require any specific therapy. More severe acidosis should be treated with adequate fluid administration and repletion of fluid deficit.[46] Ultimately, metabolic and respiratory acidosis do not resolve until the underlying cause of instability is directly addressed. Inborn errors of the metabolism are rare but should always be considered if a baby has unexplained shock, hypoglycemia, acidosis, or encephalopathy; expert consultation should be sought.

A number of antepartum, intrapartum and neonatal conditions predispose babies to impaired glucose homeostasis (**Box 4**). Impaired glucose production and subsequent hypoglycemia are common findings in postresuscitation management, fueling concerns that neuroglycopenia may have detrimental effects on brain function and development. The optimal level of plasma glucose during stabilization is unknown, as even low, physiologic levels are concerning if babies have neurologic instability, as might occur in HIE. Although healthy breastfed babies may have plasma glucose levels of 30 to 40 mg/dL at 1 to 2 hours of age, clinicians tend to target higher levels in sick newborns: American Academy of Pediatrics guidelines favor levels higher than 40 mg/dL in these babies, achieved using intravenous glucose infusions.[47] A failure to respond to up to 100 mL/kg per day of 10% dextrose intravenously should prompt consultation with a neonatologist.

Box 4
Risk factors for hypoglycemia after birth

Hyperinsulinemic states

    Infants of mothers with diabetes mellitus

    Congenital genetic (rarely known at birth)

    Macrosomia especially if Beckwith Wiedemann syndrome is suspected

Large for gestational age

    May reflect undiagnosed maternal diabetes

Intrauterine growth restriction

Prematurity or late-prematurity

Perinatal stress

    Sepsis

    Shock

    Asphyxia

    Hypothermia

Polycythemia

Maternal therapy with beta blockers

Hyperbilirubinemia is common, but a rare cause of instability, and best addressed by preventative measures and early detection using protocols.

Fluid Homeostasis

Healthy babies breastfeed shortly after birth and with increasing frequency subsequently. Urine output is minimal on day 1 while the only intake is colostrum. Healthy babies lose approximately 10% of their body weight over the first 3 days or so of age while breastfeeding is established. They regain their birth weight in approximately a week.

Clinical assessment of fluid status starts with assessment of cardiovascular stability. Dehydration is virtually never present at birth. It is a significant cause of infant death worldwide, however, and may be a contributing cause if a baby requires resuscitation on admission at a few days of age. Care providers should recognize the signs of severe dehydration: babies may be shocked, neurologically unstable, and present with sunken fontanel or poor skin turgor. There may be greater than 15% weight loss. In situations of cardiovascular compromise, fluid resuscitation is lifesaving. Maintenance fluids are usually required for glucose homeostasis, unless there are significant ongoing losses.

Thermoregulation

Normal term and late preterm babies maintain body temperature when held skin-to-skin by their parents; no technology is required. Unstable babies are at risk for both hyperthermia and hypothermia. Those who need resuscitation or are postresuscitation may require care under an overhead warmer, in a room with an ambient temperature of 25°C.[18] The baby needing resuscitation should be dried immediately after birth and the wet linens removed, unless extremely preterm, in which case a plastic wrap should be used. A skin probe with servocontrolled warmth is recommended if the baby spends more than 10 minutes under a radiant warmer. Alternatively, the baby should be transferred to a servocontrolled incubator. Body temperature, usually axillary, should be checked at regular intervals. During the stabilization period, attention should be paid to ensuring that the infant remains warm, recognizing that heat loss occurs via the following 4 mechanisms:

1. Radiation. The infant will radiate heat to colder objects in the environment. This includes windows and walls, especially in colder climates.
2. Convection. Heat is lost to moving air, so avoiding drafts or ventilation ducts is important.
3. Evaporation. Infants should be dried after birth to prevent evaporative heat loss.
4. Conduction. Direct loss to the surface on which the baby is lying, unless it is kept warm also.

Infection

Although improvements in perinatal care have led to marked reductions in the incidence of infection at birth, particularly among term infants, sepsis neonatorum remains a major problem worldwide. Health care providers should familiarize themselves with the risk factors for infections and local policies relating to prevention, such as Group B streptococcal prevention protocols. Septicemia, pneumonia, and meningitis commonly present with cardiorespiratory instability and depression at birth, so risk factors for infection are often identified among babies requiring resuscitation at birth. The signs and reported symptoms of infection may mimic many of the conditions described in the preceding sections.

The most investigated cause of early-onset sepsis in the newborn is Group B Streptococcus (GBS). Maternal risk factors that predict GBS disease include maternal colonization, intrapartum fever higher than 38°C, evidence of maternal chorioamnionitis, and rupture of the membranes for longer than 18 hours. Premature birth (especially without another explanation) and birth weight less than 2500 g are also associated risks.

Neonatal infection may present as bacteremia, viremia, pneumonia, or meningitis. Even local skin infections, such as omphalitis, will rapidly develop systemic involvement. Although affected infants may initially be asymptomatic, most cases present soon after birth. Clinical signs commonly include respiratory distress of variable severity, sometimes associated with persistent pulmonary hypertension. There are often more generalized signs, such as irritability, decreased perfusion, hypotension, and temperature instability. It may be difficult to differentiate early signs of sepsis from those seen in RDS, TTN, or HIE. As a result, infection should be considered when evaluating an infant with cardiorespiratory or neurologic instability.

When sepsis is suspected, evaluation includes a blood culture and CBC. Neutropenia or thrombocytopenia support the diagnosis of infection, and changes in values may reflect improvement or development of coagulopathy.[48] Unfortunately, the CBC is poorly predictive of infection and should not be used in isolation to decide whether a baby has an infection. Additional evaluation of the symptomatic infant may include measurement of plasma glucose levels because hyperglycemia may be a sign of sepsis, and blood gases so that any associated metabolic acidosis may be identified. With abnormal neurologic signs or a high index of suspicion, cerebrospinal fluid should be obtained by lumbar puncture to exclude meningitis (unless cardiorespiratory instability contradicts the procedure). After the first few days of age, urine culture should be considered (by catheter or bladder tap).

Antibiotic therapy should be administered, with the choice of agents determined by the most likely organisms and local sensitivities. Typically causative organisms include GBS, *Escherichia coli* and other gram-negative organisms, and *Listeria monocytogenes*; most of these organisms are sensitive to ampicillin and gentamicin. Antibiotics continue until cultures are negative and the baby is asymptomatic, or until a specific organism is identified,[49] at which time the therapy can be appropriately tailored.

If there is a strong suspicion of a particular causative organism, based on maternal evaluation, the choice of antibiotic agents should reflect this. In some situations, antiviral treatments are indicated.

Surgical Emergencies

There are a number of conditions that may require surgery soon after birth that require stabilization. They may affect any organ system. Most severe surgical anomalies are diagnosed antenatally during routine maternal ultrasound examination. It is important to arrange for consultation with a surgeon before delivery and to develop a plan for delivery in a center familiar with management of these conditions.

Respiratory and cardiac anomalies have been discussed previously. Abnormalities of the gastrointestinal tract consist of obstructions, masses, and abdominal wall defects. Polyhydramnios occurs in about 1 of 1000 births. When identified, prenatal ultrasound examination may lead to a specific surgical diagnosis, in particular esophageal atresia (often associated with tracheoesophageal fistula). Antenatal ultrasound may also detect diaphragmatic hernia and abdominal wall defects. Proximal dilatation of the bowel is often a sign of intestinal obstruction owing to stenosis or atresia. Meconium peritonitis is also diagnosed by ultrasonography, appearing as areas of calcification scattered through the abdomen: the result of antenatal perforation of the intestinal tract, usually in association with anatomic (intestinal atresia) or functional (meconium ileus) intestinal obstruction. Fetal ascites is mostly frequently attributable to cardiac failure in utero, sometimes associated with intrathoracic mass effects from tumors.

Management of most abdominal surgical emergencies start with cardiorespiratory stabilization, followed by specific management of the lesion with gastric drainage, covering open lesions to prevent infection and water loss, and intravenous fluids. Feeds are usually held. Chest and abdominal radiographs with a nasogastric or orogastric tube in place may be diagnostic of many lesions.

Renal anomalies are common, but only the most severe result in a baby who requires stabilization. When bilateral, hydronephrosis or renal dysplasia in a fetus may be a sign of serious anomalies of the urinary tract, with renal dysfunction or posterior urethral valves.

Babies with neural tube defects are usually stable at birth, but may require surgical intervention soon after. Care should be taken to protect the area and avoid contamination.

A variety of disorders may be diagnosed after birth based on presenting symptoms. Respiratory distress, as noted previously, may result from such disorders as choanal atresia, esophageal atresia with or without tracheoesophageal fistula, congenital lobar emphysema, and cystic adenomatoid malformation of the lung. Esophageal atresia should be suspected in a baby with excessive secretions or saliva. Bilious emesis, while unusual immediately after birth, should raise suspicion of intestinal obstruction, in particular malrotation and possible volvulus. This should be rapidly evaluated, as it can be a life-threatening anomaly.

Other disorders are evident on physical examination immediately after birth, including imperforate anus, possible testicular torsion, or abdominal mass lesions. In all of these cases, further care will depend on surgical evaluation.

RESOURCE-SPECIFIC ISSUES RELATING TO STABILIZATION
Human Resources and Training

Like neonatal resuscitation, stabilization of the newborn is a team sport that includes many players. Frontline staff should receive training in the evaluation-decision-action cycles of stabilization, no differently from the evaluation-decision-action cycles of resuscitation.

Training should be relevant to the work environment of the provider, whether in a rural community or in an advanced care institution. Clear lines of communication are vital when help is needed. Important team attributes, such as leadership, assignment of roles, preparation, and debriefing should be focused on during orientation and training. Simulation may be used as a learning tool in environments where babies rarely need resuscitation and stabilization. There is no reason to stop a resuscitation simulation just because the baby has started breathing: teams can be challenged to evaluate the need for stabilization, decide what to, and act on their decisions.

Institutional Resources and Equipment

Transport to and birth in an institution with the appropriate level of care is essential to good perinatal outcomes. Effective stabilization is facilitated by institutional recognition of the importance of adequate resources. In addition to staff training, institutions should evaluate their readiness to deal with an unstable newborn. The ACoRN Program uses an institutional needs assessment to enable the evaluation process. Important questions include the following:

- Is there a designated area for stabilization?
- Is there designated equipment, including a servocontrolled warmer?

- Is there appropriate neonatal monitoring, including oximetry, blood pressure monitoring?
- Are critical diagnostic tests available 24/7, including plasma glucose, blood gases, and radiography?
- Are important therapies available, such as blended oxygen and air, or prostaglandin?
- Is there support for families?

Referral and Transport

Most institutions, and units within institutions, have limitations on the levels of care they can provide to a sick baby. When these limits are reached, clear lines of communication are required to access consultation and to prepare for transfer. Staff should be orientated to these pathways.

Supporting Families and Staff

The human cost of caring for a sick baby is substantial, for both parents and caregivers, especially in environments where illness is not expected. It is important to keep families informed of the progress of their child, and to provide an explanation of the nature and risks of their child's illness. Allowing parents to see, touch, or hold their baby may be reassuring.

Following a difficult resuscitation or stabilization, staff may feel supported by debriefing. If a diagnosis is confirmed after transfer, they may be helped by feedback from the referral center. Positive experiences and successes should be reinforced, and, perhaps, shared with other team members through simulation.

RESEARCH OPPORTUNITIES AND GAPS

Surprisingly, comprehensive neonatal stabilization has been a poorly researched field. Scientists have focused on specific components of stabilization, such as resuscitation, shock, seizures, and hypoglycemia. When put together into one process, stabilization is a complex set of evaluation-decision-action cycles that require critical thinking and prioritization. It is often performed by teams of individuals with disparate skill sets and experience. It is often complicated by a lack of a diagnosis, and interaction between organ systems that impair focus on one area of concern.

Significant gaps in the science, in keeping with the *evaluation-decision-action* process, include the following:

- The validation of *evaluation* parameters (such as normal blood pressure and plasma glucose)
- The establishment and validation of evidence-based *decision*-trees, protocols, and algorithms
- The study of clinical interventions and the effectiveness of *action* during stabilization
- The educational and implementation science behind optimizing stabilization in many differing institutions and environments

A shift in the focus of research from resuscitation to the "resuscitation-stabilization" continuum is long overdue.

SUMMARY

Worldwide, many causes of neonatal death can be addressed by effective resuscitation followed by effective stabilization. The American Academy of Pediatrics[50] and Health Canada[51] state that all hospitals should be able to resuscitate and stabilize babies of all gestational ages. To meet these guidelines, institutions need to train and resource their staff to address the resuscitation-stabilization continuum.

A systematic clinical approach to babies who need stabilization requires repeated evaluation-decision-action cycles with a strong grounding in clinical examination and the knowledge of common presentations. During the process of stabilization, clear lines of communication should be accessed between team members and with parents, and transfer to a more advanced level of care should be considered or planned.

More research is needed to optimize processes of stabilization, as well as appropriate educational and implementation methodologies.

REFERENCES

1. Liu L, Johnson HL, Cousens S, et al, Child Health Epidemiology Reference Group of WHO and UNICEF. Global, regional, and national causes of child mortality: an updated systematic analysis for 2010 with time trends since 2000. Lancet 2012; 379(9832):2151–61.
2. Central Statistical Agency of Ethiopia. Ethiopian welfare monitoring survey 2011 summary report, 27th April 2012. Available at: http://www.csa.gov.et/docs/wms_summary_report.pdf. Accessed June 24, 2012.
3. Feng XL, Guo S, Hipgrave D, et al. China's facility-based birth strategy and neonatal mortality: a population-based epidemiological study. Lancet 2011; 378(9801):1493–500.
4. Frazier MD, Werthammer J. Post-resuscitation complications in term neonates. J Perinatol 2007;27(2):82–4.
5. Committee on Infectious Diseases, Committee on Fetus and Newborn, Baker CJ, Byington CL, Polin RA. Policy statement—Recommendations for the prevention of perinatal group B streptococcal (GBS) disease. Pediatrics 2011;128(3):611–6.
6. Lee SK, Zupancic JA, Pendray M, et al, Canadian Neonatal Network. Transport risk index of physiologic stability: a practical system for assessing infant transport care. J Pediatr 2001;139(2):220–6.
7. The CRIB (clinical risk index for babies) score: a tool for assessing initial neonatal risk and comparing performance of neonatal intensive care units. The International Neonatal Network. Lancet 1993;342(8865):193–8.
8. World Health Organization, United Nations Population Fund, UNICEF, The World Bank. Pregnancy, childbirth, postpartum and newborn care. A guide for essential practice. Available at: http://www.who.int/maternal_child_adolescent/documents/924159084x/en/index.html. Accessed June 19, 2012.
9. UNICEF India. Integrated Management of Neonatal and Childhood Illness. Available at: http://www.unicef.org/india/health_6725.htm. Accessed June 19, 2012.
10. Bhandari N, Mazumder S, Taneja S, et al, IMNCI Evaluation Study Group. Effect of implementation of Integrated Management of Neonatal and Childhood Illness (IMNCI) programme on neonatal and infant mortality: cluster randomised controlled trial. BMJ 2012;344:e1634.
11. University of Virginia. Perinatal Continuing Education Program. Available at: http://www.healthsystem.virginia.edu/internet/pcep/bkgd.cfm. Accessed June 19, 2012.
12. The S.T.A.B.L.E. Program. Available at: http://www.stableprogram.org/index.php. Accessed June 19, 2012.
13. ACoRN. Available at: http://www.acornprogram.net/. Accessed June 19, 2012.
14. Kattwinkel J, Nowacek G, Cook LJ, et al. A regionalized perinatal continuing education programme: successful adaptation to a foreign health care system and language. Med Educ 1997;31(3):210–8.

15. Harris JK, Yates B, Crosby WM. A perinatal continuing education program: its effects on the knowledge and practices of health professionals. J Obstet Gynecol Neonatal Nurs 1995;24(9):829–35.
16. Singhal N, Lockyer J, Fidler H, et al. Acute Care of At-Risk Newborns (ACoRN): quantitative and qualitative educational evaluation of the program in a region of China. BMC Med Educ 2012;12(1):44.
17. Schuchat A, Zywicki SS, Dinsmoor MJ, et al. Risk factors and opportunities for prevention of early-onset neonatal sepsis: a multicenter case-control study. Pediatrics 2000;105(Pt 1):21–6.
18. American Academy of Pediatrics and American Heart Association. Textbook of neonatal resuscitation. 6th edition. In: Kattwinkel J, editor. Elk Grove Village, IL: American Academy of Pediatrics; 2011.
19. McIntire DD, Leveno KJ. Neonatal mortality and morbidity rates in late preterm births compared with births at term. Obstet Gynecol 2008;111(1):35–41.
20. Ma XL, Xu XF, Chen C, et al, National Collaborative Study Group for Neonatal Respiratory Distress in Late Preterm or Term Infants. Epidemiology of respiratory distress and the illness severity in late preterm or term infants: a prospective multi-center study. Chin Med J (Engl) 2010;123(20):2776–80.
21. Saugstad OD, Speer CP, Halliday HL. Oxygen saturation in immature babies: revisited with updated recommendations. Neonatology 2011;100(3):217–8 [Epub 2011 Jul 15].
22. Guglani L, Lakshminrusimha S, Ryan RM. Transient tachypnea of the newborn. Pediatr Rev 2008;29(11):e59–65.
23. Teune MJ, Bakhuizen S, Gyamfi Bannerman C, et al. A systematic review of severe morbidity in infants born late preterm. Am J Obstet Gynecol 2011; 205(4):374.e1–9 [Epub 2011 Jul 20].
24. Rojas-Reyes MX, Morley CJ, Soll R. Prophylactic versus selective use of surfactant in preventing morbidity and mortality in preterm infants. Cochrane Database Syst Rev 2012;(3):CD000510.
25. Singh N, Hawley KL, Viswanathan K. Efficacy of porcine versus bovine surfactants for preterm newborns with respiratory distress syndrome: systematic review and meta-analysis. Pediatrics 2011;128(6):e1588–95 [Epub 2011 Nov].
26. Willson DF, Notter RH. The future of exogenous surfactant therapy. Respir Care 2011;56(9):1369–86.
27. Aziz N, Cheng YW, Caughey AB. Neonatal outcomes in the setting of preterm premature rupture of membranes complicated by chorioamnionitis. J Matern Fetal Neonatal Med 2009;22(9):780–4.
28. Lapointe A, Barrington KJ. Pulmonary hypertension and the asphyxiated newborn. J Pediatr 2011;158(Suppl 2):e19–24.
29. Konduri GC, Kim UO. Advances in the diagnosis and management of persistent pulmonary hypertension of the newborn. Pediatr Clin North Am 2009;56(3): 579–600.
30. Fanaroff AA. Meconium aspiration syndrome: historical aspects. J Perinatol 2008; 28:53–7.
31. Singh BS, Clark RH, Powers RJ, et al. Meconium aspiration syndrome remains a significant problem in the NICU: outcomes and treatment patterns in term neonates admitted for intensive care during a ten-year period. J Perinatol 2009; 29(7):497–503.
32. Kotecha S, Barbato A, Bush A, et al. Antenatal and postnatal management of congenital cystic adenomatoid malformation. Paediatr Respir Rev 2012;13(3): 162–71.

33. Barber M, Blaisdell CJ. Respiratory causes of infant mortality: progress and challenges. Am J Perinatol 2010;27(7):549–58.

34. Smith J, Schumacher RE, Donn SM, et al. Clinical course of symptomatic spontaneous pneumothorax in term and late preterm newborns: report from a large cohort. Am J Perinatol 2011;28(2):163–8 [Epub 2010 Aug 10].

35. Keane JF, Fyler DC, Lock JE. Nadas' pediatric cardiology. 2nd edition. Philadelphia: Hanley and Belfus; 2006.

36. Rein AJ, Omokhodion SI, Nir A. Significance of a cardiac murmur as the sole clinical sign in the newborn. Clin Pediatr 2000;39(9):511–20.

37. Penny DJ, Shekerdemian LS. Management of the neonate with symptomatic congenital heart disease. Arch Dis Child Fetal Neonatal Ed 2001;84(3):F141–5.

38. Zubrow AB, Hulman S, Kushner H, et al. Determinants of blood pressure in infants admitted to neonatal intensive care units: a prospective multicenter study. J Perinatol 1995;15:470–9.

39. Fanaroff JM, Fanaroff AA. Blood pressure disorders in the neonate: hypotension and hypertension. Semin Fetal Neonatal Med 2006;11(3):174–81.

40. Jones JG, Smith SL. Shock in the critically ill neonate. J Perinat Neonatal Nurs 2009;23(4):346–54.

41. Selway LD. State of the science: hypoxic ischemic encephalopathy and hypothermic intervention for neonates. Adv Neonatal Care 2010;10(2):60–6.

42. Shah PS. Hypothermia: a systematic review and meta-analysis of clinical trials. Semin Fetal Neonatal Med 2010;15(5):238–46.

43. Shankaran S, Laptook AR, Ehrenkranz RA, et al. Whole-body hypothermia for neonates with hypoxic-ischemic encephalopathy. N Engl J Med 2005;353(15): 1574–84.

44. Sheth RD, Hobbs GR, Mullett M. Neonatal seizures: incidence, onset, and etiology by gestational age. J Perinatol 1999;19(1):40–3.

45. Seshia SS, Huntsman RJ, Lowry NJ, et al. Neonatal seizures: diagnosis and management. Zhongguo Dang Dai Er Ke Za Zhi 2011;13(2):81–100.

46. Aschner JL, Poland RL. Sodium bicarbonate: basically useless therapy. Pediatrics 2008;122(4):831–5.

47. Committee on Fetus and Newborn, Adamkin DH. Postnatal glucose homeostasis in late-preterm and term infants. Pediatrics 2011;127(3):575–9.

48. Newman TB, Puopolo KM, Wi S, et al. Interpreting complete blood counts soon after birth in newborns at risk for sepsis. Pediatrics 2010;126(5):903–9.

49. Puopolo KM, Eichenwald EC. No change in the incidence of ampicillin-resistant, neonatal, early-onset sepsis over 18 years. Pediatrics 2010;125(5):e1031–8.

50. Stark AR, American Academy of Pediatrics Committee on Fetus and Newborn. Levels of neonatal care. Pediatrics 2004;114(5):1341–7.

51. Health Canada. Family-Centred Maternity and Newborn Care: National Guidelines. Ottawa: Canada; 2000. Available at: http://www.phac-aspc.gc.ca/hp-ps/dca-dea/publications/fcm-smp/index-eng.php. Accessed June 28, 2012.

Hypoxic-ischemic Encephalopathy and Novel Strategies for Neuroprotection

Seetha Shankaran, MD

KEYWORDS

- Hypothermia • Neonatal hypoxic-ischemic encephalopathy
- Neurodevelopmental outcome • Term infants

KEY POINTS

- Hypothermia is neuroprotective for neonatal hypoxic ischemic encephalopathy.
- The neuroprotective effects persist to childhood.
- The future of optimizing hypothermia therapy with adjuvant agents to further reduce death and disability holds promise.

INTRODUCTION

Neonatal encephalopathy due to hypoxic ischemia (HI) occurs in 1.5 (95% confidence interval [CI], 1.3–1.7) per 1000 live full-term births. About 15% to 20% of affected newborns die in the postnatal period, and an additional 25% will sustain childhood disabilities.[1] The presence of abnormal neurologic examination results in the first few days of life highly predicts a brain insult in the perinatal period. Neonates with mild encephalopathy usually do not have an increased risk of motor or cognitive deficits. Neonates with severe encephalopathy have a high risk of death (up to 85%) and an increased risk of cerebral palsy (CP) and mental retardation among survivors. Neonates with moderate encephalopathy have significant motor deficits, fine motor disability, memory impairment, visual or visuomotor dysfunction, increased hyperactivity and delayed school readiness.[2–6] The essential criteria suggested as prerequisites to a diagnosis of a hypoxic-ischemic insult resulting in moderate or severe encephalopathy in term infants include the following: metabolic acidosis with a cord pH of less than 7.0 or a baseline deficit of 12 mmol/L or more, early onset of encephalopathy, multisystem organ dysfunction, and exclusion of other causes such as coagulation, metabolic and genetic disorders, or maternal trauma.[7]

Wayne State University School of Medicine, Division of Neonatal/Perinatal Medicine, Children's Hospital of Michigan and Hutzel Women's Hospital, 3901 Beaubien, #4C19, Detroit, MI 48201, USA
E-mail address: sshankar@med.wayne.edu

Clin Perinatol 39 (2012) 919–929
http://dx.doi.org/10.1016/j.clp.2012.09.008   perinatology.theclinics.com

PATHOPHYSIOLOGY OF BRAIN INJURY DUE TO HI

The pathophysiology of brain injury secondary to HI is associated with 2 phases: primary and secondary energy failure based on characteristics of the cerebral energy state documented in both preclinical models and human infants (**Box 1**).[8–11] Primary energy failure is characterized by reductions in cerebral blood flow and oxygen substrates. High-energy phosphorylated compounds such as ATP and phosphocreatine are reduced, and tissue acidosis is prominent. Primary energy failure is associated with an "excitotoxic-oxidative cascade"[12,13] with excessive stimulation of neurotransmitter receptors and membrane depolarization, which mediates an increase in intracellular calcium levels and osmotic dysregulation.[14] Intracellular calcium activates neuronal nitric oxide synthase, leading to the release of the oxygen free radical nitric oxide, which can disrupt mitochondrial respiration. Signals released from damaged mitochondria lead to apoptosis or programmed cell death as long as energy supplies persist, but exhaustion of these supplies leads to cell necrosis. Apoptosis can also be triggered by the activation of caspase enzymes. Resolution of HI within a specific time interval reverses the decrease in the levels of high-energy phosphorylated metabolites and intracellular pH and promotes recycling of neurotransmitters. If the injury is severe, the cascade of events results in a second interval of energy failure in the mitochondria, in which the brain's energy supplies decrease over 24 hours.[15] Secondary energy failure differs from primary energy failure in that the declines in the levels of phosphocreatine and ATP are not accompanied by brain acidosis.[10] The pathogenesis of secondary energy failure involves continuation of the excitotoxic-oxidation cascade, apoptosis, inflammation and altered growth factor levels, and protein synthesis.[13]

The interval between primary and secondary energy failure represents a latent phase that corresponds to a therapeutic window. The duration of the window was noted to be approximately 6 hours in near-term fetal sheep treated with hypothermia initiated at varying intervals following timed HI injury.[16,17] Subsequent research has noted that cell death in the brain exposed to HI is delayed over several days to weeks after an injury, and apoptosis and necrosis continue depending on the region and severity of the injury.[13]

Box 1
Mechanisms of damage in the fetal/neonatal model of hypoxia-ischemia

Primary energy failure

- Decrease in CBF, O_2 substrates, high-energy phosphate compounds

- Excitotoxic-oxidative cascade

- Loss of ionic homeostasis across membranes, entry of intracellular calcium, mitochondrial disruption, brain acidosis, apoptosis followed by necrosis

Secondary energy failure

- Continuation of excitotoxic-oxidative cascade

- Activation of microglia—inflammatory response

- Activation of caspase proteins

- Reduction in levels of growth factors, protein synthesis

- Apoptosis–necrosis continuum

Abbreviation: CBF, cerebral blood flow.

Current Therapies for Neonatal Hypoxic-ischemic Encephalopathy

Before the introduction of neuroprotective therapies, the management of neonates with hypoxic-ischemic encephalopathy (HIE) was limited to supportive intensive care, including resuscitation in the delivery room followed by stabilization of hemodynamic and pulmonary disturbances (hypotension, metabolic acidosis, and hypoventilation), correction of metabolic disturbances, (glucose, calcium, magnesium and electrolytes), treatment of seizures, and monitoring for multiorgan dysfunction.

Diagnosis of Encephalopathy

A detailed history regarding the pregnancy and intrapartum period reflecting events leading to compromised blood or oxygen supply to the fetus should be obtained. These events include placental abruption, amniotic fluid embolism, tight nuchal cord, cord prolapse/avulsion, maternal hemorrhage (placental abruption/accreta), trauma or cardiorespiratory arrest, uterine rupture, and acute severe and sustained fetal decelerations. A history of maternal elevation of temperature increases the risk of neonatal encephalopathy. A careful neurologic examination needs to be performed to diagnose encephalopathy. Laboratory evaluations that should be performed include placental pathology to evaluate for the presence of infection. Amplitude-integrated electroencephalography (aEEG) when performed at less than 6 hours of age has been found to highly predict early childhood outcome.

EVIDENCE FOR HYPOTHERMIA FOR NEUROPROTECTION
Preclinical Studies

There is established evidence in fetal and neonatal animal models, and across species, that cooling by a depth of 4°C to 6°C versus controls has been neuroprotective while being well tolerated.[13,18–20] The duration of cooling in these studies varied from 3 to 72 hours, and each study compared a specific depth of cooling with controls. Hypothermia is neuroprotective by inhibiting many steps in the excitotoxic-oxidative cascade, including inhibiting the increase in brain lactic acid, glutamate, and nitric oxide concentrations and epileptic activity (**Box 2**). In addition, hypothermia inhibits protease activation, mitochondrial failure, free radical damage, lipid peroxidation, and inflammation. Hypothermia has been shown to decrease brain energy use,

---

Box 2
Mechanism of action of hypothermia

Hypothermia is protective at critical cellular and vascular sites of cerebral injury in fetal/ neonatal model of HI

- Reduces cerebral metabolism; prevents edema and loss of membrane potential

- Decreases energy use

- Reduces/suppresses cytotoxic AA accumulation and NO

- Inhibits PAF, inflammatory cascade

- Suppresses free radical activity and lipid peroxidation

- Attenuates secondary energy failure

- Inhibits apoptosis and necrosis

- Reduces extent of brain injury

Abbreviations: AA, amino acid; NO, nitric oxide; PAF, platelet activating factor.

prolong the latent phase, reduce infarct size, decrease neuronal cell loss, retain sensory motor function, and preserve hippocampal structures.[21–23] Increased protection is noted with increasing depth of temperature (up to 28°C). None of the studies comparing different depths of temperature with controls have documented adverse effects except a decrease in heart rate. Optimal neuroprotection by hypothermia may occur at different temperatures in the cortical and deep gray matter.[24]

There are data that hypothermia may be protective of other organ systems; hypothermia reduced cardiac troponin 1 and was associated with fewer ischemic lesions.[25] On the other hand, hypothermia to a greater depth may be detrimental; cooling to 30°C from a baseline of 38.4°C is associated with metabolic derangements and higher rate of death and cardiac arrest than cooling to 33.5°C.[26] In addition, neuroprotective effects are reversible; resuscitation of the neonatal rat model with 100% oxygen increases brain injury and counteracts the neuroprotective effect of hypothermia.[27]

Hypothermia for Neuroprotection: Clinical Trials

Six major randomized controlled trials (RCTs) of hypothermia for neonatal HIE have been published, enrolling infants born at greater than or equal to 36 weeks or greater than or equal to 35 weeks gestation, within the therapeutic window of 6 hours. Each of these trials are summarized briefly: the number of infants enrolled, type of cooling (head or whole body), inclusion criteria and percentage of mild encephalopathy enrolled, source of core temperature monitoring, any exclusions from analysis, and primary and predefined secondary outcomes.

The CoolCap study involved 234 term infants with moderate or severe encephalopathy and abnormal aEEG, either cooled to a rectal temperature of 34°C to 35°C for 72 hours or kept under conventional care. The primary outcome was death or severe disability at 18 months.[28] Data were unavailable for 16 infants (7%). Death or disability occurred in 66% conventional care and 55% cooled group (adjusted odds ratio [OR] [95% CI] 0.61 [0.34–1.09], $P = .10$). Predefined subgroup analysis suggested that head cooling had no effect in infants with the most severe aEEG changes but was beneficial in infants with less severe aEEG changes.

The National Institute of Child Health and Human Development (NICHD) RCT of whole-body hypothermia for neonates with HIE[29] was preceded by an animal study of feasibility and a pilot study. Term infants ($n = 208$) with moderate or severe encephalopathy were randomly assigned to whole-body cooling to an esophageal temperature of 33.5°C for 72 hours or usual care. The primary outcome was death or moderate or severe disability at 18 months. Data were unavailable for 3 infants (1%). Death or severe disability occurred in 62% of the usual care group and 44% of the hypothermia group (relative risk [RR] [95% CI] 0.72 [0.54–0.95], $P = .01$).

The Total Body Hypothermia for Neonatal Encephalopathy (TOBY) trial[30] enrolled 325 infants with moderate or severe encephalopathy and an abnormal aEEG. Infants were randomly assigned to whole-body hypothermia to a rectal temperature of 33°C to 34°C for 72 hours or usual care. The primary outcome was death or severe neurodevelopmental disability at 18 months. Data were unavailable for 2 infants (<1%). Death or severe disability occurred in 53% of the usual care group and 45% of the hypothermia group (RR 0.86 [0.68–1.07], $P = .17$). Predefined secondary outcomes of survival without disabilities were significantly higher in the cooled group compared with the usual care group. The rate of CP was lower, and improved mental and psychomotor indices were noted in the hypothermia group as compared with the usual care group, all $P<.05$.

The fourth trial was a selective head cooling or usual care RCT in China, in which 256 infants were enrolled with encephalopathy.[31] The cooling group was maintained at

34°C nasopharyngeal and rectal temperatures for 72 hours. The primary outcome was death or severe disability at 18 months. There were 21 postrandomization exclusions, and of the remainder, 21% and 19% had mild encephalopathy in the hypothermia and usual care groups, respectively. Data were unavailable for 41 infants (16% of analyzed or 24% of recruited cohort). The primary outcome occurred in 49% control and 31% hypothermia group infants (OR 0.47 [0.26–0.84, P = .01]).

The European Network RCT[32] enrolled 129 infants with moderate or severe encephalopathy and an abnormal aEEG. In the whole-body hypothermia group, a rectal temperature of 33°C to 34.0°C was maintained. All infants received morphine (0.1 mg/1 g) infusions. The primary outcome was death or disability at 18 months. Data on 18 infants (14%) were not available. Death or severe disability occurred in 51% of the hypothermia group and 83% in the normothermia group (OR, 0.21 [0.09–0.54], P = .001).

The most recent RCT published is the Infant Cooling Evaluation (ICE) trial[33] (n = 221). Whole-body cooling was initiated at the referral hospital after clinical diagnosis of encephalopathy, and rectal temperatures were monitored. The primary outcome was death or major disability at 24 months. Mild encephalopathy was noted in 15% of the hypothermia group and 23% of control infants. Data were unavailable for 13 (6%) infants. The primary outcome occurred in 51% of the hypothermia group and 66% of control infants (RR, 0.77 [0.62–0.98]). The mortality rate was significantly reduced, whereas survival free of disability was increased in the hypothermia group compared with the control group.

Recent systematic reviews and meta-analyses have demonstrated that hypothermia improves survival and neurodevelopmental outcome at 18 months among term infants with moderate or severe HIE.[34,35]

BRAIN IMAGING EVIDENCE OF NEUROPROTECTION

The TOBY trial evaluated neonatal magnetic resonance images (MRI) from 131 of 325 (40%) trial participants.[36] Hypothermia was associated with a reduction in the number of lesions in the basal ganglia or thalamus (OR, 0.36 [0.15–0.84, P = .02]), white matter (OR, 0.30 [0.12–0.77, P = .01]), and abnormal posterior limb of the internal capsule (OR, 0.38 [0.17–0.85, P = .02]). Cooled infants had more normal scans and fewer scans that predicted 18-month neuromotor abnormalities. The accuracy of prediction of death and disability by MRI was 0.84 (0.74–0.94) in the cooled group and 0.81 (0.71–0.91) in the control group.

The NICHD Neonatal Research Network (NRN) examined neonatal MRI scans of 136 of 208 (65%) trial participants.[37] The infants were characterized based on the pattern of injury on the MRI findings. Normal scans were noted among 52% of the hypothermia group and 35% of the control group (P = .06). Cerebral infraction was noted among fewer infants in the hypothermia compared to control group (P = .02) in addition to anterior limb of the internal capsule abnormality (P = .05) and posterior limb of internal capsule injury (P = .06). The MRI brain injury pattern correlated with the outcome of death or disability and with disability in survivors at 18 months. Each point increase in the severity of the pattern of brain injury was independently associated with a twofold increase in the odds of death or disability.

CHILDHOOD OUTCOMES AFTER HYPOTHERMIA
Six- to Eight-Year Outcomes After Hypothermia for Neonatal Encephalopathy

The CoolCap study investigators evaluated whether outcomes at 18 to 22 months predicted functional outcomes at 7 to 8 years among 62 of 135 surviving children from the trial.[38] Measures of self-care, mobility, and cognitive function were assessed by the WeeFIM parent questionnaire. Functional outcome at 7 to 8 years was associated with the 18-month assessments; this was noted among children with favorable and adverse outcomes.

The NICHD NRN trial evaluated cognitive, attention and executive, and visuospatial function; neurologic outcomes; and physical and psychosocial health, with data available among 190 of 208 trial participants.[39] The primary outcome of death or IQ less than 70 was noted among 47% of the hypothermia group children and 62% of the control group children ($P = .06$). Secondary outcomes included a mortality rate of 28% and 44% ($P = .04$), death or CP of 41% and 60% ($P = .02$), and death and severe disability of 41% and 60% ($P = .03$) in the hypothermia and control groups, respectively. These data extend support for the use of hypothermia for neonatal HIE.

CLINICAL APPLICATION OF COOLING

Secondary analyses of the trials have provided important information applicable to the clinical aspects of providing hypothermia therapy. A scoring system using clinical and laboratory values at less than 6 hours of age developed within the NICHD trial of whole-body hypothermia revealed correct classification rates for death and disability at 18 months (78%) and death alone (71%). Severe encephalopathy predicted death and disability at 67% and 73%, respectively, whereas classification and regression tree models had correct classification rates of 80% and 77%, respectively.[40] Severe HIE (at <6 hours of age) and an abnormal aEEG (at <9 hours of age) were related to death and disability at 18 months in univariate analysis in another report, whereas severe HIE alone predicted outcome in the multivariate analysis. The addition of the aEEG pattern to HIE stage did not add to the predictive value of the model; area under the curve changed from 0.72 to 0.75 ($P = .19$).[41] The importance of serial neurologic examinations during the study intervention period is highlighted in a study demonstrating that at 24 and 48 hours, infants in the hypothermia group had less severe encephalopathy than infants in the control group. Persistence of severe encephalopathy at 72 hours increased the risk of death and disability after controlling for the treatment group. The discharge examination improved the predictive value of the stage of HIE at less than 6 hours for death and disability.[42] None of the trials to date have an adequate sample size to examine the effect of hypothermia separately on moderate and severe encephalopathy; however, a consistent trend in the decrease in frequency of disability in both moderate and severe encephalopathy was noted in the NICHD trial in the hypothermia group as compared with the control group.[43]

The CoolCap trial has reported better outcomes with treatment with hypothermia: lower encephalopathy grade at random assignment, lower birth weight, greater aEEG amplitude, and absence of seizures.[44] Infants with persistent moderate encephalopathy on day 4 had a more favorable prognosis compared with those on standard care.[45]

The TOBY trial has noted that more infants with severely abnormal aEEG died or had severe disability at 18 months.[30] Both the NICHD trial and the TOBY trial have reported that time to randomization and time to initiate cooling did not have an effect on the outcome at 18 months.[30,43] Clinical seizures and severe encephalopathy at random assignment in the NICHD trial was noted to be associated with death and disability or mental development index less than 70 at 18 months of age in the univariate analysis; when controlling for treatment and stage of encephalopathy, seizures no longer had an independent effect on the outcome.[46] In another secondary analysis evaluating early blood gas parameters and ventilation with outcome among NICHD trial participants, both minimum P_{CO_2} and cumulative P_{CO_2} (<35 mm Hg) at less than 12 hours of age were associated with increased risk of death or disability at 18 months.[47]

Two of the trials have noted that elevated temperatures (among control group infants) were associated with an increased risk of death and disability.[44,48] Among cooled infants, infants at lower birth weight are at risk for decreases in temperature to less than 32.0°C, both during induction and maintenance of cooling.[49] Phenobarbital administered before cooling in the NICHD trial resulted in lower target esophageal temperatures during the induction phase.[50]

Safety of Hypothermia

The safety of hypothermia as neuroprotection has been reported in the trials to date.[28–33,43] No increase in persistent pulmonary hypertension, use of inhaled nitric oxide, or need for extracorporeal membrane oxygenation has been noted among cooled infants compared with infants who received standard care. No increases in metabolic disturbances or cardiac arrhythmia have been reported.[43] Hypothermia is currently being recommended by health care policy makers (American Heart Association Guidelines for Cardiopulmonary Resuscitation and Emergency Cardiovascular Care and the International Consensus on Cardiopulmonary Resuscitation and Emergency Cardiovascular Care Science with Treatment Recommendations), stating that during the postresuscitation period in greater than or equal to 36-week gestation neonates with evolving moderate or severe encephalopathy, hypothermia should be offered in the context of clearly defined protocols similar to published trials.[51,52]

KNOWLEDGE GAPS IN HYPOTHERMIA THERAPY
Cooling During Transport

Hypothermia administered during transport of high-risk infants with possible or established encephalopathy has been associated with overcooling.[53] The benefit of cooling during transport has not been demonstrated; earlier time to cooling has not been shown to affect outcome.[30,43] Hypothermia during transport of high-risk infants should be conducted only with targeted core temperature monitoring; servocontrolled devices may soon be available.[54]

Cooling of Preterm Infants

There are currently no evidence-based data on the benefits of cooling for HI for infants less than or equal to 36 weeks gestation age; this is an area that needs to be investigated.[55] One RCT is ongoing, evaluating hypothermia as neuroprotection for late preterm infants (NCT00620711).

Cooling of Infants Presenting after more than 6 Hours of Age

There is evidence of ongoing brain injury beyond the 6-hour therapeutic window; hence hypothermia as therapy for infants with moderate/severe HIE who present after 6 hours of birth is being evaluated (NCT0061477).

Pharmacokinetics of Medications During Hypothermia

Pharmacokinetic parameters are altered during hypothermia therapy.[56] Morphine levels have been noted to increase.[57] Gentamicin levels are not affected during cooling.[58] Phenobarbital and topiramate accumulate during hypothermia therapy.[59] The effects of hypothermia on drug metabolism, clearance, and response have been reviewed.[60]

FUTURE OF HYPOTHERMIA

The rate of death or disability following hypothermia at 33°C to 34°C for 72 hours for neonatal HIE is unacceptably high and ranges from 31% to 55% in the published trials. Hence, optimizing cooling strategies further or adjuvant therapies are needed. Preclinical studies have noted that cooling to a depth of 5°C may be more protective than cooling to a depth of 3°C. In addition, because injury is ongoing, a duration of cooling for more than 72 hours may be more protective that cooling for 72 hours. The NICHD is currently evaluating an optimizing cooling strategy by examining a greater depth of cooling (32.0°C) and longer duration of cooling (120 hours) to decrease death and disability at 18 months (NCT01192776).

Hypothermia Plus Adjuvant Therapies

Hypothermia plus adjuvant therapies have been extensively reviewed in 2 publications.[61,62] Based on the preclinical studies, ongoing trials in neonates include inhaled xenon and cooling (NCT01545271 and NCT00934700), safety of erythropoietin (NCT00719407), darbepoetin and hypothermia (NCT0147105), and topiramate plus hypothermia (NCT01241019). The use of human cord blood for the hypoxic-ischemic neonate is also being investigated. A recent review highlights the approaches to this therapy.[63]

In summary, hypothermia for neonatal HIE is an effective therapy with a number needed to treat of only 6 infants. The safety of hypothermia has been clearly demonstrated. The neuroprotective effects noted at 18 months of age persist to childhood. The future of optimizing hypothermia therapy with additional adjuvant agents to reduce death and disability to a greater extent than current hypothermia therapy alone holds promise.

REFERENCES

1. Kurinczuk JJ, White-Koning M, Badawi N. Epidemiology of neonatal encephalopathy and hypoxic-ischaemic encephalopathy. Early Hum Dev 2010;86:329–38.
2. Shankaran S, Woldt E, Koepke T, et al. Acute neonatal morbidity and long-term central nervous system sequelae of perinatal asphyxia in term infants. Early Hum Dev 1991;25:135–48.
3. Robertson CM. Long term follow-up of term infants with perinatal asphyxia. In: Stevenson DK, Benitz WE, Sunshine P, editors. Fetal and neonatal brain injury. 3rd edition. New York, NY: Cambridge University; 2003. p. 829–58.
4. De Vries LS, Jongmans MJ. Long-term outcome after neonatal hypoxic-ischemic encephalopathy. Arch Dis Child Fetal Neonatal Ed 2010;95:F220–4.
5. Marlow N, Rose AS, Rands CE, et al. Neuropsychological and educational problems at school age associated with neonatal encephalopathy. Arch Dis Child Fetal Neonatal Ed 2005;90:F380–7.
6. Gonzalez FF, Miller SP. Does perinatal asphyxia impair cognitive function without cerebral palsy? Arch Dis Child Fetal Neonatal Ed 2006;91:454–9.
7. American College of Obstetricians and Gynecologists and the American Academy of Pediatrics. Criteria required to define an acute intrapartum hypoxic event as sufficient to cause cerebral palsy. Neonatal encephalopathy and cerebral palsy: defining the pathogenesis and pathophysiology. ACOG 2003:73–80.
8. Hope PL, Costello AM, Cady EB, et al. Cerebral energy metabolism studied with phosphorus NMR spectroscopy in normal and birth-asphyxiated infants. Lancet 1984;2:366–70.

9. Azzopardi D, Wyatt JS, Cady EB, et al. Prognosis of newborn infants with hypoxic-ischemic brain injury assessed by phosphorus magnetic resonance spectroscopy. Pediatr Res 1989;25:445–51.
10. Lorek A, Takei Y, Cady EB, et al. Delayed ("secondary") cerebral energy failure after acute hypoxia-ischemia in the newborn piglet: continuous 48-hour studies by phosphorus magnetic resonance spectroscopy. Pediatr Res 1994;36:699–706.
11. Blumberg RM, Cady EB, Wigglesworth JS, et al. Relation between delayed impairment of cerebral energy metabolism and infarction following transient focal hypoxia-ischaemia in the developing brain. Exp Brain Res 1997;113:130–7.
12. Johnston MV, Trescher WH, Ishida A, et al. Neurobiology of hypoxic-ischemic injury in the developing brain. Pediatr Res 2001;49:735–41.
13. Johnston MV, Fatemi A, Wilson MA, et al. Treatment advances in neonatal neuroprotection and neurointensive care. Lancet Neurol 2011;10:372–82.
14. Cross JL, Meloni BP, Bakker AJ, et al. Modes of neuronal calcium entry and homeostasis following cerebral ischemia. Stroke Res Treat 2010;2010:316862.
15. Hagberg H, Mallard C, Rousset CI, et al. Apoptotic mechanisms in the immature brain: involvement of mitochondria. J Child Neurol 2009;24:1141–6.
16. Gunn AJ, Gunn TR, de Haan HH, et al. Dramatic neuronal rescue with prolonged selective head cooling after ischemia in fetal lambs. J Clin Invest 1997;99: 248–56.
17. Gunn AJ, Bennet L, Gunning MI, et al. Cerebral hypothermia is not neuroprotective when started after postischemic seizures in fetal sheep. Pediatr Res 1999; 46(3):274–80.
18. Busto R, Dietrich WD, Globus MY, et al. Small differences in intraischemic brain temperature critically determine the extent of ischemic neuronal injury. J Cereb Blood Flow Metab 1987;6:729–38.
19. Colbourne F, Corbett D. Delayed and prolonged post-ischemic hypothermia is neuroprotective in the gerbil. Brain Res 1994;654:265–72.
20. Thoresen M, Bågenholm R, Løberg EM, et al. Posthypoxic cooling of neonatal rats provides protection against brain injury. Arch Dis Child Fetal Neonatal Ed 1996;74:F3–9.
21. Laptook AR, Corbett RJ, Sterett R, et al. Modest hypothermia provides partial neuroprotection when used for immediate resuscitation after brain ischemia. Pediatr Res 1997;42(1):17–23.
22. Laptook AR, Corbett RJ, Sterett R, et al. Quantitative Relationship between brain temperature and energy utilization rate measured in vivo using P and H magnetic resonance spectroscopy. Pediatr Res 1995;38(6):919–25.
23. O'Brien FE, Iwata O, Thornton JS, et al. Delayed whole body cooling to 33 to 35°C and the development of impaired energy generation consequential to transient cerebral hypoxia-ischemia in the newborn piglet. Pediatrics 2006;117(5):1549–58.
24. Iwata O, Thornton JS, Sellwood MW, et al. Depth of delayed cooling alters neuroprotection pattern after hypoxia-ischemia. Ann Neurol 2005;58:75–87.
25. Liu X, Tooley J, Løberg EM, et al. Immediate hypothermia reduces cardiac troponin I after hypoxic-ischemic encephalopathy in newborn pigs. Pediatr Res 2011;70(4):352–6.
26. Kerenyi A, Kelen D, Faulkner SD, et al. Systemic effects of whole-body cooling to 35°C, 33.5°C, and 30°C in a piglet model of perinatal asphyxia: implications for therapeutic hypothermia. Pediatr Res 2012;71(5):573–82.
27. Dalen ML, Liu X, Elstad M, et al. Resuscitation with 100% oxygen increases injury and counteracts the neuroprotective effect of therapeutic hypothermia in the neonatal rat. Pediatr Res 2012;71(3):247–52.

28. Gluckman PD, Wyatt J, Azzopardi DV, et al. Selective head cooling with mild systemic hypothermia after neonatal encephalopathy: multicenter randomised trial. Lancet 2005;365:663–70.

29. Shankaran S, Laptook AR, Ehrenkranz RA, et al. Whole-body hypothermia for neonates with hypoxic-ischemic encephalopathy. N Engl J Med 2005;353: 1574–84.

30. Azzopardi DV, Strohm B, Edwards AD, et al. Moderate hypothermia to treat perinatal asphyxial encephalopathy. N Engl J Med 2009;361:1349–58.

31. Zhou WH, Cheng GQ, Shao XM, et al. Selective head cooling with mild systemic hypothermia after neonatal hypoxic-ischemic encephalopathy: a multicenter randomized controlled trial in China. J Pediatr 2010;157:367–72, 372.e1–3.

32. Simbruner G, Mittal RA, Rohlmann F, et al. Systemic hypothermia after neonatal encephalopathy: outcomes of neo.nEURO.network RCT. Pediatrics 2010; 126(4):e771–8.

33. Jacobs SE, Morley CJ, Inder TE, et al. Whole-body hypothermia for term and near-term newborns with hypoxic-ischemic encephalopathy: a randomized controlled trial. Arch Pediatr Adolesc Med 2011;165:692–700.

34. Tagin MA, Woolcott CG, Vincer MJ, et al. Hypothermia for neonatal hypoxic ischemic encephalopathy: an updated systematic review and meta-analysis. Arch Pediatr Adolesc Med 2012;166:558–66.

35. Edwards AD, Brocklehurst P, Gunn AJ, et al. Neurological outcomes at 18 months of age after moderate hypothermia for perinatal hypoxic ischaemic encephalopathy: synthesis and meta-analysis of trial data. BMJ 2010;340:c363.

36. Rutherford M, Ramenghi LA, Edwards AD, et al. Assessment of brain tissue injury after moderate hypothermia in neonates with hypoxic-ischaemic encephalopathy: a nested substudy of a randomised controlled trial. Lancet Neurol 2010;9:39–45.

37. Shankaran S, Barnes PD, Hintz SR, et al. Brain injury following trial of hypothermia for neonatal hypoxic-ischemic encephalopathy. Arch Dis Child 2012. [Epub ahead of print].

38. Guillet R, Edwards AD, Thoresen M, et al. Seven- to eight-year follow-up of the CoolCap trial of head cooling for neonatal encephalopathy. Pediatr Res 2012; 71(2):205–9.

39. Shankaran S, Pappas A, McDonald SA, et al. Childhood outcomes after hypothermia for neonatal encephalopathy. N Engl J Med 2012;366:2085–92.

40. Ambalavanan N, Carlo WA, Shankaran S, et al. Predicting outcomes of neonates diagnosed with hypoxemic-ischemic encephalopathy. Pediatrics 2006;118(5): 2084–93.

41. Shankaran S, Pappas A, McDonald SA, et al. Predictive value of an early amplitude integrated electroencephalogram and neurologic examination. Pediatrics 2011;128:e112–20.

42. Shankaran S, Laptook AR, Tyson JE, et al. Evolution of encephalopathy during whole body hypothermia for neonatal hypoxic-ischemic encephalopathy. J Pediatr 2012;160. 567–572.e3.

43. Shankaran S, Pappas A, Laptook AR, et al. Outcomes of safety and effectiveness in a multicenter randomized, controlled trial of whole-body hypothermia for neonatal hypoxic-ischemic encephalopathy. Pediatrics 2008;122:e791–8.

44. Wyatt JS, Gluckman PD, Liu PY, et al. Determinants of outcomes after head cooling for neonatal encephalopathy. Pediatrics 2007;119(5):912–21.

45. Gunn AJ, Wyatt JS, Whitelaw A, et al. Therapeutic hypothermia changes the prognostic value of clinical evaluation of neonatal encephalopathy. J Pediatr 2008;152:55–8, 58.e1.

46. Kwon JM, Guillet R, Shankaran S, et al. Clinical seizures in neonatal hypoxic-ischemic encephalopathy have no independent impact on neurodevelopmental outcome: secondary analyses of data from the neonatal research network hypothermia trial. J Child Neurol 2011;26(3):322–8.
47. Pappas A, Shankaran S, Laptook AR, et al. Hypocarbia and adverse outcome in neonatal hypoxic-ischemic encephalopathy. J Pediatr 2011;158:752–758.e1.
48. Laptook A, Tyson J, Shankaran S, et al. Elevated temperature after hypoxic-ischemic encephalopathy: a risk factor for adverse outcome. Pediatrics 2008;122:491–9.
49. Shankaran S, Laptook AR, McDonald SA, et al. Temperature profile and outcomes of neonates undergoing whole body hypothermia for neonatal hypoxic-ischemic encephalopathy. Pediatr Crit Care Med 2012;13(1):53–9.
50. Sant'Anna G, Laptook AR, Shankaran S, et al. Phenobarbital and temperature profile during hypothermia for hypoxic-ischemic encephalopathy. J Child Neurol 2012;27(4):451–7.
51. Kattwinkel J, Perlman JM, Aziz K, et al. Neonatal resuscitation: 2010 American Heart Association Guidelines for cardiopulmonary resuscitation and emergency cardiovascular care. Pediatrics 2010;126(5):e1400–13.
52. Perlman JM, Wyllie J, Kattwinkel J, et al. Neonatal resuscitation: 2010 International Consensus on cardiopulmonary resuscitation and emergency cardiovascular care science with treatment recommendations. Pediatrics 2010;126(5): e1319–44.
53. Fairchild K, Sokora D, Scott J, et al. Therapeutic hypothermia on neonatal transport: 4-year experience in a single NICU. J Perinatol 2010;30(5):324–9.
54. Kendall GS, Kapetanakis A, Ratnavel N, et al. Passive cooling for initiation of therapeutic hypothermia in neonatal encephalopathy. Arch Dis Child Fetal Neonatal Ed 2010;95(6):F408–12.
55. Higgins RD, Raju T, Edwards AD, et al. Hypothermia and other treatment options for neonatal encephalopathy: an executive summary of the Eunice Kennedy Shriver NICHD workshop. J Pediatr 2011;159:851–858.e1.
56. Zanelli S, Buck M, Fairchild K. Physiologic and pharmacologic considerations for hypothermia therapy in neonates. J Perinatol 2011;31(6):377–86.
57. Róka A, Melinda KT, Vásárhelyi B, et al. Elevated morphine concentrations in neonates treated with morphine and prolonged hypothermia for hypoxic ischemic encephalopathy. Pediatrics 2008;121(4):e844–9.
58. Liu X, Borooah M, Stone J, et al. Serum gentamicin concentrations in encephalopathic infants are not affected by therapeutic hypothermia. Pediatrics 2009; 124(1):310–5.
59. van den Broek MP, Groenendaal F, Egberts AC, et al. Effects of hypothermia on pharmacokinetics and pharmacodynamics: a systematic review of preclinical and clinical studies. Clin Pharmacokinet 2010;49(5):277–94.
60. Filippi L, la Marca G, Cavallaro G, et al. Phenobarbital for neonatal seizures in hypoxic ischemic encephalopathy: a pharmacokinetic study during whole body hypothermia. Epilepsia 2011;52(4):794–801.
61. Robertson NJ, Tan S, Groenendaal F, et al. Which neuroprotective agents are ready for bench to bedside translation in the newborn infant? J Pediatr 2012; 160(4):544–552.e4.
62. Cilio MR, Ferriero DM. Synergistic neuroprotective therapies with hypothermia. Semin Fetal Neonatal Med 2010;15(5):293–8.
63. Pimentel-Coelho PM, Rosado-de-Castro PH, da Fonseca LM, et al. Umbilical cord blood mononuclear cell transplantation for neonatal hypoxic-ischemic encephalopathy. Pediatr Res 2012;71(4 Pt 2):464–73.

The Delivery Room of the Future
The Fetal and Neonatal Resuscitation and Transition Suite

Neil N. Finer, MD[a],*, Wade Rich, RRT, CCRC[a],
Louis P. Halamek, MD, FAAP[b], Tina A. Leone, MD[c]

KEYWORDS

- Delivery room • Fetal-neonatal resuscitation and transition suite • Human factors
- Human performance • Neonatal resuscitation • Resuscitation room

KEY POINTS

- Adequate space for all members to operate during complex resuscitations must be provided to the neonatal resuscitation team.
- Current technology allows for the generation of multiple streams of real-time physiologic data during neonatal resuscitation.
- Raw physiologic data must be translated into coherent interpretable information to be useful during resuscitation.
- Human factors analysis will play an increasingly important role in the design and testing of the devices and techniques used to conduct safe, effective, and efficient resuscitation of the newborn.

INTRODUCTION

Compare a contemporary neonatal ICU (NICU) with one from the 1970s. Present-day NICUs are filled with modern technology, consisting of radiant warmers that become incubators with the flip of a switch, servo-controlled ventilators capable of measuring

Financial Disclosures: Dr. Halamek is a consultant to Laerdal Medical, Inc.

Conflicts: There are no conflicts of interest to report.

Dr Halamek's effort was sponsored in part by the Endowment for the Center for Advanced Pediatric and Perinatal Education at Packard Children's Hospital at Stanford.

[a] Division of Neonatology, Department of Pediatrics, UC San Diego Medical Center, UC San Diego School of Medicine, 402 Dickinson Street, MPF 1-140, San Diego, CA 92103, USA;
[b] Fellowship Training Program in Neonatal-Perinatal Medicine, Division of Neonatal and Developmental Medicine, Department of Pediatrics, Center for Advanced Pediatric and Perinatal Education, Stanford University School of Medicine, 750 Welch Road, Suite 315, Palo Alto, CA, USA; [c] Neonatal-Perinatal Medicine Training Program, UC San Diego Medical Center, UC San Diego School of Medicine, 402 Dickinson Street, MPF 1-140, San Diego, CA 92103, USA
* Corresponding author.
E-mail address: nfiner@ucsd.edu

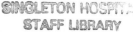

tiny tidal volumes and displaying that information continuously at the bedside, intravenous pumps that accurately deliver miniscule doses of powerful medications, monitors with multiple color-coded real-time data streams that also store hours and days worth of information, communication systems that allow immediate discussion between bedside staff and neonatologists, and video cameras that allow parents to view their newborn via the Internet 24 hours per day.

Now think about a "modern" delivery room (DR). Most DRs are designed around the welfare of the pregnant patient and the comfort of the health care professionals (HCPs) making up the obstetric team. There may or may not be sufficient space dedicated to resuscitation of the newborn; in some DRs resuscitations are performed within a few feet of the mother. Not only is the amount of space typically restricted, so is the amount and quality of the technology that is consigned to the newborn. In many ways, the neonatal team continues to be limited to the same tools (their eyes, ears, and hands) that they have used for decades. The technology available in DRs has changed very little over the last 20 years. Individual centers have developed sophisticated monitoring systems[1,2] but, in general, with the exception of a pulse oximeter, the DRs in most hospitals today look very much like they did before the surfactant era, functioning as little more than a repository for aging equipment from the NICU. Published reviews have found significant variability in what types of equipment are used worldwide.[3–5] In addition, despite the current era of ever-increasing facilitated communication, the DR often remains an isolated venue.

The authors' vision for the Fetal and Neonatal Resuscitation and Transition Suite of the future involves the development of user-friendly, highly interactive monitors and other devices characterized by artificial intelligence to guide decision-making; efficient modular warming environments; improved systemic communication abilities; audiovisual recording systems capable of generating high-definition video of every resuscitation; and well-trained, highly competent HCPs who actively participate in regular debriefings and maintain their cognitive, technical and behavioral skills through highly realistic simulations that involve all members of their multidisciplinary team.

Let us first examine the physical space where most newborns are resuscitated. Some institutions use "pass-through" windows that allow for resuscitation and stabilization of infants to occur in the NICU. Most delivery hospitals use a corner of the actual DR, and a few (about 15%) have a dedicated resuscitation room.[5] Basic requirements for a resuscitation room include the following: the ability to control the temperature of the room independent of the room where the mother is cared for so that it can be increased as needed to maintain normothermia in even the most immature infants, sufficient space to house the equipment and supplies needed for multiple births and accommodate up to three adult HCPs at each bedside, adjustable lighting, electrical and gas (air and oxygen) outlets, and the capability for both storage of continuous data streams on secure servers and wireless transmission of that same data including all monitor and video signals. The room should also have a hands-free phone or similar communication device as an aid to immediately and easily summon assistance, and all communications should be remotely monitored from a central communication station in the NICU to allow for complete two-way communication and enhanced situational awareness by NICU staff of the events taking place in the resuscitation room.

Proper therapy for the newborn in transition requires an understanding of the patient's dynamic physiology. Parameters that should be readily available include the ECG, pulse oximetry (SPO2), end-tidal carbon dioxide, tidal volume, co-oximetry with hemoglobin measuring capability, patient temperature, room temperature, and time. The capability to measure cerebral oxygen delivery and consumption is also important and will become standard of care in the near future. In addition such a room in a tertiary or quaternary facility should be equipped with dedicated portable cardiac and general purpose ultrasound machines replete with a variety of transducers, a transilluminator, and a built-in portable radiograph machine with an extendable arm. A video-laryngoscope and bronchoscope should also be available with all video capable of being displayed on a large flat-panel display in full view of the resuscitation team. A central monitor programmed to record and store all of the parameters noted previously and display selected trends should be placed in a location easily visible by all members of the resuscitation team. There should be at least one overhead high-definition video camera to record team activity; this video feed should be integrated into the data stream that is displayed on the central monitor. The current resuscitation-transition room at the University of California San Diego Medical Center (UCSD) already has the capability of providing almost all of the above functionality. In addition, at UCSD, portable ultrasound is used in the resuscitation room for a variety of situations, including diagnosis of congenital cardiac disease, detection of air (pneumothoraces) and fluid (ascites) accumulations, and confirmation of proper tube and line placements.

Transition from the intrauterine environment to the DR radiant warmer during resuscitation and then to the transport unit for transfer to the NICU after stabilization involves a significant amount of connecting and disconnecting of sensors, cables, tubes, and lines. In addition to being a very inefficient use of time, this process creates multiple opportunities for potentially serious errors. This could be greatly simplified by the use of a "pod" that can be moved from the DR radiant warmer to the transport unit, then to the bed in the NICU, by simply sliding it out of one bed and into another. This type of device is currently used to transfer infants from an incubator to an MRI scanner without ever actually being removed from the incubator section of the transport unit and for air transport where space is severely limited and cannot accommodate a full-size incubator. To eliminate this inefficient and unsafe aspect of patient transport, a docking module that is intrinsic to the pod easily and quickly links to a receptacle in the radiant warmer or incubator, and incorporates all of the wires and tubes conveying the electrical signals from the leads and probes on the patient to all of the monitors and monitors, infusions from pumps to the intravenous lines placed within the patient, and any other devices as needed.

NICUs are replete with visual and auditory cues to alert HCPs to changes in patient status. Much of the monitoring equipment currently available does not function well during the transition from fetus to neonate in the first minutes of life and, as a result, those caring for newborns are often forced to silence those alarms in the DR. The Fetal and Neonatal Resuscitation and Transition Suite of the future will include devices that integrate physiologic data obtained from standard patient monitors with a resuscitation timeline to provide real-time cues to the members of the resuscitation team, thereby enhancing the timeliness and appropriateness of their interventions. Ideally, this system will be small, inexpensive, and easily installed in any area where newborn resuscitation takes place. Of course such a system should not be seen as a replacement for human intelligence and critical thinking during resuscitation. Any data that elicit a prompt for action would need to be confirmed as accurate before team members intervene based on the prompt.

Recommendations for the monitoring of infants at birth are moving from rudimentary methods based on direct clinical examination that have been found to be subjective and inaccurate[6,7] to more direct physiologic measurements using devices similar to those in the NICU. This requires an environment with dedicated wiring to secure data servers that securely store video, analog, and digital data from multiple systems in multiple rooms. Monitors should be specifically designed and purpose-built for such an environment. This will necessitate innovations in alarm algorithms that are appropriate for the

DR environment, such as automatic alarm silencing during the first minute and dynamic alarm limits for parameters that change over time, such as SPO2 values during the first 10 minutes of life. As an example of this type of innovative design, the Transitional Oxygen Targeting System (TOTS) has been developed at UCSD based on the work of Dawson and colleagues[8] (**Fig. 1**). TOTS generates a graphic display of prespecified high and low hemoglobin oxygen saturation limits, as well as a real-time display of hemoglobin oxygen saturation and administered supplemental oxygen values to assist resuscitation team members by providing them with a visual indicator of the effectiveness of their resuscitative efforts. Currently this system is capable of simply displaying the patient's SPO2 against the curves indicating high and low acceptable values. To more easily determine whether the SPO2 is within the target range, additional cues such as variable loudness, pitch, brightness, and color will need to be incorporated. Similarly, the heart rate alarm might be programmed to automatically silence for rates less than 60 beats per minute in the first 60 seconds, with the limits and the alarm volume gradually increasing over time based on normative data curves.[9]

As the number and type of monitoring devices in the DR increase, the need to incorporate all of this information into a single display that is visible to the entire team and is easily and quickly understood becomes critical. A flat-screen monitor mounted on the visual center of the radiant warmer provides enough surface area to effectively display SPO2 normative curves (as in TOTS), ECG, temperature, and time (**Fig. 2**). Multiparameter bedside monitors may be modified for this purpose or multichannel analog data acquisition systems can be interfaced to a standalone computer to generate the same tracings. During review sessions at UCSD, six channels of analog data are displayed as indicated in **Fig. 3**. The integration of these parameters onto a single display screen facilitates pattern recognition of not only current events but also trends over time.

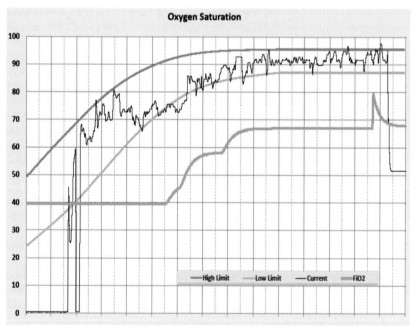

Fig. 1. The Transitional Oxygen Targeting System (TOTS) developed at UCSD.

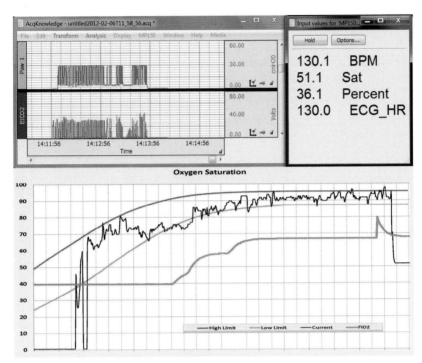

Fig. 2. Flat-screen monitor display of SaO2 normative curves (bottom, as in TOTS), airway pressure, end tidal CO2 graphic display (top left), ECG, pulse rate from oximeter, SpO2, percent inspired oxygen and ECG derived HR. Digital display (top right).

An area requiring intense investigation is the application of human factors engineering to patient monitoring.[10–12] Patient data must be presented in a manner in which it can be easily detected, assimilated, interpreted, and acted on. Therefore, one cannot simply study just the patient or just the technology, but also must critically examine how the human beings responsible for delivering care to the patients interface with that technology.[13] The design of patient monitors, specifically the display parameters and alarms, is a critical element in enabling HCPs to recognize and respond to abnormalities and changes in patient physiology. Simply providing more data will not necessarily translate into more useful information. What patient data are best recognized as a numerical display versus a waveform? What sizes, colors, and fonts of the numbers and what widths, textures, and hues of the waveforms produce optimal human performance? The same types of questions need to be asked of alarms and prompts. What is the ideal pitch and volume of an alarm that will allow it to grab the attention of those at the bedside most quickly? Should the pitch and volume vary over time or in response to changes in the physiologic variables themselves? Should prompts consist of visual or auditory cues? For those prompts that are best delivered via visual cues, what sizes and colors facilitate the most effective response by the members of the resuscitation team? For those prompts that are found to be optimally delivered by auditory cues, should mechanical tones or voice prompts be used? If tones are used, what is the best pitch and volume? If voice prompts are indicated, should the voice be male, female, or synthetic? Another key question involves the number of data points, data streams, and prompts that can be accurately processed by human beings working under the time pressure inherent in resuscitation.

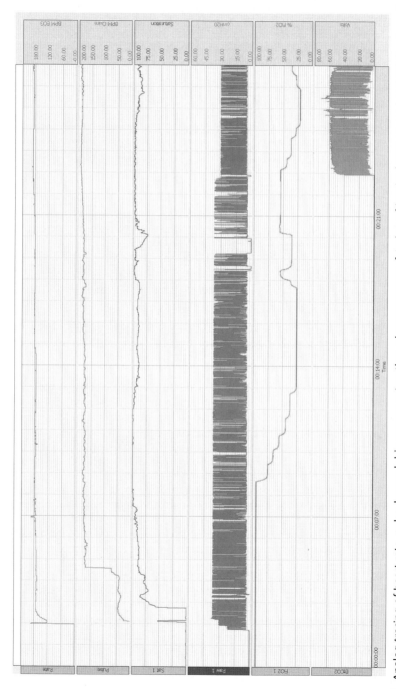

Fig. 3. Analog tracing of heart rate, pulse, hemoglobin oxygen saturation, airway pressure, fraction of inspired oxygen, and end-tidal carbon dioxide.

Thus, there are a tremendous number of questions to be answered to design the ideal monitoring technology for use during newborn resuscitation.

Communication among members of the resuscitation team is an element of performance that is critical to good patient outcomes. Communication at the bedside is primarily verbal, although nonverbal communication, in terms of hand signals, nods, and eye movements, also plays a role. Currently there is no standard methodology by which resuscitation team members communicate. The authors believe that a standardized, validated lexicon should be developed for resuscitation situations in health care; the system used in the commercial aviation industry for succinct transmission of information between aircraft crews and air traffic controllers is a suitable model for this purpose. In addition to the communication occurring among resuscitation team members in the DR, direct auditory and visual communication between those in the DR and the NICU will ensure that the NICU team is fully prepared for the eventual transport and arrival of the patient.

Selection and training of the human beings who make up the neonatal resuscitation team and who will be required to function at a high level in this intense environment will need also to be modeled after the type of training used in other industries in which there is substantial risk to human life. In most of these industries, frequent objective

---

Box 1
Steps in the initial selection and ongoing training of resuscitation team members at LPCH and CAPE

Step 1: Base appointment to the neonatal resuscitation team on performance

- Number of team members and team composition to be determined by NICU leadership
- Selection to team based on performance, experience, and motivation
- All team members must meet objective performance markers
- Experience and motivation will be critically evaluated

Step 2: Train resuscitation team members to the highest standards

- Undergo highly realistic simulation-based multidisciplinary team training in the management of challenging DR resuscitation situations, such as extreme prematurity, multiple gestation, multiple congenital anomalies, hydrops fetalis, congenital heart block, pneumothorax, ascites, death in the DR, initiation of comfort care, and so forth
- Participate in regular drills conducted in labor and delivery in collaboration with obstetric team members to enhance communication skill in intense, dynamic, and time-pressured situations
- Participate in constructive, objective debriefings of all simulation-based activities

Step 3: Record and debrief real resuscitations

- Record all challenging resuscitations
- Constructively and objectively debrief actual resuscitations in a manner that is protected under the appropriate state code of evidence

Step 4: Using data from real resuscitations, simulate areas of weakness

- Integrate these specific simulations into regular drills

Step 5: Evaluate effect of these interventions on safety, quality, and risk outcomes

- Facilitate active communication and collaboration among those delivering care, those responsible for training and simulation, and the professionals in the departments of patient safety, quality assurance, and risk management

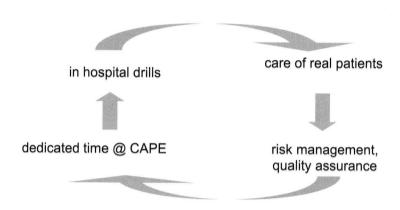

Fig. 4. The Packard Circle of Safety, a method for linking safety and simulation to address system and human weaknesses and improve the safety, effectiveness, and efficiency of patient care.

assessment and ongoing simulation-based learning is the standard for acquisition and maintenance of skill. Selection of the "best" and ensuring their ongoing optimal level of performance requires a comprehensive approach (**Box 1**). Resuscitation team members should be selected to and retained on the team based on objective performance criteria. Simulation-based learning should be an integral component of their initial preparation, as well as their ongoing learning. This should be complemented with regular review of their performance during real resuscitations so that any weaknesses can be readily identified and addressed. Such reviews should consist of objective, constructive, confidential debriefings of videos of their activities in the DR. The coupling of detailed reviews of real-life performance with simulations designed to address the weaknesses discovered from such reviews will provide the opportunity to enhance patient safety in a manner that is highly effective. This is the process that is being implemented at the Center for Advanced Pediatric and Perinatal Education (CAPE) and Lucile Packard Children's Hospital (LPCH) at Stanford (**Fig. 4**).

SUMMARY

The Fetal and Neonatal Resuscitation and Transition Suite of the future will be marked by several innovations in the design and standardization of the physical space and the monitoring and communication technologies that will facilitate optimal human performance in that domain. Although the patient will continue to be at the center of this process, increasing attention will be devoted to analysis of this environment from a human factors viewpoint, addressing ways in which to enhance the acquisition, maintenance, and application of the cognitive, technical, and behavioral skills of the members of the resuscitation team.

REFERENCES

1. Carbine DN, Finer NN, Knodel E, et al. Video recording as a means of evaluating neonatal resuscitation performance. Pediatrics 2000;106(4):654–8.
2. Schmolzer GM, Kamlin OC, Dawson JA, et al. Respiratory monitoring of neonatal resuscitation. Arch Dis Child Fetal Neonatal Ed 2010;95(4):F295–303.
3. Mitchell A, Niday P, Boulton J, et al. A prospective clinical audit of neonatal resuscitation practices in Canada. Adv Neonatal Care 2002;2(6):316–26.
4. Trevisanuto D, Doglioni N, Ferrarese P, et al. Neonatal resuscitation of extremely low birthweight infants: a survey of practice in Italy. Arch Dis Child Fetal Neonatal Ed 2006;91(2):F123–4.
5. Leone TA, Rich W, Finer NN. A survey of delivery room resuscitation practices in the United States. Pediatrics 2006;117(2):e164–75.
6. O'Donnell CP, Kamlin CO, Davis PG, et al. Clinical assessment of infant colour at delivery. Arch Dis Child Fetal Neonatal Ed 2007;92(6):F465–7.
7. Voogdt KG, Morrison AC, Wood FE, et al. A randomised, simulated study assessing auscultation of heart rate at birth. Resuscitation 2010;81(8):1000–3.
8. Dawson JA, Kamlin OF, Vento M, et al. Defining the reference range for oxygen saturation for infants after birth. Pediatrics 2010;125:e1340–7.
9. Dawson JA, Kamlin CO, Wong C, et al. Oxygen saturation and heart rate during delivery room resuscitation of infants <30 weeks' gestation with air or 100% oxygen. Arch Dis Child Fetal Neonatal Ed 2009;94(2):F87–91.
10. Walsh T, Beatty PC. Human factors errors and patient monitoring. Physiol Meas 2002;23:R111–32.
11. Gosbee J. Human factors engineering and patient safety. Qual Saf Health Care 2002;11:352–4.
12. Gawron VJ, Drury CG, Fairbanks RJ, et al. Medical error and human factors engineering: where are we now? Am J Med Qual 2006;21:57–67.
13. Hunt EA, Nelson KL, Shilkofski NA. Simulation in medicine: addressing patient safety and improving the interface between healthcare providers and medical technology. Biomed Instrum Technol 2006;40:399–404.

The Mathematics of Morality for Neonatal Resuscitation

William Meadow, MD, PhD[a],*, Joanne Lagatta, MD, MA[b],
Bree Andrews, MD, MPH[a], John Lantos, MD[c]

KEYWORDS

- Resuscitation • Neonatal ethics • Neonatal outcomes • Prognostication
- Distributive justice

KEY POINTS

- This article introduces data regarding three separate aspects of the morality of resuscitation for neonatal infants: money, outcomes, and predictive ability.
- There are no credible financial arguments against neonatal ICU (NICU) care for infants born at the border of viability.
- NICU care for extremely low birth weight infants is particularly cost-effective when compared with medical interventions in adults, even when post-NICU care is included in the calculations.
- For parents who view starting NICU intervention as a worthwhile option, counseling about resuscitation as a function of gestational age seems to have limited support from the data.
- Antenatal and delivery room predictions are inadequately accurate, and prediction at the time of discharge is too late. Abnormal head ultrasound and a health care professional's intuition that the child will "die before discharge" may offer a positive predictive value of greater than 95% for the combined outcome of death or survival with neurodevelopmental impairment.

INTRODUCTION

Most neonates do not need resuscitation. A bit of drying, a slap on the butt, and they are good to go. Some neonates unexpectedly need resuscitation. Their antenatal histories yield no hint that at the time of birth they will need extra efforts to get them going. There are almost no ethical dilemmas for these infants. They need resuscitation and they receive it.

However, some babies, predictably, are born at a time when it is not clear whether physicians should offer, perform, deny, or accede to resuscitative efforts. These babies are born extremely prematurely, at the border of neonatal viability.

[a] The University of Chicago, Chicago, IL, USA; [b] Medical College of Wisconsin, Wauwatosa, WI, USA; [c] Children's Mercy Hospital, Kansas City, MO, USA
* Corresponding author. Department of Pediatrics, The University of Chicago, 5815 South Maryland Avenue, Chicago, IL 60637.
E-mail address: wlm1@uchicago.edu

Clin Perinatol 39 (2012) 941–956
http://dx.doi.org/10.1016/j.clp.2012.09.013
0095-5108/12/$ – see front matter © 2012 Elsevier Inc. All rights reserved.

Resuscitation of these babies provokes passionate debates and disagreements. This article discusses the data that underlie these debates.

The issues that arise for doctors are different from those facing parents or policy makers. Doctors might want to know the data on the likelihood that resuscitative efforts will be successful. How many infants in similar conditions responded to resuscitative efforts? Of those that survived, how many were in the hospital for months at enormous expense? How many had poor long-term outcomes?

A public policy-maker might want to know how many such babies were born, how much their treatment cost (initially and long-term), and how these expenses compare with other public health expenses, either in children or adults. A public policy-maker might want to know if money spent to prevent preterm birth would lead to lower overall costs.

Parents want to know the answer to only one question, "What will happen to the baby?" It would not help to know that, of 100 similar babies, 50 die and half the survivors have neurocognitive problems. Parents want to know what will happen to their baby and they want to know as early as possible in the baby's treatment course so that they can make the right decision at the right time.

Data are available that speak to the morality of neonatal resuscitation from the perspective of what is sometimes called evidence-based ethics. This article discusses three lines of evidence concerning the morality of neonatal resuscitation: money, outcomes, and predictability.

FINANCIAL CONSIDERATIONS FOR NEONATAL RESUSCITATION

Approximately 4 million babies are born each year in the United States. Approximately 3 million people die. Approximately 1% of 4 million, or 40,000 infants, are born each year weighing less than 1000 g (extremely low birthweight [ELBW], roughly 28 weeks gestation). Of the 4 million births, 0.6% (24,000) die. Half die of complications of prematurity. The other half die of congenital anomalies. Those babies raise a set of complicated issues that are related to, but not identical to, the issues raised by premature babies. This article focuses only on premature babies.

The first financial consideration regarding resuscitation for extremely premature infants is the percentage of neonatal ICU (NICU) resources expended on ELBW infants are devoted to infants who will die in the NICU compared with the resources devoted to infants who will survive to be discharged. **Fig. 1** depicts data from the University of Chicago hospitals.[1,2] At the higher ELBWs (eg, >800 g), mortality is so low (<20%) that most NICU expenses (closely approximated by NICU bed-days) are devoted to infants who survive to discharge.

The surprising feature of **Fig. 1** is that even at the lower end of the ELBW distribution (birthweight 450–600 g) at which survival is less than 50%, most NICU expenses (>80%) are still expended on infants who will survive to discharge, as opposed to those infants who will die in the NICU. This occurs because doomed infants die relatively quickly (median day of death is <7days), because the smallest and the sickest die sooner, and because survivors stay in the NICU for an extended time.

This is not the case in the adult medical ICU (MICU). There, the relationship between ultimate survival and overall cost is the inverse of the relationship that holds in the NICU.[3,4] **Fig. 2** presents comparable data for the NICU and adult MICU, contrasting survival and expenses devoted to nonsurvivors, for patients with low, moderate, or high risk of dying in the hospital. The data are striking. In the NICU, at every risk of death, only a small percentage of resources are expended on doomed infants; most NICU bed-days are occupied by patients who will be discharged, independent of their initial risk of dying.

"Wasted" Resources and Mortality vs Birth Weight

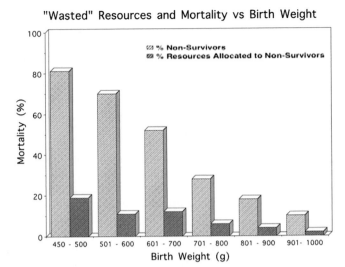

Fig. 1. Mortality and resources devoted to nonsurvivors as a function of gestational age. At all gestational ages, independent of the likelihood of mortality, more dollars are devoted to infants who will survive than those who will die.

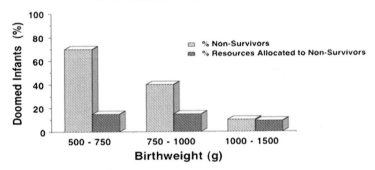

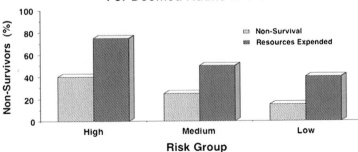

Fig. 2. Comparison of mortality and resources devoted to nonsurvivors for the NICU versus MICU. In contrast to the NICU, for adults in the MICU proportionally more dollars are devoted to patients who will not survive, at all risk groups.

In the adult MICU, the phenomenon is reversed. For every risk group, more money is directed to patients who will die in hospital than to those who will be discharged. The mean and median length of stay for MICU nonsurvivors is higher than for MICU survivors, at every risk group. Moreover, as was noted previously, of the 3 million people who die in the United States each year, only 24,000, or approximately 1%, are neonates; the other 99% adults.

Clearly, more is spent, both absolutely and relatively, on dying MICU patients than on dying NICU patients. This remains true, even if long-term costs of impaired NICU survivors are included.[5] NICU costs have been estimated at between $5000 and $10,000 per quality-adjusted life-year, whereas comparable adult procedures cost roughly ten times more.[3] The individual patients who stay the longest in the NICU mostly survive, whereas the individual patients who stay longest in the MICU mostly die. And there are 100 times more dying adults than there are dying neonates. Consequently, if policy makers seek evidence-based algorithms for rationing care, starting with the least cost-effective care (instead of more cost-effective alternatives) the MICU (instead of the NICU) is the place to start. Saving 500-g premature babies is far more cost-effective than saving 85-year-old adults. If any cost-savings at the end-of-life are sought, they can be found in adult MICUs, not in NICUs.

OUTCOMES OF NEONATAL RESUSCITATION

There are only four possible outcomes after birth of an extremely premature infant. The groups include: (1) the infant cannot be resuscitated but, instead, receive comfort care (these infants are not discussed further); (2) the infant can be resuscitated in the delivery room, be admitted to the NICU, but die at some point during their NICU care; (3) the infant can be resuscitated, survive to NICU discharge, and experience neurodevelopmental impairment (NDI); or (4) the infant can be resuscitated, survive to NICU discharge, and be neurologically intact. In this article, NDI is defined by a mental development index (MDI) score or a psychomotor developmental index (PDI) score that is less than 70 on the Bayley-II scale of infant development.

Moral calculations of the value of a short trial in the NICU, even in situations where survival is unlikely, depend on the value (positive or negative) assigned to each of the four outcome groups. If survival is the desired outcome, then "good" outcomes are calculated as the ratio of all survivors (groups 3 and 4) to all births (groups 1–4). If "intact" survival is the only desirable outcome, then good outcomes are the ratio of "intact survivors" (group 4) to all births (groups 1–4). However, one more moral calculation is conceivable. Many parents report that they feel better if they gave their baby a chance, if they opted to try resuscitation, even if it fails, than they feel if they did not even try. For such parents, trying and failing in the NICU (group 2) is better than not trying (group 1). For such parents, good outcomes are calculated as the ratio of intact survivors (group 4) to all survivors (groups 3 and 4). These differing moral weightings lead to very different conclusions about the worth of NICU resuscitation as a function of gestational age for extremely premature infants.

Fig. 3 displays a subset of data obtainable from the National Institute of Child Health and Human Development (NICHD) calculator published in 2008.[6] The x-axis presents gestational age divided into small for gestational age (SGA) and appropriate for gestational age groups, and the y-axis presents survival. The point to be made is familiar: survival is strongly dependent on gestational age between 22 and 25 weeks. Fig. 4 superimposes intact survival (ie, survival with both MDI and PDI >70) as a function of gestational age. The point is clear that intact survival is lower than overall survival, and depends strongly on gestational age. Fig. 5 superimposes one more outcome,

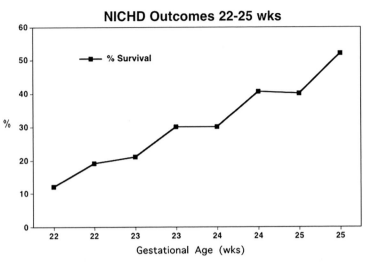

Fig. 3. Likelihood of survival versus gestational age for infants weighing less than 600 g from the NICHD online calculator. Survival depends strongly on gestational age.

which is the percentage of NICU survivors who survive intact. Two points are clear. First, the percentage of survivors who survive intact is much higher than the percentage of all births who survive intact. Second, the percentage of intact survivors is relatively independent of gestational age.

This phenomenon can also be seen in other countries. In **Figs. 6** and **7**, data from Britain[7] and France[8] reveal that outcomes for NICU survivors measured at 6 years of age, and 7 to 9 years of age, have the same lack of dependence on gestational age.

In sum, moral calculations of the value of neonatal resuscitation depend strongly on the valence assigned to two different types of dying in the NICU. If dying without

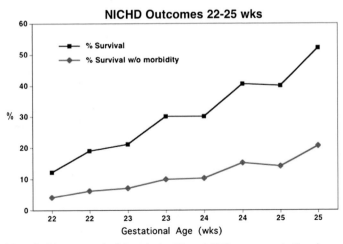

Fig. 4. Likelihood of intact survival (survival with out NDI) versus gestational age for infants weighing less than 600 g from the NICHD online calculator. Intact survival depends strongly on gestational age.

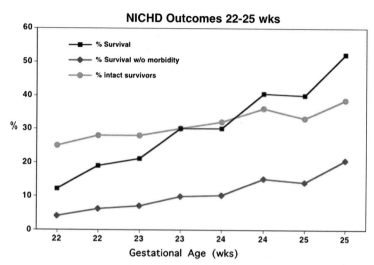

Fig. 5. Percentage of survivors who will be neurodevelopmentally intact versus gestational age for infants weighing less than 600 g from the NICHD online calculator. Percentage of intact survivors does not depend strongly on gestational age.

resuscitation and dying after failed resuscitation are equivalent, then good outcomes vary strongly as a function of gestational age. Many more babies die at lower gestational ages. If, however, dying after resuscitative efforts is better than dying without such efforts, that is, if "giving our child a chance" matters to parents and if the worst

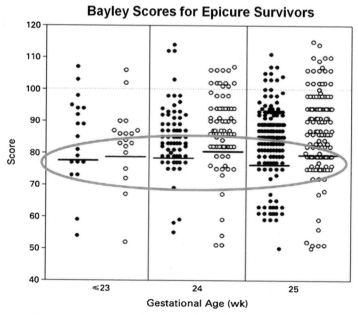

Fig. 6. Bayley II scores versus gestational age for infants born in the United Kingdom enrolled in the EPICURE study. The scores do not depend strongly on gestational age.

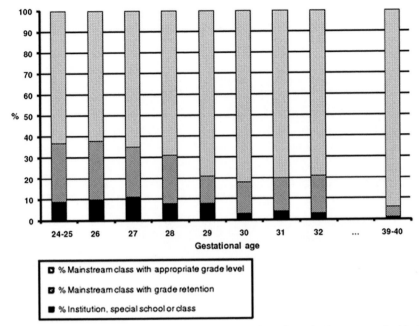

Fig. 7. Type of schooling versus gestational age for infants born in France enrolled in the Epipage study. The scores do not depend strongly on gestational age.

outcome is not death but impaired survival, then the likelihood of a good outcome does not depend much on gestational age. At every gestational age between 23 and 26 weeks, the percentage of survivors with neurodevelopmental problems is about the same.

This leads to a problem with no obvious solution. If the major concern is survival of an infant with NDI, then the gestational age to be most concerned about from the standpoint of neonatal resuscitation is not 23 to 24 weeks but, instead, 25 to 26 weeks (**Fig. 8**), precisely because so many more infants will survive as gestational age increases, whereas intactness of survivors does not vary much as gestational age increases. Currently there are no ethical alternatives to resuscitation when confronted with infants born at 25 to 26 weeks gestation. As for the pain and suffering of the children themselves during their time in the NICU, it is, to our mind, most reasonable for the parents to be the judge of whether, and when, NICU intervention is ever, or still, worth it.

PREDICTING THE OUTCOME OF NEONATAL RESUSCITATION

When predicting outcomes of neonatal resuscitation for parents, the only two things that matter are timing and positive predictive value. **Fig. 9** presents a complex timeline illustrating this point. Four time points are illustrated.[9,10] The first is when many, probably most, neonatal decisions about resuscitation for infants born extremely prematurely are discussed before the infant's birth during an antenatal consultation. The data available antenatally (gestational age, SGA status, antenatal steroids, twinning, and gender), either from the local institution or using the NICHD calculator,[5] are used to predict either overall survival or intact survival for a population of infants born sharing the same features. These data inform and constrain the conversations

Absolute number of NICU survivors with moderate to severe
neuro-developmental disability
(NICHD data)

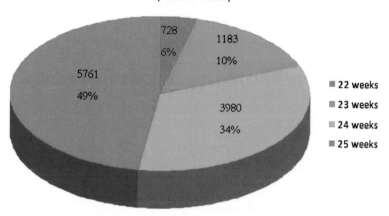

Fig. 8. Percent of all infants born less at than 26 weeks gestation who survive with NDI versus gestational age. Most survivors with NDI are born at higher gestational age, precisely because survival depends strongly on gestational age, whereas the percentage of survivors who will be impaired does not.

between the parents, obstetricians, and neonatologists regarding the appropriateness of resuscitation for the infant.

The second time point is immediately after delivery, in the minutes while the infant lies in the delivery room suite. Here, in addition to confirming gestational age, SGA, twinning, and gender, the neonatologist also learns the Apgar scores: how the infant looks at birth (Apgar at 1 minute) and how the infant responds to initial resuscitation (Apgar at 5 minutes). Although scant data exist correlating Apgar scores to ultimate outcomes (mortality or morbidity) in the ELBW population, many neonatologists

Outcome prediction in neonatology:
a proposed timeline

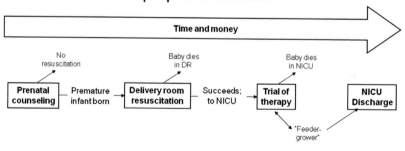

Fig. 9. Timeline for outcome prediction for infants. Four possible opportunities for counseling are presented. ACS, antenatal corticosteroids; BPD, bronchopulmonary dysplasia; CP, cerebral palsy; GA, gestational age; ROP, retinopathy of prematurity; SNAP, Score for Neonatal Acute Physiology.

seem to value this information and use it to influence the initiation, or duration, of their delivery room resuscitative efforts.[11]

The relevant third time point for predicting the outcome of neonatal resuscitation is during the NICU stay. To be ethically relevant (ie, to envision a clinical course distinct from continuing intervention, such as extubation and palliative care), optimally, data will be obtained while the child is requiring mechanical ventilation. Several predictive data variables could be used, including individual occurrences such as sepsis or necrotizing enterocolitis or intraventricular hemorrhage; composite scores of abnormal physiology such as Score for Neonatal Acute Physiology, Score for Physiology and Perinatal Extension (SNAPPE), or Clinical Risk Index for Babies; or something less tangible, but no less real, such as the health care professional's intuition of impending demise (see later discussion).

The final time point for predicting the outcome of neonatal resuscitation is at NICU discharge when the most is known about the condition of the baby; however, it is too late to do much about it. That is, other than attempting to optimize postdischarge early intervention, there is nothing to withdraw, and no alternative to continued support for the infant at home.

These data illustrate the reasons why antenatal counseling is so imprecise. Antenatal counseling suffers from the inevitable uncertainty associated with statistical descriptions of the outcomes of populations (as opposed to individuals) born at the border of viability (roughly 22–26 weeks gestation). Moreover, in the authors' experience, parents desire prognostic information about their baby, not about 100 more-or-less similar babies.

This uncertainty does not go away in the delivery room where the infant is weighed, examined for congenital anomalies, and assessed for responses to initial resuscitative efforts. Although neonatologists often describe making assessments in the delivery room about the usefulness or futility of further interventions,[11] none of these assessments has been shown to predict either death or future NDI in any helpful way.

The authors believe that the best time to predict the outcome of neonatal resuscitation for individual infants, and to counsel their parents accordingly, occurs while the infant is in the NICU, on a ventilator. At that time, there are still choices to be made about life-sustaining treatment. The ventilator can be withdrawn. If the decision is made too soon, the prognostic uncertainty is too great. If the decision is delayed (eg, until NICU discharge), although there may be improved prognostic accuracy[12] there is no longer any treatment to withhold or withdraw.

During the first days after NICU admission, while an infant remain on mechanical ventilation, the physician can determine more robust predictors of outcome than those that are available in the delivery room. These predictors come in two categories: hard data available in algorithms and soft data available from the clinical judgments of health care professionals.

Consider algorithms first. Algorithms award points for physiologic derangements; the more abnormal the respirations, blood pressure, or electrolytes, the higher the score. Because patients who die are clearly more physiologically deranged than patients who live, it is perfectly reasonable to assume that, over time, serial illness severity scores will diverge, growing ever higher for patient populations who are on the path to die, and growing lower for patient populations whose physiology is improving and who will eventually survive. As **Fig. 10** demonstrates, this perfectly reasonable expectation is completely wrong. **Fig. 10** plots the SNAPPE-II scores of two populations of infants born weighing less than 1000 g at the University of Chicago. One population will eventually die in the NICU and the other population will survive to NICU discharge.[13] Several points are apparent. First, at the time of birth, eventual

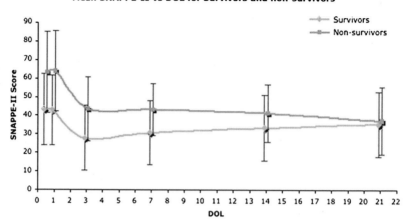

Fig. 10. Serial SNAPPE-II scores versus day of life (DOL) for NICU survivors and nonsurvivors. Over time, serial SNAPPE-II scores become less, not more, able to distinguish survivors from nonsurvivors.

nonsurvivors do have higher SNAPPE-II scores than survivors, as would be anticipated by the definition of SNAPPE-II. However, and more importantly for this argument, over time the differences between the SNAPPE-II scores of the nonsurviving population and the scores for those infants who survive converge; they do not diverge.

How can this be? How do the illness severity scores of the two populations grow closer, not farther apart, over time? The answer is simple – the sickest infants, those with the highest SNAPPE-II scores and most likely to die, do die, quickly, lowering the SNAPPE-II scores of the residual population of non-survivors. Consequently, even though the surviving infants' SNAPPE-II scores also improve, the overall distance between the two populations narrows. Serial illness severity scores will be of no help in counseling parents of infants who have been resuscitated.

Clinical judgment, on the other hand, is criticized as imprecise and as simply masking an implicit algorithm that could be better analyzed if it could be made explicit. Most clinicians recognize, however, that some things are hard to define, even if you "know them when you see them." The authors have tested the predictive power of clinical judgment.

At the University of Chicago, over the past 14 years, we have assessed the predictive power of the clinical judgments of health care professionals (registered nurses, neonatal nurse practitioners, residents, fellows, attending physicians). Each day that a child remains on mechanical ventilation, we ask one simple question, "Do you think this infant is going to survive to be discharged, or die in the NICU?" We limit the question to concern only infants who require mechanical ventilation precisely because the parents have an ethically available option, which is extubation and palliative care.

Our first finding is a simple one. Sixty percent of babies are never predicted to "die before discharge" by any health professional in the NICU (**Fig. 11**). Another 15% are predicted to die by only one person on 1 day of ventilation, 10% are predicted to die by more than one person, and 15% have at least 1 day of unanimous predictions of death before discharge.

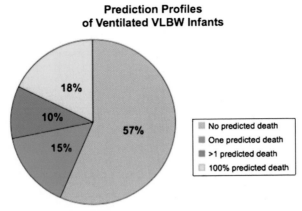

**Prediction Profiles
of Ventilated VLBW Infants**

- No predicted death
- One predicted death
- >1 predicted death
- 100% predicted death

Fig. 11. Prediction profiles for ventilated very low birth weight (VLBW) NICU infants. Most ventilated NICU infants are never predicted to die by any caretaker on any day.

Of the 60% of infants who were never predicted to die, not surprisingly, almost all survived to NICU discharge. However, of the 40% of infants who received at least one prediction of death before discharge, nearly half of these infants survived.[13] This is not very good predictive power.

Perhaps more success can be had from attempting to predict a combined outcome, either death in the NICU or NDI, defined as MDI or PDI less than 70 on the Bayley II score at 24 months of corrected age. It turns out that serial algorithms (SNAPPE-II scores) are very unhelpful at distinguishing the population of infants who will either die or survive with NDI from those infants who will survive unscathed. How accurate are clinical judgments of death before discharge in predicting the combined outcome of death or NDI?

Fig. 12 presents these data; they are some of the most illuminating in this article.[10] The figure presents the likelihood of the combined outcome of either death or NDI on the y-axis as a function of predictive features on the x-axis. The two predictors displayed are head ultrasound (HSU) results (normal, grade 1, grade 2, grade 3 or 4, periventricular leukomalacia) and caretaker clinical judgments of death before discharge (none, one, more than one on at least 1 day, or at least 1 day with a unanimous prediction of death). Several points are apparent from **Fig. 12**. First, considering the gray bars (all patients in each HUS group), there is an increased risk of death or NDI as HUS results worsen. This is not a surprise.

More importantly, the predictive value for the combined adverse outcomes of death or NDI increases when clinical judgments (the colored bars) are added to each HUS group. That is, clinical judgments and HUS results each add predictive power over using either one alone. Moreover, for infants with moderate or severe HUS abnormality who have even 1 day of corroborated prediction of death before discharge, the positive predictive value of death or NDI is at least 96%. The likelihood that these infants will be alive without NDI at 2 years of age is less than 4%. That, the authors argue, warrants a conversation with significant ethical import.

Moreover, for each HUS group, having never had a prediction of death before discharge improves the likelihood of a normal outcome. This, too, is an important conversation to have.

How does the combination of HUS and clinical judgments during the NICU stay compare with using gestational age at the time of birth to predict outcomes for ELBW infants? **Fig. 13** reveals several important comparisons. Again the y-axis is

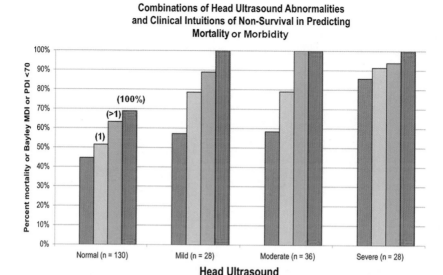

Fig. 12. Predictive power of the combination of HUS abnormalities and health care professional judgments that the infant will "die before discharge" for the outcome of death or survival with NDI. The positive predictive value of death or NDI exceeds 95% for infants with a corroborated prediction of death and an abnormal HUS.

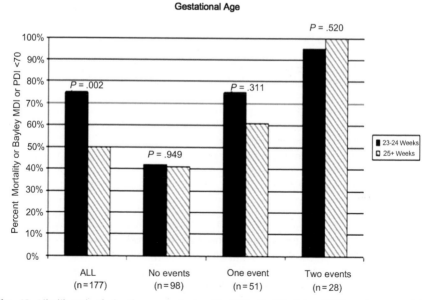

Fig. 13. Likelihood of death or survival with NDI stratified by NICU trajectory, either abnormal HUS or caretaker judgments that the infant will "die before discharge." The predictive power of gestational age disappears when infants are stratified by events that occur in the NICU.

likelihood of either death or NDI, while the x-axis now displays 177 patients as a function of both gestational age and the number of adverse events in the NICU (either abnormal HUS, prediction of death before discharge, both, or neither). The first comparison (left-most columns) is the simplest. Infants who are 23 to 24 weeks gestation are more likely to have an adverse outcome (either death or NDI) than infants who are 25 to 27 weeks gestation. This is not news.

However, what is news is in the comparison of the three groups of columns to the right. Infants who are 23 to 24 weeks gestation are compared with infants who are 25 to 27 weeks gestation if they have had zero, one, or two events (ie, either a prediction of death before discharge or an abnormal HUS). Two points are clear, one simple and the other more profound. First, infants who have had two events are more likely to have an adverse outcome than infants who have had one event, who, in turn, are more likely to do poorly than infants who have had neither an abnormal HUS nor a prediction of death. That, again, is not surprising.

However, the second comparison is remarkable. For each group of patients (zero, one, or two adverse events) there is no distinction comparing infants born at 23 to 24 weeks gestation with those born at 25 to 27 weeks gestation. In other words, although younger gestation infants are more likely to have one of these two adverse events (the left-most columns), once there are either or both of the adverse events (abnormal HUS or prediction of death), gestational age drops out as a predictive factor. Also, the positive predictive value for infants with both abnormal HUS and a prediction of death for the combined outcome of death or survival with NDI is greater than 95%, independent of gestational age.

This predictive accuracy is approaching the kind of power that parents are asking for when health care practitioners counsel them about whether or not to resuscitate their infants at the time of delivery. Now parents can be offered two aspects of information that are unavailable at birth: (1) the individualized trajectory for their particular baby, not 100 more-or-less similar babies; and (2) the knowledge that the predictive value of either death or survival with NDI for infants with both abnormal HUS and a prediction of death before discharge is over 95%, about as high as medical certainty is likely to ever achieve.

This comparison, between what is known before birth and what is learned in the NICU, is captured nicely in **Fig. 14**, which displays the time course of gaining knowledge about the likely outcomes of individual infants after their resuscitation. A good outcome increases along the y-axis and, again, two major groups of infants are displayed: 23 to 24 weeks gestation versus 25 to 27 weeks gestation.

At birth, it is clear that infants born at 25 to 27 weeks gestation have roughly a 50% likelihood of survival without NDI, significantly higher than the 25% likelihood for infants born at 23 to 24 weeks gestation. This phenomenon has been documented by many other groups. However, as **Fig. 14** makes clear, it does not take long for the infants born at 25-plus weeks gestation to receive their "hits." That is, within roughly a week, most infants born at 25-plus weeks gestation who will go on to die or survive with NDI will have "declared themselves," allowing health care practitioners to discuss this with their parents. Again, those infants born at 25-plus weeks gestation will have the same likelihood of a bad outcome (>95%) as infants born at 23 to 24 weeks gestation who also two bad prognostic predictors.

In contrast, as **Fig. 14** also reveals, for infants born at 23 to 24 weeks gestation, it will take between 2 and 3 weeks for their good clinical course to declare itself. By roughly day 21 of life, the likelihood of a good outcome for an infant born at 23 to 24 weeks gestation, who has neither an abnormal HUS nor a prediction of death before discharge, becomes as good as the outcome for infants born at 25 to 27 weeks gestation.

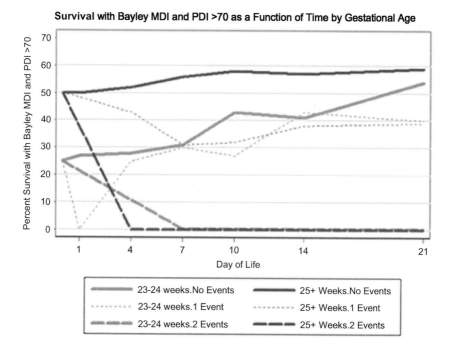

Fig. 14. Likelihood of intact survival as a function of day of life for infants with zero, one, or two events in the NICU (either abnormal HUS or caretaker intuition of death before discharge). Less than 1 week is needed to clarify the likely outcome for infants born at more than 25 weeks gestation. For infants born at 23 to 24 weeks gestation, 3 weeks are needed to clarify their likely outcome.

In both cases, for infants who develop abnormal HUS or predictions of death and for infants who do not, more is learned about their likely outcome during their NICU stay than could have possibly been predicted at the time of delivery. This powerful effect of the passage of time on the prognostic capability is, the authors argue, the most important ethical contribution health care practitioners can make to the process of parental decision-making for infants born at the threshold of viability.

Here is an analogy. Traditionally, when betting on baseball games one has to place a bet before the game starts. One can take into account factors such as team records, starting pitchers, home field advantage, but one is obligated to make a decision before the first pitch. This, the authors argue, is analogous to decision-making before delivery, where gestational age, SGA status, antenatal steroids, twins, and gender are the factors the parents can take into account before they decide to place their bet on resuscitation, or not.

But what if the betting rules were changed? What if one could continue to place bets while learning information about the game while the innings passed—analogous to resuscitating a baby at birth and then learning about the baby's course while ventilated in the NICU? One could become a better bettor as time went on. **Fig. 15** presents data from 411 major league baseball games, plotting the likelihood of winning eventually as a function of whether a team was leading at the end of a particular inning.[14] It is clear that, at the beginning of the game, the likelihood of betting success is roughly 50-50. However, by the end of the eighth inning, the team that is leading wins 94% of the time.

Here, then, is the claim, in its boldest framing. If one bets on the baseball game while it is still going on, one does a lot better than if forced to bet using the pre-game line.

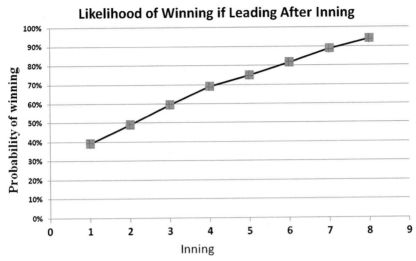

Fig. 15. Likelihood of eventually winning if a baseball team is leading at the end of each inning.

The same option should be allowed for the parents of extremely low gestation age newborns.

SUMMARY

This article discusses ethical issues surrounding the resuscitation of infants who are at great risk to die or survive with significant morbidity. The authors have chosen not to take a philosophic approach; that is, we have not spoken much about autonomy, beneficence, paternalism, or best-interests. Rather, we have chosen to address data. Specifically, we have introduced data regarding three separate aspects of the morality of resuscitation for these infants: money, outcomes, and prediction.

We have demonstrated that there are no credible financial arguments against NICU care (including post-NICU costs) for infants born at the border of viability. Instead, the NICU is a bargain in terms of dollars devoted to infants who will survive to discharge as opposed to die in hospital. Moreover, the NICU is particularly cost-effective when compared with medical interventions in adults, such as adult MICUs or other widely-accepted adult procedures.

We have noted that, of the four possible outcomes after birth (comfort care, death in the NICU, survival with NDI, survival without NDI), gestational age influences some (death in the NICU) much more than others (percentage of survivors with NDI). Consequently, for parents who view "giving their child a chance" by starting NICU intervention as a worthwhile option, counseling about resuscitation as a function of gestational age appears to have limited support from the data.

Finally, we have noted that prediction is possible at four stages of the resuscitation process: before birth (antenatal counseling), in the delivery room, in the NICU while the child remains on the ventilator (when there are ethical alternatives to continued NICU intervention, namely extubation and palliative care), and at the time of discharge. We have presented data suggesting that antenatal and delivery room predictions are inaccurate, and predictions at the time of discharge are too late. Rather, we suggest that learning about individual infants from data collected during the trajectory of their own NICU experience (specifically, abnormal HUS and a health care professional's intuitions that the child will "die before discharge") can offer a positive predictive value of greater than 95% for the combined outcome of death or survival with neurodevelopmental impairment. This predictive value is worth talking about.

The authors end with this plea. We need more study of parental attitudes, both about infants who die in the NICU and infants who survive with NDI. We also need to continue to search for better predictors of infant outcome, while infants remain on ventilators and ethical alternatives exist. We owe this to our colleagues, our patients, and their parents.

REFERENCES

1. Meadow WL, Lantos JD, Reimschisel T, et al. Distributive justice across generations: epidemiology of ICU care for the very young and the very old. In Hageman J and Freed G eds; Ethical issues in Neonatal Intensive Care. Clin Perinatol 1996; 23:597–608.
2. Buchh B, Graham N, Harris B, et al. Neonatology has always been a bargain—even when we weren't very good at it. Acta Paediatr 2007;96:659–63.
3. Lantos JD, Meadow WL. Costs and end-of-life care in the NICU: lessons for the MICU? J Law Med Ethics 2011;39(2):194–200.
4. Meadow WL, Hall J, Frain L, et al. Some are old, some are new, life and death in the ICU. Semin Perinatol 2003;27:471–9.
5. Behrman RE, Butler AS, editors. Preterm birth: causes, consequences, and prevention. Institute of Medicine (US) Committee on Understanding Premature Birth and Assuring Healthy Outcomes; chapter 12: societal costs of preterm birth. Washington, DC: National Academies Press (US); 2007.
6. Tyson J, Parikh N, Langer J, et al. Intensive care for extreme prematurity—moving beyond gestational age. N Engl J Med 2008;358:1672–81.
7. Marlow N, Wolke D, Bracewell MA, et al. Neurologic and developmental disability at six years of age after extremely preterm birth. N Engl J Med 2005;352(1):9–19. Available at: http://www.nejm.org/doi/full/10.1056/NEJMoa041367. Accessed October 9, 2012.
8. Larroque B, Ancel PY, Marchand-Martin L, et al. Special care and school difficulties in 8-year-old very preterm children: the Epipage cohort study. PLoS One 2011; 6(7):e21361. Available at: http://www.plosone.org/article/info%3Adoi%2F10.1371% 2Fjournal.pone.0021361#pone.0021361-Larroque1. Accessed October 9, 2012.
9. Meadow W, Lagatta J, Andrews B, et al. Just in time: ethical implications of serial predictions of mortality and morbidity for ventilated premature infants. Pediatrics 2008;121:732–40.
10. Lagatta J, Andrews B, Caldarelli L, et al. Early neonatal intensive care unit therapy improves predictive power for the outcomes of ventilated extremely low birth weight infants. J Pediatr 2011;159(3):384–91.
11. Singh J, Fanaroff J, Andrews B, et al. Resuscitation in the "gray zone" of viability: determining physician preferences and predicting infant outcomes. Pediatrics 2007;120(3):519–26.
12. Schmidt B, Asztalos EV, Roberts RS, et al. Impact of bronchopulmonary dysplasia, brain injury, and severe retinopathy on the outcome of extremely low-birth-weight infants at 18 months: results from the trial of indomethacin prophylaxis in preterms. JAMA 2003;289(9):1124–9.
13. Meadow WL, Frain L, Ren Y, et al. Serial assessment of mortality in the neonatal intensive care unit by algorithm and intuition: certainty, uncertainty, and informed consent. Pediatrics 2002;109:878–86.
14. Meadow W, Meadow X, Tanz RR, et al. The power of a trial of therapy–football as a proof of concept. Acta Paediatr 2011;100(2):167–9.

Index

Note: Page numbers of article titles are in **boldface** type.

A

Abdominal wall defects, 881–883
Accelerations, in fetal heart rate, 755–756
Acidosis, 911–912
AcoRN (Acute Care of at-Risk Newborns), 903–906
Air, versus oxygen therapy, 805–807
Airway obstruction
 congenital, 877–879
 in ventilation, 860–861
American Academy of Pediatrics
 on chest compression, 834–839
 on meconium aspiration, 821–823
American College of Obstetricians and Gynecologists
 on meconium aspiration, 821–823
 workshop on electronic fetal heart rate monitoring, 754
American Heart Association
 on chest compression, 834–839
 on meconium aspiration, 821–823
Amnioinfusion, for meconium aspiration syndrome, 820–821
Anemia, cord clamping timing and, 892–893
Angiotensin, adaptation of, in transition from intrauterine to extrauterine life, 773
Antepartum surveillance, of fetal compromise, 758–762
Asphyxia
 chest compression for, **833–842**
 end organ injury in, **785–802**
 medications for, **843–855**
Asystole
 chest compression for, **833–842**
 medications for, **843–855**
Atophoric dysplasia, 883–884
Atrial septal defect, 875–876

B

Bags, for ventilation, 859
Baseline, in fetal heart rate, 755
Biophysical profile and modified biophysical profile, 759–760
Body temperature
 monitoring of, in preterm infants, 864–865
 stabilization of, 912
Bradycardia
 chest compression for, **833–842**

http://dx.doi.org/10.1016/S0095-5108(12)00122-4
0095-5108/12/$ – see front matter © 2012 Elsevier Inc. All rights reserved.
perinatology.theclinics.com

Bradycardia (*continued*)
  intrapartum, 763–764
  medications for, **843–855**
Brain, injury of. *See also* Hypoxic-ischemic encephalopathy.
  cellular biology of, 787–789
Breathing
  assessment of, 905–908
  cord clamping timing and, 892
  in transition from intrauterine to extrauterine life, 776–780
Bronchopulmonary dysplasia, 858, 862–863
Bronchopulmonary malformations, 876–877

c

Carbon dioxide levels, in organ injury, 796
Cardiac arrest, medications for, **843–855**
Cardiac compression, **833–842**
Cardiogenic shock, stabilization for, 908–909
Cardiovascular system
  adaptations of, in transition from intrauterine to extrauterine life, 775–776
  insufficiency of, 908–909
Catecholamines, adaptation of, in transition from intrauterine to extrauterine life,
  771–773
Cervical lymphatic malformations, 877–879
Chest compression, **833–842**
Clamping, of umbilical cord, timing of, **889–890**
Clinical risk index for babies (CRIB), 903
Communication, in resuscitation team, 937
Compression, cardiac, **833–842**
Congenital anomalies, **871–887**
  abdominal wall defects, 881–883
  airway obstruction, 877–879
  delivery timing and mode in, 874
  encephalocele, 879–881
  heart disease, 874–876
  intrathoracic masses, 876–877
  maternal complications in, 873–874
  multidisciplinary approach to, 871–872
  myelomeningocele, 879–881
  prenatal issues in, 872–874
  skeletal dysplasia, 883–884
Congenital high airway obstruction syndrome, 878–879
Continuous positive airway pressure, for preterm infants, 863–864
Contraction stress test, 760
CoolCap study, 922–924
Coronary perfusion pressure, epinephrine effects on, 845
Cortisol levels, adaptation of, in transition from intrauterine to extrauterine life, 770–771
CRIB (Clinical risk index for babies), 903
Cricoid pressure, for meconium aspiration prevention, 827
Cystic adenomatoid malformation, 876–877
Cystic hygromas, 877–879

D

Darbopoietin, with hypothermia, 926
Decelerations
    in fetal heart rate, 756–757
    intrapartum, 763–764
Dehydration, 912
Diaphragmatic hernia, 876–877
Dopamine, adaptation of, in transition from intrauterine to extrauterine life, 771–773
Doppler velocimetry, 761
Ductus arteriosus closure, 775

E

Education
    for resuscitation team, 937–938
    for stabilization, 903–904, 914
Encephalocele, 879–881
Encephalopathy
    hypoxic-ichemic, **919–929**
    stabilization for, 909–911
End organ injury, **785–802**
    blood glucose control in, 797
    brain, 787–789
    cell death mechanisms in, 788–790
    circulatory changes causing, 786–787
    fluid therapy for, 796
    kidney, 790
    liver, 790
    long-term consequences of, 794
    management of, 794–797
    mitochondria role in, 788–789
    myocardium, 789–790
    noncirculatory factors in, 787–788
    oxygen for, 795
    pathology of, 793–794
    perfusion maintainence for, 796
    risk factors for, 794–795
    supportive care for, 795–796
    systemic, 790–793
    targeted therapy for, 797
Endocrine adaptations, in transition from intrauterine to extrauterine life, 770–774
Energy failure, in hypoxic-ischemic encephalopathy, 920
Energy metabolism, adaptation of, in transition from intrauterine to extrauterine life, 774
Epinephrine
    adaptation of, in transition from intrauterine to extrauterine life, 771–773
    for resuscitation, 844–847
Erythropoietin, with hypothermia, 926
Ethical issues, in resuscitation, **941–956**
    financial considerations and, 942–944
    outcomes and, 944–947
    prediction and, 947–955

Eunice Kennedy Shriver National Institute of Child Health and Human Development, workshop on electronic fetal heart rate monitoring, 754–755
European Association of Perinatal Medicine, cord clamping statement of, 891
European Network trials, on hypothermia, 923

F

Family support, in stabilization, 915
Fentanyl, for meconium aspiration prevention, 827
Fetal and Neonatal Resuscitation and Transition Suite, of future, **931–939**
Fetal compromise, **753–768**
    antepartum surveillance of, 758–762
    intrapartum monitoring of, 762–765
    monitoring of, 754–758
    physiology of, 754
Fetal heart rate
    classification of, 757–758
    interpretation of, 754–757
    intrapartum monitoring of, 762–765
Fetal movement assessment, 759
Financial considerations, in resuscitation, 942–944
Flow-inflating bags, for ventilation, 859
Fluid therapy, 796, 912

G

Gastric suction, for meconium aspiration prevention, 827
Gastrointestinal anomalies, 881–883, 913–914
Gastroschisis, 881–883
Glucose control, 797, 911
Guidelines for Perinatal Care, on meconium aspiration, 823

H

Heart
    compression of, **833–842**
    congenital disease of, 874–876, 908–909
    injury of, cell death mechanisms in, 789–790
Heat loss, 912
Hemorrhage, postpartum, cord clamping timing and, 895
Hernia, diaphragmatic, 876–877
Hyperbilirubinemia, 912
Hyperglycemia
    organ injury in, 797
    stabilization for, 911
Hypoglycemia
    organ injury in, 797
    stabilization for, 911
Hypoplastic left heart syndrome, 875–876
Hypothermia
    for hypoxic-ischemic encephalopathy, **919–929**
    for neurologic disorders, 910

for organ injury, 797
    prevention of, 864–865
Hypoxia-ischemia
    end organ injury in, **785–802**
    stabilization for, 909–910
Hypoxic-ischemic encephalopathy, **919–929**
    diagnosis of, 921
    hypothermia for, 921–923
        adjuvant therapies with, 926
        clinical applications of, 924–925
        evidence for, 921–923
        future of, 926
        imaging after, 923
        knowledge gaps in, 925
        mechanism of action of, 921
        medications used with, 925
        outcomes of, 923–924
        safety of, 925
    incidence of, 929
    pathophysiology of, 920

I

Infections, stabilization in, 912–913
Integrated Management of Neonatal and Childhood Illnesses, 903–904
International Committee on Cardiopulmonary Resuscitation, on meconium aspiration, 821–823
International Liaison Committee on Resuscitation
    chest compression guidelines of, 834–839
    cord clamping statement of, 891
    on body temperature, 864–865
    on epinephrine resuscitation, 844–847
    on respiratory support, 858–864
    recommendations of, 805–811
Intrapartum compromise, monitoring for, 762–765
Intrathoracic masses, congenital, 876–877
Intubation
    for meconium aspiration, 823–827
    for preterm infants, 863–864
Iron deficiency anemia, cord clamping timing and, 892–893

K

Kidney
    anomalies of, 914
    injury of, cell death mechanisms in, 790

L

Laerdal resuscitator, 859
Liver, injury of, cell death mechanisms in, 790

Lung
    adaptation of, in transition from intrauterine to extrauterine life, 776–780
    congenital malformations of, 907–908
    injury of, in preterm infants, 779–780, 862–863

M

Malformations. *See* Congenital anomalies.
Masks, for ventilation, of preterm infants, 858–860
Mattresses, for hypothermia prevention, 864–865
Meconium-stained amniotic fluid and meconium aspiration syndrome, **817–831**
    epidemiology of, 818–819
    history of, 817–818
    management of, 820–827
    pathophysiology of, 820
    significance of, 819–820
    stabilization needs in, 907
Medications, for resuscitation, **843–855**
    case study of, 844
    epinephrine, 844–847
    vasopressin, 848–850
    versus nonpharmacologic alternatives, 850–851
Meningitis, 912–913
Metabolism
    adaptations of, in transition from intrauterine to extrauterine life, 774–775
    instability of, 911–912
Micrognathia, airway obstruction in, 877–879
Milking, of umbilical cord, 894–895
Mitochondria, in cell death, 788–789
Monitoring
    in future delivery rooms, 932–937
    of fetal compromise, **753–768**
Morality, for resuscitation. *See* Ethical issues.
Mortality
    prediction of, 947–955
    reduction of, stabilization for, **901–918**
Myelomeningocele, 879–881
Myocardium, injury of, cell death mechanisms in, 789–790

N

Nasal prongs, for ventilation, of preterm infants, 858–859
National Institute of Child Health and Human Development
    hypothermia study of, 922–924
    survival calculator of, 944–947
National Resuscitation Program, on meconium aspiration, 821–823
Neural tube defects, 879–881, 914
Neurodevelopmental impairment, ethical issues with, 944–954
Neurological disorders, stabilization for, 909–911
Neuroprotection, for hypoxic-ischemic encephalopathy, **919–929**
Nonstress test, 759
Norepinephrine, adaptation of, in transition from intrauterine to extrauterine life, 771–773

O

Observation, for stabilization needs, 903, 905
Omphalocele, 881–883
Osteogenesis imperfecta, 883–884
Outcomes, of resuscitation, 944–947
Oxygen therapy, **803–815**
    disadvantages of, 807–808
    for organ injury, 795
    history of, 803–805
    in chest compression, **833–842**
    new recommendations for, 811–812
    physiologic principles of, 805
    pulmonary vascular resistance and, 808–810
    research needs for, 812
    toxicity of, 804, 807–808
    versus air therapy, 805–807

P

Packard Circle of Safety, 938
Perfusion, maintenance of, in organ injury, 796
Perinatal Continuing Education Program, 903–904
Persistent pulmonary hypertension of the newborn, 907
Physical space, in future delivery rooms, 932
Pierre Robin syndrome, 879
Placenta, blood flow in, interruption of, end organ injury in, **785–802**
Pneumonia, 907, 912–913
Pneumothorax, 907–908
Polycythemia, cord clamping timing and, 893, 897
Polyethylene bags, for hypothermia prevention, 864–865
Positive pressure ventilation, for preterm infants, 859–864
Pregnancy, childbirth, postpartum, and newborn care guide, 903–904
Preterm infants
    cord clamping timing and, 893–894
    hypothermia for, 925
    lung injury in, 779–780
    resuscitation of, **857–869**
        body temperature monitoring in, 864–865
        ethical issues in, **941–956**
        respiratory support in, 858–864
Priestly, Joseph, 803–804
Pulmonary hypertension, persistent, of newborn, 907
Pulmonary vascular resistance, oxygen therapy and, 808–810
Pulse oximetry, intrapartum, 764

R

Referral, for stabilization, 915
Renin, adaptation of, in transition from intrauterine to extrauterine life, 773
Respiratory distress, stabilization for, 905–908

Respiratory distress syndrome, 907
Respiratory support. *See also* Ventilation.
    for preterm infants, 858–864
        airway obstruction in, 859–860
        continuous positive airway pressure for, 863–864
        devices for, 859
        interfaces for, 858–859
        mask ventilation, 859
        routine intubation for, 863–864
        sustained inflation in, 862–863
        tidal volume in, 860, 862
Resuscitation
    care after, **901–918**
    chest compression in, **833–842**
    ethical issues in, **941–956**
    fetal surveillance and, **753–768**
    future developments in, **931–939**
    hypoxic-ischemic encephalopathy in, **919–929**
    injury prevention and, **785–802**
    intrauterine, 762–765
    medications for, **843–855**
    of infants with anomalies, **871–887**
    of meconium-stained infant, **817–831**
    of preterm infants, **857–869**
    oxygen in, 795, **803–815**
    statistics for, 942–944
    transition physiology and, **769–783**
    umbilical cord clamping in, **889–900**
Retinopathy of prematurity, 804

S

Samson resuscitator, 859
Score for Neonatal Acute Physiology Score for Physiology and Perinatal Extension (SNAPPE), 949
Seizures, neonatal, 910–911
Self-inflating bags, for ventilation, 859
Sendivogius, Michal, 803–804
Septicemia, 912–913
Shock, stabilization for, 908–909
Sinusoidal pattern, in fetal heart rate, 757
Skeletal dysplasia, 883–884
SNAPPE (Score for Neonatal Acute Physiology Score for Physiology and Perinatal Extension), 949–951
Society for Maternal-Fetal Medicine, workshop on electronic fetal heart rate monitoring, 754
Society of Obstetricians and Gynaecologists of Canada, cord clamping statement of, 891
Stabilization, **901–918**
    education programs for, 903–904
    in cardiovascular insufficiency, 908–909
    in fluid imbalance, 912

in infections, 912–913
in metabolic instability, 911–912
in neurologic instability, 909–911
in respiratory distress, 905–908
in surgical emergencies, 913–914
in thermoregulation problems, 912
observation in, 903, 905
recognizing need for, 902–903
research needs in, 915
resource issues in, 914–915
vital signs for, 902–903
S.T.A.B.L.E. Program, 903–904
Streptococcal infections, 912–913
Suctioning, for meconium aspiration, 823–827
SUPPORT trial, for ventilation, 863–864
Surfactant
    for preterm infants, 863–864
    lung adaptation and, 778–779
Surgical emergencies, 913–914
Survival, prediction of, 947–955
Sustained inflation, for preterm infants, 862–863

T

Tachycardia, intrapartum, 763
Tachypnea, transient
    in transition from intrauterine to extrauterine life, 777
    of newborn, 906
Tachysystole, intrapartum, 764
Temperature
    monitoring of, 864–865
    stabilization of, 912
Thermoregulation
    adaptation of, in transition from intrauterine to extrauterine life, 774–775
    need for, 912
Three-tier system, for fetal heart rate tracings, 757–758
Thyroid hormones, adaptation of, in transition from intrauterine to extrauterine life, 773–774
Tidal volume, in ventilation, 860, 862
TOBY (Total Body Hypothermia for Neonatal Encephalopathy) study, 922–924
Topiramate, with hypothermia, 926
Total Body Hypothermia for Neonatal Encephalopathy (TOBY) study, 922–924
T-pieces, for ventilation, of preterm infants, 859
Training. See Education.
Transient tachypnea of newborn, 906
Transition, from intrauterine to extrauterine life, **769–783**
    adaptations in
        cardiovascular, 775–776
        endocrine, 770–774
        lung, 776–780
        metabolic, 774–775
Transitional Oxygen Targeting System, 934

Transport
    cooling during, 925
    for stabilization, 914–915
    in future delivery rooms, 933
Triage, for resuscitation needs, 902–903
TRIPS (transport risk index of physiologic stability), 903
Two-thumb method, for chest compression, 836–837

U

Ultrasound, for congenital anomalies, 872–873
Umbilical cord, clamping of, early versus delayed, **889–900**
    comparison of, 890
    future research needs for, 897
    historical view of, 889–890
    in preterm infants, 893–894
    in term newborns, 892–893
    maternal outcomes and, 895
    milking of, 894–895
    physiologic rationale for, 890–892
    unresolved issues in, 896
UNICEF, World Health Organization, 903–904
University of California San Diego Medical Center resuscitation-transition room, **931–939**
Uterine activity, in fetal heart rate monitoring, 755

V

Variability, in fetal heart rate, 755, 764
Vasopressin, for resuscitation, 848–850
Ventilation
    for organ injury, 795–796
    for preterm infants, 858–864
    in chest compression, **833–842**
Vital signs, for stabilization, 902–903

W

World Health Organization
    cord clamping statement of, 891
    stabilization programs of, 903–904

X

Xenon inhalation, with hypothermia, 926

United States
Postal Service

Statement of Ownership, Management, and Circulation
(All Periodicals Publications Except Requestor Publications)

1. Publication Title	2. Publication Number								3. Filing Date
Clinics in Perinatology	0	0	1	-	7	4	4	4	9/14/12

4. Issue Frequency	5. Number of Issues Published Annually	6. Annual Subscription Price
Mar, Jun, Sep, Dec	4	$273.00

7. Complete Mailing Address of Known Office of Publication *(Not printer) (Street, city, county, state, and ZIP+4®)*

Contact Person

Elsevier Inc.
360 Park Avenue South
New York, NY 10010-1710

Stephen R. Bushing

Telephone *(Include area code)*

215-239-3688

8. Complete Mailing Address of Headquarters or General Business Office of Publisher *(Not printer)*

Elsevier Inc., 360 Park Avenue South, New York, NY 10010-1710

9. Full Names and Complete Mailing Addresses of Publisher, Editor, and Managing Editor *(Do not leave blank)*

Publisher *(Name and complete mailing address)*

Kim Murphy, Elsevier, Inc., 1600 John F. Kennedy Blvd. Suite 1800, Philadelphia, PA 19103-2899

Editor *(Name and complete mailing address)*

Kerry Holland, Elsevier, Inc., 1600 John F. Kennedy Blvd. Suite 1800, Philadelphia, PA 19103-2899

Managing Editor *(Name and complete mailing address)*

Sarah Barth, Elsevier, Inc., 1600 John F. Kennedy Blvd. Suite 1800, Philadelphia, PA 19103-2899

10. Owner *(Do not leave blank. If the publication is owned by a corporation, give the name and address of the corporation immediately followed by the names and addresses of all stockholders owning or holding 1 percent or more of the total amount of stock. If not owned by a corporation, give the names and addresses of the individual owners. If owned by a partnership or other unincorporated firm, give its name and address as well as those of each individual owner. If the publication is published by a nonprofit organization, give its name and address.)*

Full Name	Complete Mailing Address
Wholly owned subsidiary of	1600 John F. Kennedy Blvd., Ste. 1800
Reed/Elsevier, US holdings	Philadelphia, PA 19103-2899

11. Known Bondholders, Mortgagees, and Other Security Holders Owning or Holding 1 Percent or More of Total Amount of Bonds, Mortgages, or Other Securities. If none, check box ☐ None

Full Name	Complete Mailing Address
N/A	

12. Tax Status *(For completion by nonprofit organizations authorized to mail at nonprofit rates) (Check one)*
The purpose, function, and nonprofit status of this organization and the exempt status for federal income tax purposes:
☐ Has Not Changed During Preceding 12 Months
☐ Has Changed During Preceding 12 Months *(Publisher must submit explanation of change with this statement)*

PS Form 3526, September 2007 (Page 1 of 3 (Instructions Page 3)) PSN 7530-01-000-9931 PRIVACY NOTICE: See our Privacy policy in www.usps.com

13. Publication Title	14. Issue Date for Circulation Data Below
Clinics in Perinatology	September 2012

15. Extent and Nature of Circulation			Average No. Copies Each Issue During Preceding 12 Months	No. Copies of Single Issue Published Nearest to Filing Date
a. Total Number of Copies *(Net press run)*			1871	1770
b. Paid Circulation (By Mail and Outside the Mail)	(1)	Mailed Outside-County Paid Subscriptions Stated on PS Form 3541. *(Include paid distribution above nominal rate, advertiser's proof copies, and exchange copies)*	1205	1094
	(2)	Mailed In-County Paid Subscriptions Stated on PS Form 3541 *(Include paid distribution above nominal rate, advertiser's proof copies, and exchange copies)*		
	(3)	Paid Distribution Outside the Mails Including Sales Through Dealers and Carriers, Street Vendors, Counter Sales, and Other Paid Distribution Outside USPS®	390	386
	(4)	Paid Distribution by Other Classes Mailed Through the USPS (e.g. First-Class Mail®)		
c. Total Paid Distribution *(Sum of 15b (1), (2), (3), and (4))*			1595	1480
d. Free or Nominal Rate Distribution (By Mail and Outside the Mail)	(1)	Free or Nominal Rate Outside-County Copies Included on PS Form 3541	64	50
	(2)	Free or Nominal Rate In-County Copies Included on PS Form 3541		
	(3)	Free or Nominal Rate Copies Mailed at Other Classes Through the USPS (e.g. First-Class Mail)		
	(4)	Free or Nominal Rate Distribution Outside the Mail (Carriers or other means)		
e. Total Free or Nominal Rate Distribution *(Sum of 15d (1), (2), (3) and (4))*			64	50
f. Total Distribution *(Sum of 15c and 15e)*			1659	1530
g. Copies not Distributed *(See instructions to publishers #4 (page #3))*			212	240
h. Total *(Sum of 15f and g)*			1871	1770
i. Percent Paid *(15c divided by 15f times 100)*			96.14%	96.73%

16. Publication of Statement of Ownership

If the publication is a general publication, publication of this statement is required. Will be printed
in the **December 2012** issue of this publication.

☐ Publication not required.

17. Signature and Title of Editor, Publisher, Business Manager, or Owner	Date
[signature] Stephen R. Bushing – Inventory/Distribution Coordinator	September 14, 2012

I certify that all information furnished on this form is true and complete. I understand that anyone who furnishes false or misleading information on this form or who omits material or information requested on the form may be subject to criminal sanctions (including fines and imprisonment) and/or civil sanctions (including civil penalties).

PS Form 3526, September 2007 (Page 2 of 3)

Moving?

Make sure your subscription moves with you!

To notify us of your new address, find your **Clinics Account Number** (located on your mailing label above your name), and contact customer service at:

Email: journalscustomerservice-usa@elsevier.com

800-654-2452 (subscribers in the U.S. & Canada)
314-447-8871 (subscribers outside of the U.S. & Canada)

Fax number: 314-447-8029

Elsevier Health Sciences Division
Subscription Customer Service
3251 Riverport Lane
Maryland Heights, MO 63043

*To ensure uninterrupted delivery of your subscription, please notify us at least 4 weeks in advance of move.

ELSEVIER